American Health Policy

American Health Policy

Critical Issues for Reform

Edited by Robert B. Helms

The AEI Press

Publisher for the American Enterprise Institute
WASHINGTON, D.C.

1993

Distributed to the Trade by National Book Network, 15200 NBN Way, Blue Ridge Summit, PA 17214. To order call toll free 1-800-462-6420 or 1-717-794-3800. For all other inquiries please contact the AEI Press, 1150 Seventeenth Street, N.W., Washington, D.C. 20036 or call 1-800-862-5801.

Library of Congress Cataloging-in-Publication Data
American health policy : critical issues for reform / edited by Robert B. Helms.
    p. cm.
Includes bibliographical references.
  ISBN 0-8447-3818-2.—ISBN 0-8447-3819-0 (pbk.)
  1. Medical policy—United States. 2. Medical care, Cost of—United States. 3. Insurance, Health—United States. I. Helms, Robert B.
RA395.A3A527 1992
362.1'0973—dc20
                                                                        92-22281
                                                                            CIP

    3 5 7 9 10 8 6 4

The AEI Press
Publisher for the American Enterprise Institute
1150 17th Street, N.W., Washington, D.C. 20036

Contents

LIST OF TABLES

LIST OF FIGURES

Contributors

ROBERT B. HELMS is resident scholar and director of health policy studies at the American Enterprise Institute. Before coming to AEI he was the executive director of the American Pharmaceutical Institute. Mr. Helms has served as the assistant secretary for planning and evaluation and the deputy assistant secretary for health policy in the Department of Health and Human Services.

HENRY J. AARON is director of the Economic Studies Program at the Brookings Institution. He has also served as assistant secretary for planning and evaluation at the Department of Health, Education, and Welfare, and he chaired the 1979 Advisory Council on Social Security. He is the author or editor of numerous books, including *Serious and Unstable Condition: Financing America's Health Care.*

MICHAEL D. BROMBERG has been the executive director of the Federation of American Health Systems since 1969. Previously he served as a member of the National Advisory Commission on Catastrophic Illness. This commission's report was the foundation for legislation to protect elderly patients against financial ruin from catastrophic illnesses. Mr. Bromberg is also an attorney.

STUART M. BUTLER is vice president and director of Domestic and Economic Policy Studies at the Heritage Foundation. In March 1990 he was appointed commissioner of Housing Secretary Jack Kemp's Advisory Commission on Regulatory Barriers to Affordable Housing. Mr. Butler is the author of *Out of the Poverty Trap* and the coauthor of *A National Health System for America.*

ROBERT M. CRANE is Kaiser Permanente's senior vice president for national accounts and public relations. Prior to joining Kaiser Permanente, Mr. Crane served as deputy commissioner for Program and Policy Development of the New York State Department of Health and director of its Office of Health Systems Management. He also has experience on the

U.S. House of Representatives' Subcommittee on Health and the Environment and with the Department of Health, Education, and Welfare.

PATRICIA M. DANZON is Celia Moh Professor of Health Care Management and Insurance at the Wharton School, University of Pennsylvania. Her research activities include applying microeconomics to markets for health care and insurance, social insurance, law, and economics. Ms. Danzon is on the editorial boards of the *Journal of Health Economics* and the *Journal of Risk and Insurance*.

KAREN DAVIS is executive vice president of the Commonwealth Fund. From 1983 until 1992 she was chairman of the Department of Health Policy and Management in the School of Hygiene and Public Health at Johns Hopkins University. She is a member of the Physician Payment Review Commission and the Maryland Governor's Commission on Health Care Policy and Financing. Ms. Davis is the author of *Health Care Cost-Containment; Health and the War on Poverty: A Ten Year Appraisal;* and *National Health Insurance: Benefits, Costs, and Consequences.*

WILLIAM J. DENNIS is senior research fellow at the NFIB Foundation, an affiliate of the National Federation of Independent Business, where he has directed research activities for the past fourteen years. Mr. Dennis is the author or coauthor of several monographs and reports, including the *Quarterly Economic Report for Small Business, Monthly Economic Update, Small Business and Banks: The United States, Small Business Employee Benefits, New Business in America,* and *To Increase Small Business Productivity.*

BRYAN E. DOWD is associate professor in the division of health services research and policy at the University of Minnesota. Mr. Dowd has written extensively on the areas of health care cost and insurance. Among his latest works are "Cost Function Analysis of Medicare Policy: Are Rural Reimbursement Limits for Home Health Agencies Sufficient?" with John Nyman and "Evaluating Exclusionary Interventions" with Roger Feldman for the *Journal of Health Economics.*

DAVID DRANOVE is associate professor of management and strategy and of health services management at Northwestern University's Kellogg Graduate School of Management. His research activities focus on the health care industry and related industries, and he is on the editorial boards of the *Journal of Health Economics* and the *Journal of Medical Practice Management.*

DAVE DURENBERGER was elected to the U.S. Senate in 1978. Senator Durenberger has emerged as a leader in the Senate on health care and environmental protection, serving on the two principal committees dealing with health care policy—Finance, and Labor and Human Resources. He is also a member of the Senate's Environment and Public Works Committee and the Special Senate Committee on Aging.

ROGER FELDMAN is professor of health services research and economics at the University of Minnesota. Mr. Feldman was senior staff economist for health policy and economics at the President's Council of Economic Advisers, and was the lead author of a chapter in the 1985 *Economic Report of the President*. He has directed one of the four national research centers sponsored by the Health Care Financing Administration. Mr. Feldman is a regular contributor to professional journals in health services research and economics, and he is on the editorial boards of several journals.

H. E. FRECH III is professor of economics at the University of California at Santa Barbara. His current research focuses on health economics, and he is writing a book entitled *Competition and Monopoly in Medical Care*. He is editor of the AEI publication *Regulating Doctors' Fees: Competition, Benefits, and Controls under Medicare*.

BILL GRADISON was elected to the House of Representatives in 1974. He is a member of the House Ways and Means and Budget Committees. On the Ways and Means Committee, he is the ranking member of the Health Subcommittee. Representative Gradison is chairman of the House Wednesday Group, and he is also chairman of the Economic Roundtable of the American Enterprise Institute. Recently he served as vice chairman of the U.S. Bipartisan Commission on Comprehensive Health Care (the Pepper Commission).

WARREN GREENBERG is professor of health economics and of health care sciences and senior fellow at the Center for Health Policy Research at George Washington University. He is the author of numerous articles on the economics of health care, and he is the author or editor of nine books. Mr. Greenberg's latest book is entitled *Competition, Regulation, and Rationing in Health Care*.

CLARK C. HAVIGHURST is the William Neal Reynolds Professor of Law at Duke University and has taught at Duke since 1964. His areas of concentration include antitrust law, economic regulation, and health care law and policy. Mr. Havighurst is the author of the book *Deregulating the Health Care Industry* and of a law school casebook, *Health Care Law and Policy*. He is also a member of the Institute of Medicine of the National Academy of Sciences and of its Board of Health Care Services.

GAIL A. JENSEN is associate professor at Wayne State University, jointly appointed in the Economics Department and the University's Institute of Gerontology. Her research has focused on the premium consequences of group health insurance provisions, the nature of employer initiatives to contain health-benefit costs, the dynamics of health insurance among older adults, the effects of state regulations on employers' insurance offerings, and the scope of corporate health benefits for retirees.

STANLEY B. JONES is a private consultant to insurers, providers, and private foundations on competitive private health insurance markets and on the roles of public policy in improving these markets. He was a founding partner of the Washington consulting firm Health Policy Alternatives, Inc., and he has served as vice president for Washington representation of the Blue Cross-Blue Shield Association and as staff director of the Senate Health Subcommittee.

KARLYN H. KEENE is editor of *The American Enterprise* magazine and is resident fellow at the American Enterprise Institute. Before joining AEI she was research director for a public relations firm. Ms. Keene has written on many public opinion topics, including the gender gap, the political impact of the baby boom generation, and views about the federal government's role in our society.

RICHARD KRONICK is assistant professor in the Department of Community and Family Medicine at the University of California at San Diego, and health policy consultant for health plans, employers, and government agencies. Mr. Kronick has held posts with the Commonwealth of Massachusetts, serving as assistant director of the Office of Health Policy in the Executive Office of Human Services and as director of policy and reimbursement of the Medicaid Division, Department of Public Welfare.

SANDER M. LEVIN was elected to the House of Representatives in 1982 and currently serves on the House Ways and Means Committee, with assignments on the Health and Human Resources subcommittees. He is also a member of the Select Committee on Children, Youth, and Families. Representative Levin served in the Michigan State Senate for six years, where he was chairman of the Labor Committee, vice chairman of the Education Committee, and a member of the Judiciary and Administrative Rules Committee.

HAROLD S. LUFT is professor of health economics and associate director of the Institute for Health Policy Studies at the University of California, San Francisco. Mr. Luft is a member of the Institute of Medicine of the

National Academy of Sciences. His research has covered a wide range of areas, including health maintenance organizations, competition among hospitals, studies of medical care utilization, and adverse selection in multiple-option health insurance settings. His most recent book is *Hospital Volume, Physician Volume, and Patient Outcomes: Assessing the Evidence*.

CATHERINE G. MCLAUGHLIN is associate professor at the University of Michigan's School of Public Health. She is currently the principal investigator on "Survey and Analysis of the Small Business Health Insurance Market," a project funded by the Robert Wood Johnson Foundation.

JACK A. MEYER is founder and president of New Directions for Policy, a research and policy organization in Washington, D.C. Mr. Meyer is also founder and president of the Economic and Social Research Institute. He is a former assistant director of the U.S. Council on Wage and Price Stability and consultant in residence at the Organization for Economic Cooperation and Development in Paris, France. Mr. Meyer is the author of a comprehensive report on the U.S. social welfare system entitled *The Common Good: Social Welfare and the American Future*.

DONALD W. MORAN joined Lewin/ICF in 1985 as vice president. Mr. Moran is a former executive associate director for budget and legislation at the Office of Management and Budget. He also served as associate director for Human Resources, Veterans, and Labor at the Office of Management and Budget, where he directed OMB policy analysis and budget review for the Department of Health and Human Services, the Veterans Administration, and other related agencies.

MICHAEL A. MORRISEY is professor in the Department of Health Care Organization and Policy at the University of Alabama at Birmingham (UAB), acting director of the Lister Hill Center for Health Policy at UAB, and deputy editor of the health services research journal *Medical Care*. Mr. Morrisey was formerly assistant director and senior economist with the Hospital Research and Educational Trust, the research affiliate of the American Hospital Association.

NEIL NEWHOUSE is partner and cofounder of Public Opinion Strategies, a national public opinion and polling firm established in April 1991. Before this, Mr. Newhouse joined the Wirthlin Group in 1984 and eventually headed the company's political division. Mr. Newhouse has also worked in the survey research division and the local elections campaign division of the Republican National Committee. He presently serves on the board of the Campaign Management Institute of American University.

G. ROBERT O'BRIEN is executive vice president of the CIGNA Corporation. He directs CIGNA's public position regarding national health policy. For the past seven years, Mr. O'Brien was president of the CIGNA Employee Benefits Companies, which include group insurance, managed health, dental and mental health care, and case management activities. He is also chairman of the Healthcare Leadership Council.

MARK V. PAULY is Bendheim Professor of Health Care Systems, Public Management Insurance, and Economics at the Wharton School, University of Pennsylvania. He is chairman of the Department of Health Care Systems and former executive director of the Leonard Davis Institute of Health Economics. He is a member of the Institute of Medicine and principal investigator of an evaluation of the Pew National Dental Foundation Program for the Pew Foundation.

CARL J. SCHRAMM is the president of the Health Insurance Association of America (HIAA). Prior to joining HIAA, Mr. Schramm served on the U.S. Labor Department Commission studying pension and benefits issues in the nation's coal industry. He also served as a special adviser on health care policy to the assistant secretary for policy of the U.S. Department of Labor, and was the Robert Wood Johnson Foundation health policy fellow at the National Academy of Sciences' Institute of Medicine.

DEBORAH STEELMAN practices law in the fields of employee benefits, health care, and environment. She also volunteered as the chair of the 1991 Advisory Council on Social Security, a statutory, voluntary, private-sector panel whose charter focused on health care financing and retirement policy. Ms. Steelman was the director of domestic policy of the 1988 George Bush for President Campaign and has served as associate director of the Office of Management and Budget, deputy assistant to President Reagan, director of intergovernmental affairs at the EPA, and legislative director to the late Senator John Heinz.

C. EUGENE STEUERLE is senior fellow at the Urban Institute and author of a weekly column, "Economic Perspective," for *Tax Notes* magazine. From 1987 to 1989 he was the deputy assistant secretary of the Treasury for tax analysis. In that role he directed the Treasury study *Financing Health and Long-Term Care: A Report to the President and Congress.* Between

1984 and 1986, Mr. Steuerle served as economic coordinator and original organizer of the Treasury's tax reform effort.

STEPHEN ZUCKERMAN is senior research associate at the Urban Institute and is working on several studies addressing physician and hospital payment issues. The ultimate objective of the physician research is to refine the present Medicare Volume Performance Standard policy. In addition, Mr. Zuckerman was the coauthor of a proposal aimed at refining health care financing. A recently completed project led to the development of the geographic practice cost indexes used in the Medicare Fee Schedule for physician services.

Foreword

American health policy has been and will continue to be a major political issue. This is not difficult to understand when one considers the intense personal interest of consumers in their own health status, the size of the health care sector in the U.S. economy, and the projected increases in health care expenditures in government, business, and personal budgets. But it is also a complex policy issue that is difficult for most people to understand. This is in part because, as Eugene Steuerle (chapter 14) and Mark Pauly (chapter 13) tell us, health care is financed predominately through public and tax-subsidized private insurance that hides the true cost of care from consumers.

In the midst of this complexity and misunderstanding is an intense debate about how to reform the health care system. This debate is affected by concerns about the cost of health care, access to health care services, and differences of opinion as to how traditional market forces are working in health care. It can lead to simplistic proposals for reform that receive much attention and public support without being subjected to careful analysis.

In contrast to this apparent confusion is a growing body of careful analysis about specific health policy issues. This research is being conducted by a host of scholars at academic and other institutions around the country. AEI's purpose in this volume is to present a selection of this research, to inform policy makers and others about the critical issues for reform. Fourteen chapters offer research and analysis about the performance of the private insurance sector, the problems of access and cost-containment, and the basic choices for reform. Each chapter has been subjected to evaluation by commentators with extensive experience with these issues. The chapters were presented and discussed at an AEI conference held in Washington, D.C., on October 3–4, 1991.

I would like to thank several people and institutions who have made the research presented in this volume possible. First and foremost, I want to acknowledge with deep gratitude a major grant from SmithKline Beecham Corporation and the support and encouragement of its remarkable chairman, Henry Wendt. I am also grateful for the additional generous support of the CIGNA companies, the Prudential Insurance Company of America, New York Life Insurance Company, the Principal Financial Group, and Glaxo Incorporated. We do not want anyone to think that all these firms support all the propositions put forth in this volume. We thank them for making possible the research and the expansion of the health policy debate.

While numerous people at AEI have contributed to this volume, I would like to thank especially Heather Gradison for organizing and supervising the conference, Robert Helms for planning and editing the volume, and the publications staff for its preparation and production.

CHRISTOPHER C. DEMUTH
President, American Enterprise Institute
for Public Policy Research

American Health Policy

1
Introduction

Robert B. Helms

The U.S. health care sector is receiving increasing attention as an object of dissatisfaction and as a subject of potential political action. Political figures, academics, and task forces representing a variety of interests have proposed numerous plans to reform our health care system (Blue Cross and Blue Shield Association 1991). These proposals have ranged from Canadian-style plans with extensive government financing and control to minor modifications of state insurance laws to correct perceived inequities and inefficiencies in private insurance markets. Dissatisfaction appears to be pervasive across all participants and observers of the American health care system. Almost no one defends all aspects of the present system or even argues that health care markets have the self-correcting mechanisms that can be counted on in most markets to restore both equity and efficiency.

In the midst of this growing and pervasive dissatisfaction, disagreement about what is really wrong with market incentives in health care markets is increasing. The market pessimists look both to past trends in costs and to apparent success by foreign countries to control health care costs as evidence that health care markets cannot and will not respond to market incentives. Their reform proposals call for direct government action to control more aspects of both the delivery and the financing of health care. The market optimists explain the increasing cost of health care and other malfunctions of the market as direct consequences of a perverse set of incentives created by several decades of government tax and regulatory policies. Their policy prescriptions call for changes in government tax and regulatory policies that they believe would restore the basic incentives of providers and patients to purchase and to deliver health care in a more efficient way. Health care markets would then take on more of the characteristics of efficiency and equity as in other nonhealth markets.

Even with such pervasive dissatisfaction and increasing calls for reform, the complexity of health care markets and the fundamental disagreement about what is wrong have been identified as a major block to political action. This volume attempts to inform the debate by bringing together a body of research and analysis on the critical issues in the health reform debate, especially competition in our private health insurance market and the effects of that competition on the costs of care and access to insurance coverage. The first four parts cover such topics as the ways to minimize the selection of only the best risks, the labor market effects of mandating benefits, the reasons small employers do not buy health insurance, and the difficulties of comparing administrative costs between Canada and the United States.

Part five of the volume takes a different approach by looking at the health policy reform debate from the point of view of three well-informed members of Congress and two experts on public opinion. The objective is to provide the reader with analysis of the political reality of the health reform debate, especially how the Congress may react to changing public perceptions of the underlying health policy issues discussed in the first four parts.

The following overview summarizes the fourteen essays and the commentaries. Like the volume, this overview is divided into five parts. Part one looks at what might be wrong with the present private insurance market. Part two looks at what role the private insurance sector might play in addressing the issue of access to health care. Part three addresses the difficult issue of cost containment, the issue that seems to be a major source of disagreement regarding proposals for reform. Part four analyzes the basic choices we have to reform our health care system. This part of the volume does not discuss actual proposals but analyzes the basic choices we face, especially the choice between reforming individual incentives and relying on direct government controls. Part five discusses the politics of health policy reform, especially how the Congress may react to political pressure and public opinion.

Part One: What, If Anything, Is Wrong with Private Health Insurance?

The title of part one attempts to leave open the possibility that nothing is wrong with the present functioning of our private health insurance market. As stated above, however, hardly anyone, even members of the health insurance industry, argues that nothing is wrong. Instead, the disagreement about what is wrong focuses on the changing structure in the employer-provided insurance market, especially the role of managed care and the process of competition among insurance companies to select, or avoid, high-risk enrollees.

Harold Luft, in chapter 2, analyzes why Alain Enthoven's model of competition among multiple-option health care plans has not worked as planned. He distinguishes several categories of problems—biased selection, premium-setting practices of health maintenance organizations, management difficulties, and lack of local market power in individual HMOs and employers—and explains why they have limited effective competition in medical markets. To remedy these problems, Luft recommends a system of intermediaries that would be responsible for negotiating payments with HMOs, preferred provider organizations, and fee-for-service plans. To make this system work, the intermediaries would have to develop methods of assessing the extent of biased selection among the plans and adjusting payments accordingly. The intermediaries would also collect and evaluate comparisons across plans and make the findings public. Such a system would encourage competition based on quality and true efficiency and could lead to long-run improvements in the health care system.

Richard Kronick, in chapter 3, discusses why effective managed competition does not exist in the private insurance market. "Managed competition" is defined as a system of competing health plans in which each plan manages the interactions of consumers and groups of providers to reward those providers for both quality and economy. Despite the rhetoric about competition, Kronick argues that we have not created a competitive environment in health care because of collective action problems. These problems occur when the actions of small groups or of individuals in a market appear too weak to change the entire market, even when such change would be in the collective interests of all employers. In such a situation, Kronick argues, neither small nor large employers have strong enough incentives to take on the interests of providers and to force effective competition onto the market. He presents several reasons why the growth of HMOs and other so-called managed-care organizations have not achieved the change in consumer and provider behavior that would be brought about by managed competition.

To solve the collective action problem, Kronick believes we must find some way of rewarding employers that do manage competition. In the small-employer market we face the additional problem of preventing health plans from prospering from favorable risk selection. These objectives could be met through the creation of a large purchaser that could aggregate the purchasing power of small groups. He calls such organizations health insurance purchasing corporations.

The establishment of HIPCs would require two changes in government policy, one at the federal level and the other at the state level. First, to give small employers incentives to offer health insurance through such collective organizations, federal tax policy would have to be changed to make the present exclusion of employer-provided health insurance available only to employers utilizing HIPCs. Second, state laws would have to be changed to require that insurance could be offered only to small employers through HIPC-type organizations.

Kronick goes on to discuss both the economic effect of such a market change and the political reaction against it. In his view, the creation of HIPCs would "jump-start" effective managed competition in health markets. But without such a start, we will not get real competition and will hasten the day when we turn to price control systems to regulate expenditures.

Roger Feldman and Bryan Dowd, in chapter 4, examine how biased selection and premium setting combine to affect fairness and efficiency in health insurance markets. They use standard welfare economics and microeconomic theory of consumer choice under risk to define economic efficiency and the concept or equity, or fairness.

To explain the role of biased selection in insurance markets, they analyze four possible situations depending on whether the insurer can identify members of different risk classes and whether the insurer can vary premiums by risk class. First, when insurers can identify risks and charge different premiums, the allocation of insurance becomes economically efficient as competition forces each insurer to charge a rate that just covers the cost of each risk class. But since high-risk people pay higher rates, the result is in sharp contrast to the policy maker's concept of fairness.

Second, insurers can still identify risks but, because of the policy maker's concerns about fairness, are prevented from charging different premiums to different risk classes. This leads to what is commonly called cream skimming, the practice of actively recruiting and retaining low-risk people and discriminating against high-risk people. Even when law or regulation allows some risk-based variation (for example, by age or sex), insurers have strong incentives to discover additional ways to identify the preferred low-risk people within each allowed category. This practice not only subverts the intended cross-subsidy from low risk to high risk but causes insurers (including managed-care plans) to compete by offering more services to the desired low-risk enrollees and fewer services to the high-risk enrollees. Requiring a single rate creates the possibility of leaving both high-risk and low-risk enrollees worse off than if premiums had been allowed to vary.

Third, "successful community rating" might refer to the case when insurers can neither identify risks nor charge different premiums. Such a situation can exist with only one insurer in a market, as was the case with Blue Cross plans in earlier decades. Since community rating can be viewed as a tax on healthy policyholders, it is an inefficient method to subsidize high risks. Feldman and Dowd use Bureau of the Census figures on income and medical expenditures by age to illustrate that community rating would result in subsidies from lower-income young people to higher-income older people. They also point to evidence that community rating might subsidize unhealthy practices such as smoking and result in a tax that would be borne more heavily by the uninsured.

Fourth, when insurers can charge different rates but cannot identify risks, insurance markets may either be unstable or result in inefficient and inequitable coverage. High-risk enrollees, for example, may have to pay high premiums and yet receive limited benefits; tightly managed plans may enroll mainly healthy people.

From the analysis of these four cases, the authors point out that the choice for health policy is between community rating and the competitive equilibrium that could occur when insurers can both determine risk and adjust premiums according to risk. They point out that an income transfer from low-income to high-income would be more efficient than a system of community rating that would result in the unfair subsidization of the high-risk by the low-risk. To accomplish the goals of both equity and efficiency, the authors recommend that market competition determine the correct price of health insurance benefits and that premium contributions by either public or private insurers for any health plan should be based on "the low bid for basic coverage submitted by a qualified health plan in a predefined market area."

Clark Havighurst asks a basic question: Why maintain our system of private financing of health insurance if it continues to operate in its present form? In chapter 5, Havighurst adopts the role of devil's advocate to demonstrate that private health insurance could perform a unique and useful function in the health care market. A prerequisite, however, is the resurrection of private contracts as an effective vehicle for specifying precise, enforceable rules to govern medical care in particular circumstances. Unless private contracts can be made viable instruments for expressing and implementing meaningful economic choices by consumers, Americans should stop pretending that privately financed medical care is a product of a free market. Instead, he argues, we should acknowledge that the most important decisions about health care are ultimately controlled by central authorities and that these authorities—essentially, the courts and the medical profession acting in tandem—are accountable neither to consumers in the marketplace nor to voters in the political process. A national health policy that leaves vital decisions in such hands is an invitation to runaway costs.

Havighurst concludes that unless private financing plans can somehow employ private contracts to transmit clear signals from cost-conscious consumers on the demand side of the market to providers on the supply side, a single-payer health policy may be the only reasonable one. He challenges private health insurers and other health plans to return to their function of providing cost-effective care. But failure to respond to this challenge would allow "little reason not to let them pass from the health care scene."

Commentaries and Discussion. Commentaries on these essays and on the performance of the private health insurance market were given by three individuals with substantial experience in the business of insurance: Stanley Jones, Robert O'Brien, and Carl Schramm. Jones reminds us that the U.S. health insurance industry has traditionally performed the function of processing claims on individual transactions rather than the broader function of serving as the consumer's agent for the purchase of cost-effective and quality care. With the exception of staff- and group-model HMOs, the growth of managed care arrangements has not changed the way hospitals and physicians organize and provide care. And despite publicity, employers' efforts to change the way they buy medical care has had little effect. In Jones's view, much more motivation is needed to induce the business sector to "buy smart" since the purchase of health insurance is secondary to the firms' objective of hiring and maintaining a labor force.

O'Brien of CIGNA and Schramm of the Health Insurance Association of America both argue that government must have a role in shaping health care reform. They call for federal legislation (1) to increase the role of government in covering the costs for the poor and indigent so that the private sector will not be burdened by these extra costs, (2) to reform state laws that mandate excessive types of care, and (3) to reform state anti–managed-care laws that prevent new forms of health care delivery from competing in health care markets. O'Brien points out the importance of the quality of care in the competitive process and argues that the federal government is unlikely to operate the health care system more efficiently than competing private insurance companies.

These observations engendered a lively debate about how private insurance companies compete and about the effects of managed care arrangements. This debate is summarized in the discussion section.

Part Two: What Should Be the Role for the Private Sector in Improving Access to Health Care?

One of the most misunderstood issues in the health reform debate is access to health care. While almost all of the U.S. population has access to some kind of medical care, about 15 percent of the population do not have health insurance coverage that would cover at least part of the cost of medical care. To the extent that medical care is actually provided to those without insurance, the cost of such care must be paid for directly by the individuals, absorbed as a bad debt by the hospital or physician providing the coverage, or covered by charity. Despite much rhetoric to the contrary, market conditions are highly unlikely to allow such costs to be passed on to another payer.

The fact that approximately 34 million do not have health insurance creates both practical problems in medical markets and political problems in the national debate about reform. Increasing the proportion of the population that has health insurance coverage is considered an objective of every health care reform proposal. As this part of the volume shows, however, a large proportion of the uninsured either are directly employed or are dependents of people who are employed. Many of the uninsured who work seem to be employed in small firms that do not offer health insurance to their employees despite the tax subsidies to do so. Therefore, improving access turns out to be a problem of finding ways to increase the coverage of employees in private business firms, many of which are small.

These three chapters and the commentaries look at the role of health insurance in labor markets and various ways that are being considered to increase private sector coverage. As in the previous part, the problem of biased selection and the role it plays in the competitive process leads to pessimism about the role of the private sector in correcting these problems. If the private sector is not self-correcting, the issue becomes the type of policy change that will result in increasing the proportion of people covered by insurance.

Michael Morrisey, in chapter 6, looks at the health reform proposals that attempt to increase insurance coverage by placing various types of mandates on employers. He reviews the estimates of the number of uninsured that would be affected by the mandates and the costs of these mandates. Using the concept of compensating differentials, Morrisey points out that it is unrealistic to expect that workers will be provided with benefits and wages that exceed what they are worth. Consequently, if health insurance benefits are mandated, the costs will be borne primarily by the workers themselves in the form of reduced wages or other benefits. Because of the effect of federal and state tax subsidies for health insurance, about a third of the additional cost will be borne by taxpayers in the form of reduced tax revenue. In some cases where wages cannot be adjusted, increased unemployment may result.

Reviewing studies of the adjustment of wages to changes in fringe benefits, Morrisey finds strong empirical support for the compensating differential hypothesis in recent studies showing that wages were adjusted to compensate for increases in workers' compensation insurance and pensions. He also identifies several technical and data problems with studies that have failed to find such adjustment of wages in response to increases in health insurance. He concludes that the effects of mandates are disconcerting and that

> mandates are expensive. Lots of people are affected besides those who are currently uninsured. There is a significant trade-off between exemption of small business and coverage of the uninsured. Mandates imply some shifting of employment across firms. Most important, however, mandated coverage will be predominately paid for by uninsured workers themselves.

Catherine McLaughiin addresses the issue of why small businesses do not offer health insurance and whether there is a private-sector solution. She reports on information from a Robert Wood Johnson Foundation project and a survey of 1,300 small businesses and forty-three insurers to correct some of the myths about the insurance market for small businesses.

McLaughlin reports that while health insurance is offered to small firms in most markets, some very small firms (fewer than ten employees) and some firms in specific, "redlined" industries (for example, bars, junkyards, physician offices, and detective agencies) may have difficulty finding an insurer. Firms with large numbers of part-time workers and workers with preexisting conditions also have trouble finding coverage. A lack of demand for health insurance and concerns about costs, however, seem to be the leading reasons small firms do not offer health insurance. McLaughlin reports that small business owners view health insurance as an expensive benefit that is usually not demanded by their employees and so is not necessary to attract workers. Owners also emphasize the expense of health insurance and the competitive nature of their businesses, which makes it impossible for them to afford such an extra fringe benefit.

In terms of the policy implications of this research, McLaughlin feels that policies that merely reform the small group insurance market or provide small subsidies or increased information "will not make a significant dent in the number of working uninsured." Because of the economic conditions that prevail in small business markets and labor markets, she believes that some public intervention through subsidies or mandates will be necessary "if policy makers want to reach low-income workers."

Gail Jensen, in chapter 8, looks at the effects of state regulations that prescribe the terms of coverage for employer group health insurance plans. These state "mandates" have been identified in most of the health reform proposals as an inhibiting factor to the provision of low-cost basic insurance policies and innovative managed-care plans that might otherwise be attractive to small employers. Jensen describes the extent of these regulations, considers why states pass such laws, and reviews what is known about their effects on the market for group health insurance.

Some of the principal findings presented in chapter 8 are the following:

- While some families gain access to a special mandated service, most of the population in a state is unaffected. Most of those affected work for small firms that offer modest benefits.
- Mandates often raise the price employers pay for health insurance. These costs are usually paid by workers in the form of reduced wages, reduced benefits, or reduced employment.
- Some small firms forgo health insurance altogether because of mandates.
- A serious problem of adverse selection results from continuation-of-coverage requirements that are burdensome to employers.
- State premium taxes have a strong effect on insurance choices, causing small firms to forgo coverage and larger firms to self-insure.

Jensen concludes that because of the growth of state mandates, the unintended effect of the Employment Retirement Income Security Act of exempting self-insured plans from state regulation must now be addressed as a major issue in health reform.

Commentaries. The three commentators on the issue of access have one thing in common: each tries to look at the issue from a perspective that is different from and broader than that of the authors of the three chapters.

William Dennis, who represents the small business sector, discusses ways to increase health insurance coverage among small employers, such as ending the tax exclusion for health insurance, adopting universal claims forms, and providing consumers with information on prices and outcomes. He argues that the access problem in the small-firm market is really a cost problem because the cost of health insurance is the overriding reason small firms do not offer insurance. Dennis is skeptical that small-group reform will improve access, since these proposals will likely increase the cost of insurance for small firms, especially if the ERISA preemption continues to allow the larger and lower risk groups to escape through self insurance. Play-or-pay proposals do not provide a private-sector solution, he says, because there will be strong incentives for most small firms to pay into the public insurance pool rather than offer private coverage. In sum, Dennis doubts that we have the political will to do the things necessary to improve access to health insurance in the small-employer market.

Donald Moran expresses a different kind of skepticism about improving access to health care. Using a clever musical metaphor, he points out that the issue of access continues to reappear in the usual cycle of the health policy debate but that it quickly fades as the debate turns to health care costs and arguments about control of resource allocation. As part of this cycle, the diagnosis of market failure is always followed by prescriptions for various kinds of nonmarket interventions to correct the problems.

But Moran warns that thinking we are ready for radical reform of the health care system may be an illusion. He uses the findings of Morrisey, McLaughlin, and Jensen to argue that the problems in our present system of private financing are "so intrinsic to the structure of the system as to doom to failure any halfhearted attempt at reform." And thinking that a public sector solution can solve these problems is equally unrealistic.

Stephen Zuckerman, who is also skeptical, reminds us that health care decisions by individuals have a public goods aspect to them; that is, when individuals get sick and do not have insurance or cannot pay for their care, the cost of the care they do receive involves a subsidy from someone else. In Zuckerman's view, the major issue in the health reform debate is how to provide more efficient and equitable subsidies to individuals who do not have adequate access. Consequently, he is critical of Morrisey's analysis of mandates because it does not consider how to provide additional access to those now without insurance.

Zuckerman makes four basic points in his commentary. First, present subsidies are skewed toward individuals with high incomes, so on equity grounds they should be restructured. But if the objective is to help low-income workers, it would be a mistake to subsidize only small firms since many employees of small firms are not low income.

Second, though the present system of private insurance needs reform, we should attempt to improve access by building on the system of employer-based coverage. As for reforms, he calls for correcting the abuses of present underwriting practices and of exclusions for preexisting conditions, and, despite the warnings of Feldman and Dowd, he would provide community rating, especially for small employers.

Third, Zuckerman would experiment with alternatives to the fairly rich packages of benefits now typically offered. One advantage of relaxing state mandates would be to allow market experimentation to test consumer acceptance of trading off more complete coverage for savings in the cost of insurance.

His concluding point is that cost containment should be given serious attention in health reform along with improving access. Zuckerman points out that agreement on how to control costs is unlikely. Therefore, it would be desirable to experiment with managed competition, rate controls, and explicit rationing. But no policy can be expected to work without penalties for failure; that is, if a cost-containment experiment does not work, providers should face reductions in income and legislators should have to raise taxes or cut benefits.

Part Three: What Can Reform Achieve in Health Care Cost-Containment?

Both the general public and politicians seem to have stronger concerns about the increasing cost of health care than about other issues in the health reform debate (*The American Enterprise* 1992). Most political analysts identify handling the cost of health care as the major stumbling block to a legislative compromise to reform the health care market. Central to this disagreement is the dispute about the efficacy of both traditional market incentives and government regulation. As evidenced in the four essays and the commentaries in this part of the volume, the debate about incentives versus regulation is carried out in terms of the performance of both the private and the public sector. Recent rates of growth of health care prices, total expenditures, or per capita expenditures, as illustrated in table 1-1, present major challenges to all payers of health care whether in the public or private sector. The central questions are:

1. Are health care markets self-correcting? That is, will the increasing cost of health care induce individual consumers to change the way they use health care and individual providers and payers (for example, insurance companies, employers) to change the way they provide both financial and medical services?

2. If health care markets are not self-correcting, then what kinds of policy changes are necessary to obtain the required changes in provider and consumer behavior?

3. If health care markets will not work, or cannot be made to work, then can government regulation through price, budget, or utilization controls be made to work?

Jack Meyer outlines the type of health care reform he believes will correct the basic problem of rising costs and lack of access. He emphasizes creating incentives that will direct both providers and patients toward managed-care arrangements and away from open-ended financing. Meyer gives examples of private sector activities that show real promise to improve the quality and value of health care. These examples include Honeywell's efforts to measure provider quality, efforts of business coalitions and insurance companies to purchase on the basis of value,

TABLE 1–1
HEALTH CARE PRICES AND EXPENDITURES, 1980 AND 1990

	1980	1990	Average Annual Rate of Change (percent)
Consumer price index[a]			
All items	82.4	130.7	4.7
Medical care	74.9	162.8	8.1
Gross national product (billions)	2,732	5,465	7.2
National health expenditures (billions)			
Total	238.9	643.4	10.4
As % of GNP	*8.74*	*11.77*	
Public	76.7	212.9	10.7
As % of GNP	*2.81*	*3.90*	
Private	162.1	430.4	10.3
As % of GNP	*5.93*	*7.88*	
Per capita health expenditures			
Total	1,015	2,478	9.3
Public	326	820	9.7
Private	689	1,658	9.2

a. 1982–84 = 100.
SOURCES: U.S. Bureau of the Census, *Statistical Abstract of the United States: 1991* (Washington, D.C., 1991), table 769, and U.S. Health Care Financing Administration, *Health Care Financing Review,* Fall 1991, table 6, and Winter 1991, tables 1 and 14.

and efforts of various companies to use financial incentives to increase employee use of selected, or network, providers. He reports that more aggressive management of health care benefits and the use of prevention and wellness programs are not in widespread use but show much potential to increase quality and to control costs if used by more private-sector payers.

Meyer then identifies federal tax policy, state-mandated benefits, anticompetitive regulations, and the medical malpractice system as barriers to such private-sector reform. To achieve incentive-based, market-oriented reform, Meyer proposes a combination of policy changes, including Medicaid expansion and tax credits for the poor, greater incentives for primary care physicians to participate in Medicaid, reform in the private insurance market to change underwriting practices that deny access to high-risk firms and employees, and tax incentives for small businesses to offer health insurance coverage.

Karen Davis takes a different approach to cost-containment and health care reform. Reviewing the trends in hospital and physician health costs, she concludes that several decades of relying on market forces and the competitive strategies tried in the 1980s have had little effect on costs. Davis argues that the Medicare system of paying hospitals in contrast has contained costs and that the new system of paying physicians according to resource-based relative-value fee schedules should be equally effective. She proposes that Medicare's system of payment controls be extended to all payers and that a system ensuring universal access be established. Reviewing several legislative proposals to establish universal access and all-payer payment controls, she argues that the advantages of such a system would be improved equity and access to care, administrative simplicity, and effective cost control. Davis does not think that such as approach would be a threat to the quality of care or to innovation and technological change in medicine.

David Dranove discusses the growing use of utilization review to contain health care costs. He documents the increased use of utilization review in conventional insurance plans and in managed-care plans but argues that such review is unlikely to prevent inappropriate utilization. Obstacles include a lack of definitive cost-effectiveness research and poor cost measurement. Reviewing some of the research on the effectiveness of utilization review, Dranove concludes that this research is inadequate because it focuses narrowly on total inpatient expenditures or inpatient days rather than on systemwide expenditures and outcomes. Unless utilization review adopts a more systemwide approach, it may fail as a means to improve the efficiency of health care. And, in Dranove's view, the failure of utilization review may also mean the failure of competitive strategies to reform medical markets.

Patricia Danzon, analyzing the issue of market forces versus regulation to control costs, compares the costs of administering the Canadian and U.S. health insurance systems. She addresses the broad issue of Canada as a model for U.S. health policy and the specific issue of measuring administrative costs (overhead) in both countries. Danzon's main purpose is to lay out a more appropriate conceptual framework for defining total overhead costs and to point out why existing comparisons focusing only on accounting costs are grossly misleading.

She reviews estimates of U.S. administrative costs by Woolhandler and Himmelstein (1991) and others who use similar methodology and identifies several fallacies and biases that overstate the implied inefficiency of the U.S. system. Danzon calculates that these adjustments alone reduce the 1987 overhead rate from 11.7 percent of benefit payments to 7.6 percent. She points out that much of this is still not wasted since these

13

administrative functions are providing benefits to consumers. Public insurers, as in Canada, spend less on such functions but impose hidden costs on consumers that do not appear in national accounts or simplistic accounting comparisons.

Even the much-criticized underwriting practices of private insurers and the cost of claims administration have offsetting benefits that help to reduce unnecessary care and to avoid problems of moral hazard. Similarly misleading is the assumption that the extra administrative costs are wasted when the system gives consumers more choices than those provided by a monopoly government system like Canada. Consumers with more choices do not have to undergo the hidden costs of adjusting to the more limited choices of a government-regulated system.

Danzon also analyzes the costs of public monopoly financing that may not appear in comparative studies. These, she argues, entail significant real but hidden costs, some of which correspond to the costs that private insurers incur to control moral hazard and to collect premiums. These include patient time costs that result from relying on nonprice rationing, forgone benefits due to tight budget caps for hospitals and nonoptimal investment in information systems, and contributions to pharmaceutical R&D. Danzon presents rough empirical estimates and indicates that these hidden costs may be at least as great as the observable overhead costs in the U.S. system. She concludes that "although there may well be waste in U.S. private insurance markets at present, this waste is attributable primarily to tax and regulatory factors and is not intrinsic to private health insurance."

Commentaries. The commentators on these chapters represent divergent interests and experience with cost-containment. One has experience in managing Kaiser Permanente, the largest and many would say the most successful health maintenance organization in the country. Before joining Kaiser, he oversaw the operation of New York state's all-payer rate system. Another, who heads a major hospital association, is considered by many to be one of the most informed participants and observers of health politics in Washington. And the third is an academic economist with considerable experience in research related to the cost of health care.

Robert Crane of Kaiser points out that the cost containment debate has put too much emphasis on placing controls on a nonsystem with perverse incentives and not enough emphasis on creating systems with the right incentives. Based on his experience as a regulator in New York, he is less sanguine than Karen Davis about the ability of government to manage costs. Crane believes that competition among prepaid organized systems of health care has the best chance to moderate health care costs.

He discusses several private and public policy changes that could help set the rules for this type of effective competition based on quality.

Michael Bromberg objects to several points made by Davis. He takes her to task for saying that competition was tried and failed in the 1980s. In Bromberg's view, we have never tried competition because we have never tried to create a real market that has incentives to distinguish between ineffective care and medically necessary care. He questions her assertion that diagnostic related groups were the primary influence on hospital expenditures in the 1980s. In Bromberg's view, changes in technology were a major factor in the movement of care out of hospitals into outpatient settings. He also questions the evidence on the effects of state rate setting and criticizes Davis for leaving out the effects of tax subsidies that affect the demand for care. In addition, Bromberg believes that rate setting is incompatible with managed care since rate setting takes away the incentive for managed-care plans to take risks and to compete on the basis of value.

H. E. Frech, perhaps reflecting the changing health care system in California, reminds us that what others have described as a half-empty competitive health care bucket may be at least half-full. In his view, the competitive nature of U.S. health care is changing rapidly, but many of these changes are subtle and difficult for researchers to measure. The fact that we are in transition from a more inefficient system to a more competitive and efficient system complicates the task of analyzing the effects of market changes and making comparisons between countries.

In this regard, Frech points out some confusion in earlier chapters about two distinct levels of competition. He distinguishes between plans designed to attract employers and those to attract employees. Frech believes there has been too much emphasis on choice by the employee and not enough on the more important type of competition for employers or groups. And he does not feel that competition on selection necessarily rules out competition on cost-containment. Frech objects to the assertion that independent practice associations do not really compete. He points out that IPAs and PPOs are the fastest growing insurers.

Frech views Patricia Danzon's chapter as a major new contribution to our understanding of nonprice rationing. It outlines the correct conceptual framework for comparing different health care systems and provides a direction for comparative research. He observes that policy makers in other countries are apparently aware of the hidden costs of their monopoly nonprice-rationing schemes since several other countries (the Netherlands, New Zealand, and the United Kingdom) are moving away from single-payer monopolistic systems.

In contrast, Frech is critical of the optimism that Davis expresses for a single-payer system. Based on the evidence in his volume (Frech 1991), he questions her belief that the resource-based relative value scale will increase primary care and reduce surgery. Further, Frech sees that limits on balanced billing by providers will cause access problems and hidden rationing costs of the type identified by Danzon. In addition, he argues that expenditure targets advocated by Davis have been a complete failure in Medicare and in state Medicaid programs.

In Frech's view, Medicare is a poor model for a new health policy for the United States. He does agree with Davis that U.S. health care is "overdone greatly in quantity and quality." But competitive markets have far greater potential to correct this overconsumption in an efficient way than single-payer systems that hide the true costs of rationing.

Part Four: What Are the Choices among Policies to Achieve Reform?

This part of the volume addresses the topic of health care reform from the point of view of the basic choices we face. Instead of talking about specific proposals, the authors of the chapters and the commentaries attempt to step back from the political fray and to discuss the political and economic effects of the basic approaches to reform. Using an approach of public choice economics, Mark Pauly addresses the issue of why health care reform is so difficult to achieve. Eugene Steuerle analyzes the basic choices, using the principles of public finance, while Warren Greenberg uses the Dutch experience to illustrate the opportunity for establishing a system of competing health plans. The commentaries present three divergent views about these basic choices for reform.

Mark Pauly gives reasons why years of debate about national health insurance have produced virtually no action. Despite large increases in prices, a growth in real income, and a substantial shift in demographic composition, the basic structure of Medicare, Medicaid, and private insurance established in 1965 has remained remarkably stable.

Arguing that health care reform could result in some net benefits, he lists three factors that have inhibited reform over the past twenty-five years. First, no known system distributes the net benefits among enough politically decisive groups to bring about change. Pauly looks at the distribution of income and the distribution of tastes and points out the conflicts that would result if we redistributed available health care resources and existing tax subsidies to those who do not now have coverage. He reviews the evidence on the uninsured and concludes that this group is an "atypical minority with special problems—of which being uninsured is only one." Any policy designed to help the uninsured would be inefficient and excessively expensive because no known method singles out only the uninsured.

The second inhibiting factor to reform is the inability, thus far, to design a policy that captures the net benefits of reform. Pauly discusses the difficulties of reducing the benefits of tax subsidies to employers and employees and of reducing excess payments to providers.

The third factor involves our basic distrust of politicians and bureaucrats to control the system in a way that is both efficient and to our liking. We do not see how politicians can better control costs or ration care. If we cannot see how a political change might improve the system, then our strong inclination is to stay with the status quo. Pauly concludes that the best approach to overcoming these obstacles to reform is to make the choices explicit so that all parties to the debate can clearly identify the net benefits of reform.

Eugene Steuerle analyzes health policy reform choices using the principles of public finance. He points out that health policy cannot be separated from tax policy since expenditures and taxes are just two sides of the same accounting ledger. Steuerle's computations of national health expenditures show that the usual presentations concentrating on uses of expenditures significantly understate total health expenditures. When tax subsidies and other hidden sources of financing are included, he estimates that national health expenditures for fiscal year 1992 were $768 billion, or $8,000 per household. When measured in this way, federal, state, and local governments spend approximately $390 billion (51 percent of the $768 billion total) to subsidize health care. A typical household pays directly for only about one-third of the $8,000 figure, the remainder being paid by hidden employer payments and government subsidies.

Steuerle uses this background to discuss how health expenditures have displaced other government efforts and functions. Consumers are given weak incentives to control their use of health care because of the open-ended nature of tax subsidies and government health programs.

He discusses proposals to correct the current distortions in health markets with tax credits or vouchers and play-or-pay approaches. While tax credits or vouchers are difficult to design and administer, they provide the flexibility and adaptability needed to correct individual incentives and improve equity. While play-or-pay proposals are rather blunt instruments to achieve fairness, Steuerle points out that almost all proposals, including tax credit proposals, are similar in that they impose penalties on those who do not participate in the scheme. He discusses the technical problems of administering any play-or-pay or tax credit approach but suggests that a flat surtax might be imposed on all those without health insurance with an exemption for the low-income.

Steuerle suggests that various health reform proposals have some common features, enough to bring about agreement on a system based on individual tax credits with some mandates. He suggests that a modest

17

annual voucher of $350 per person and a penalty of $387 per person for those without insurance could provide a significant incentive for purchasing health insurance and would build on the existing employer-based system.

Warren Greenberg analyzes the imperfections of the U.S. health care system and suggests that current attempts to reform the Dutch system may provide a good road map for the United States to follow. He describes the dissatisfaction with the present Dutch system and the plan for reform based on competing health plans and government payments based on case-mix adjustments.

Greenberg discusses several technical problems, such as adjusting payment for the severity of the illness and computing the optimal budget amount. Still, he argues that such a system has the potential of improving the efficiency, productivity, and equity of health care delivery and financing in both the Netherlands and the United States.

Commentaries. Henry Aaron, Stuart Butler, and Deborah Steelman provide various interesting points about both health care politics and economics. Aaron gives two reasons why he believes that the emphasis on retaining and expanding choice among insurance plans is grossly exaggerated and not well supported as an objective of health reform. First, he points out that the choices made about insurance plans are substantially different from the choices made during a serious medical problem. Aaron argues that the loss in well-being to individuals from a health plan that would impose society's judgments about the appropriate scope of health insurance would be trivial compared with the gains from preventing mistakes that people would later regret. He thinks that neither Mark Pauly nor anyone else has made the case that choice of insurance matters. His second point is that no one has properly explained why politicians are so reluctant to consider any change to the present tax subsidies for employer-provided health insurance, although he agrees with the desirability of some limitations on this subsidy. In Aaron's view, health care is such a great national problem that we should fix it without worrying about making our tax system slightly more regressive.

Stuart Butler focuses on the role that employers might play in a system that eliminates or limits the present tax subsidy to employer-provided insurance. He objects to Steuerle's characterization of tax credit proposals as being play-or-pay: he sees a fundamental difference in the role employers would play in the traditional play-or-pay proposals and in a system with tax subsidies not tied to employment. While Butler understands the political appeal of traditional play-or-pay, he points out that such proposals run into political problems when attempts are made to make them equitable for small employers.

18

But proposals that seek changes in incentives through changes in the tax treatment of health insurance also run into political problems. In Butler's view, the only way to break the impasse is by combining a limit on the tax exclusion with benefits designed to provide horizontal equity, that is, to create a new set of winners to challenge those who defend the status quo.

An extensive review of health reform was recently completed by the Advisory Council on Social Security (1991). Deborah Steelman, the chairman, reminds us that reforms of any public policies must come through politics. In her view, no structural reform can occur in health care until we put all government programs—Medicare, Medicaid, and the tax code—on the table. Steelman criticizes this volume's authors, particularly in part 4, for too much emphasis on finance and not enough on the delivery system and on lifestyle changes.

She argues that because major changes are not possible, we must start with incremental changes. These first steps toward reform must come by giving people more choices. The federal government must be more willing to experiment to give people in Medicare and Medicaid more choices about the types of plans available. Steelman does not think that establishing a definition of a basic benefit package at the federal level is politically feasible.

Part Five: The Politics of Health Policy Reform

As Deborah Steelman has reminded us, health care reform must take place in a political environment. Any particular issue or proposal for reform must be "sold" to the public and to the politicians representing them. The complexity of the health care system, as well as of the various proposals to reform it, adds uncertainty about when and how our political system can deal with these issues.

This part of the volume turns from analysis of the issues of health reform to analysis of the politics of health reform. Three experienced politicians, one from the Senate and two from the House of Representatives, and two experts on public opinion discuss the basic factors that will affect the debate about health policy reform.

Senator Dave Durenberger, a member of the Senate Finance Committee, represents Minnesota, a state that many consider in the forefront of market changes in health care. He points out that health care reform is a volatile subject since almost all of us express dissatisfaction with costs but seem satisfied with our own doctor and our own coverage. Durenberger believes four elements will be necessary for reform but points out that we have not achieved any of them as yet. First, we need a common understanding of the health care problem. Second, we need a vision for the future. Third, we need a set of proper values and a way to adjust our current values to the new set. The slowdown in our economic progress means that we cannot automatically pass on our old values to the next generation. We need a way to adjust our expectations. And fourth, we need to develop a capacity for change.

He points out that we are in a political standoff because the providers of care do not trust the Democrats in Congress. Durenberger sees the experience with the Medicare Catastrophic Coverage Act as an indication that Congress is reluctant to impose hard choices on the beneficiaries of public programs, especially the elderly. In his view, the four elements of change will come about only "when the sellers of services have incentives to provide only what the payer needs, at higher quality, for a price that better reflects the value of the service."

Congressman Bill Gradison is a member of the House Ways and Means Committee and recently served as cochairman of the Pepper Commission, a congressional attempt to recommend a direction for health policy. In his view, health care is becoming an increasingly important political issue because people are becoming concerned about the cost of care and the future of their coverage. Intensified political debate, however, may create confusion because public views are unformed about many aspects of reform. Gradison discusses how the realities of the budget and concerns about the loss of jobs create major political criticisms for play-or-pay or Canadian-style single-payer proposals. In addition, he points out how cultural factors limit our political flexibility in reshaping our health care system. In particular, Gradison mentions Americans' strong desire for first-dollar coverage and their impatience with waiting for service. He also makes the point that many health care costs are the result of "drugs, homicides, obesity, bad diets, alcoholism, smoking," and other cultural causes. Gradison concludes that "we will end up with a health care system that is distinctively American: it will be very complicated and expensive."

Congressman Sander Levin is also on the House Ways and Means Committee. Reporting on an extensive health survey in his suburban-urban district in Michigan, Levin finds that the results reflect those in national polls. His constituents generally are satisfied with their own health care but are concerned about costs. They do not support new taxes or government regulation but favor more controls on doctors and insurance companies. Levin draws two conclusions from this and other surveys: one, presidential candidates will not win or lose the election on health care; and two, health care is an important part of the underlying issue of economic security, which is an important election issue.

Karlyn Keene, editor of AEI's *American Enterprise* and an expert on public opinion, reminds us that public opinion polls are blunt instruments. They can tell us generalities about the electorate but not specifics. She applies this principle to health politics by reviewing a number of recent polls about health care issues in the light of the historical record of public responses to broader questions about people's concerns. Keene points out that while Americans strongly agree that health care is in crisis, they do not consider it their most important problem. She reports that Americans are concerned primarily about the cost of health care, but they are distrustful about expanding the power of government to regulate health care. While polls show support for program expansion, they also show concern about the tax burden. Keene concludes that the political dynamics of this issue are unknown and the public will not provide specific guidance about what the government should be doing.

Neil Newhouse, also an expert on public opinion polls, points out that the public is not well informed about health care issues and that health reform will not become a major issue until people develop a more informed opinion. In his view, Americans are frustrated about the economy and the direction of the country; this may translate into an anti-incumbent movement directed both at the president and at the Congress. In the health care area, people still look to the federal government to help solve the basic problems. Newhouse thinks that the public may be inclined to identify as villains insurance companies, doctors, and hospitals, in addition to politicians. He concludes that Americans "want the same excellent standards they have received in the past, they want to maintain access, and they want to cut costs by half."

References

Advisory Council on Social Security. *Critical Issues in American Health Care Delivery and Financing Policy.* Washington, D.C.: ACSS, December 1991.
American Enterprise, The. "Health Cares." Vol. 3, March/April 1992, pp. 85–89.
Blue Cross and Blue Shield Association. *National Health Care Reform: Organizing the Solutions.* Chicago: BCBSA, 1991.
Frech, H. E. III. *Regulating Doctors' Fees: Competition, Benefits, and Controls under Medicare.* Washington, D.C.: American Enterprise Institute, 1991.
Woolhandler, S., and D. U. Himmelstein. "The Deteriorating Administrative Efficiency of the U.S. Health Care System." *New England Journal of Medicine* 324 (1991): 1253–58.

PART ONE

What, If Anything, Is Wrong
with Private Health Insurance?

2
Problems and Prospects in Multiple-Option Health Plan Settings

Harold S. Luft

Competition has played an important role in the U.S. medical care system. Because of the widespread use of reimbursement insurance until the mid–1980s, however, competition among health care providers was often cost-increasing rather than cost-reducing. Even if competition among providers were restructured to encourage competition on the basis of price per service, the result could still be an increase in total expenditures as volume rises. Alain Enthoven and others recognized this and encouraged competition among health plans rather than among individual providers. If health plans had the responsibility for paying for all the services required by an enrolled population, they would have strong incentives to control both provider prices and volumes.

The underlying notion of this type of competition is that people would be given a choice, usually on an annual basis, to choose among a set of health plan options to provide their care for the coming year (Enthoven 1980; Enthoven and Kronick 1989, 29–37, 94–101). Plans would have to offer at least a minimum basic-benefit package and to accept all enrollees from within the enrollee pool. This would eliminate or at least reduce the ability of plans to accept only the low-risk enrollees. A plan sponsor such as an employer or public agency for Medicare and Medicaid beneficiaries would manage the open enrollment process and would offer a fixed contribution regardless of the health plan chosen. The fixed contribution would make consumers sensitive to the full marginal costs of more expensive plans. This price sensitivity, in turn, would force plans to be efficient or to be driven from the market. As a purchaser with far more expertise than an individual consumer, the sponsor would also be able to assess quality of care and eliminate poor quality programs from the list of options.

This approach to competition would have direct benefits for those choosing among the plans. They could have better coverage at lower cost because of the competitive pressures exerted by the structure of the system. Furthermore, allowing multiple plans to compete would also enable consumers to choose among health plans with different styles of care or caring. Thus consumers willing to wait a bit longer for appointments or to have a narrower panel of primary care physicians might have substantially lower premiums, while those demanding more personalized service would pay more.

This type of competition among multiple-option plans would also offer the promise of external benefits. That is, as tightly managed health plans such as HMOs garnered increasing shares of the patient pool, those physicians and hospitals in the fee-for-service oriented part of the market would adopt cost-containing mechanisms to retain their patients. Thus even without having all enrollees in HMOs, the system as a whole would enjoy major cost savings.

While this scenario is both attractive and plausible, it seems not to be unfolding exactly as anticipated (National Health Policy Forum 1991). Many reasons account for this, some of which will be examined in this chapter. Others are as yet unknown, largely because of the limited extent of the research on the workings of the medical care market. In some cases we may speculate on ways to overcome the problems. In others we may have to be content that effects of major policy changes are inherently uncertain and that promises and prognostications should be viewed with substantial skepticism. This attitude should apply, of course, to the prognostications of this author as well.

Many of the shortcomings of the multiple-option strategy are due not to the failure of the concept but to the way health policy is implemented, or rather not implemented, in the United States. That is, many of the crucial aspects of Alain Enthoven's proposal were never adopted, and had they been accepted, things may have worked out better. This chapter, however, focuses not on Enthoven's proposal per se, but rather on the problems and prospects of multiple-option health plans in addressing the question, What, if anything, is wrong with private health insurance?

Problems in Multiple-Option Settings

The ideal version of a multiple-option setting is one in which potential enrollees, usually employees of a firm, choose among a set of health plans once a year. The employees are provided with clear, descriptive material about each plan, which enables them to make relatively informed choices. Some aspects of health plans, however, cannot really be understood until they are experienced, so there is some switching among plans each year.

Over time, however, individuals gain experience with plans and learn about options from friends and neighbors, so the choices become relatively stable. The employer offers a fixed-dollar contribution, regardless of the plan chosen, so cost differences in plans are borne by the employee. This practice encourages plans to be efficient and to offer the lowest possible premiums. Individual marketing is prohibited—that is, plan representatives are not allowed to contact employees directly. Instead they submit promotional material to the employee benefit office, which distributes packets to those employees wishing to evaluate the various options. This lowers marketing costs and eliminates problems of adverse selection and screening by health plans. As plans compete on the basis of being efficient providers, they squeeze out the excess cost and utilization from health care providers. This leads to benefits not only for the enrollees of the various plans, but also for the rest of the community.

The reality of multiple-option settings seems to be substantially different. Consumers often appear ill-informed about the benefits and restrictions of various plans. From the employer's perspective, the management of the multiple-choice arrangements is far from simple and often is fraught with confusion and risk. Perhaps more important, many employers perceive multiple-option plans as increasing rather than decreasing their costs. Finally, there is little evidence that competition among plans has led to systemwide cost containment (McLaughlin 1987, 183–205; Luft, Maerki, and Trauner 1986, 625–58). In fact, there is reason to believe the increased competition among plans actually has worsened the cost problem and created access problems for the uninsured. Although this issue is beyond the scope of how well multiple-option plans work in the private insurance market, the implications of such plans for the health care system are crucially important. If such competition is seen as creating diseconomies elsewhere, at least during a transition period, then the political tolerance needed for the strategy to unfold may disappear.

In reviewing the various problems that plague the implementation of multiple-option health insurance plans, we should distinguish several main categories that will be helpful later in addressing prospects for the future. Some problems are primarily administrative and site-specific, such as those of offering a large number of health plans in the context of complex employer-employee relationships. Other problems arise from the structure of local health care markets and may be insoluble. These include the relatively small number of potential competitors, both health plans and hospitals, in any one market area. Recognizing the realistic

27

limits of competition, however, is an important first step in designing workable policies. Yet other problems arise from the very nature of competition and choice. These include biased selection among plans and the disappearance of cross-subsidization. In theory one may be able to offset these problems, but it is difficult to know whether theoretical solutions are possible and whether potential solutions are politically feasible.

Biased Selection. Substantially more research has been done on the question of biased selection than on the other issues, so it is a useful place to begin. Biased selection is a natural outcome of multiple-option plans. The only way to avoid biased selection would be for people to choose health plans for reasons unrelated to their risk of incurring medical care costs. Suppose, for example, that each health plan served a distinct geographic submarket within a broad market area over which the employee population was spread. If the need for health care among these employees was not related to location, then it would be possible to have strong preference differences among plans without biased selection.

If factors correlated with health care needs *are* differentially associated with various plans, then selection among plans is likely to be biased in that certain plans will have enrollees with above-average risks. If Plan A, for example, has a large deductible while Plan B offers first-dollar coverage, the economic incentive would be for people expecting to use medical care to choose Plan B and those who expect to be healthy to choose Plan A. Since the premiums quoted by health plans reflect both their efficiency in delivering care and their enrollees' needs for care, such selection will tend to increase the premium for Plan B in the following year relative to what it would have been without selection. In the next cycle, even more people who expect not to need care will leave Plan B because of its increased cost, leading to a spiral of premiums and selection.

Even in the best of worlds, multiple-option plans are likely to result in biased selection because plans do not differ just in terms of efficiency. Instead plans differ in coverages and delivery systems, factors important in the choice of plan and likely to be correlated with underlying expected use of medical care (Klinkman 1991, 295–330). Most fee-for-service oriented plans, for example, offer free choice of provider and combine some utilization management, such as second opinions and preadmission certification, with copayments and deductibles. Furthermore, most such plans exclude coverage of preventive services and routine physical examinations. In contrast, staff and group model HMOs tend to have minimal copayments, such as $5–10 per visit, but they cover preventive services and routine checkups. Such plans, however, limit the choice of providers to a small group of physicians in any one area, and this usually requires new enrollees to change physicians. Individual practice association HMOs take an intermediate position. They often have a wider choice of physicians and hospitals, but the provider list is still narrower than that of the fee-for-service plans. Copayments are small, but the premiums are often higher than those of the group or staff model plans.

These differences among plans may lead to biased selection, but the direction of the effects is difficult to determine a priori (Berki and Ashcraft 1980, 588–632). The absence of copayments and deductibles in HMOs, for example, is a potential attraction for people planning on using medical care (Robinson et al. 1991, 107–116). Nevertheless, people planning to use medical care are more likely to have attachments to a provider and thus to be less willing to switch into an HMO if it requires a change in physician. It is also the case that most fee-for-service plans have maximum out-of-pocket expenses, so people facing very high costs may view the traditional plan as just having a large fixed cost rather than the standard 20 percent copayment.

Biased or uneven selection of risks across plans is not a problem if the amount paid to the various plans may be adjusted to offset the differences in risk. The Health Care Financing Administration comes closest to doing this under the Medicare program in which HMOs are paid varying amounts depending on the mixture of enrollees according to age, gender, disability status, and county of residence. In spite of this system, various studies have suggested that the adjustment does not offset fully the risk differences (see, for example, Lichtenstein et al. 1991, 318–31).

Uncompensated biased selection has several deleterious consequences. First, it changes the nature of the competitive "game." In general it is far easier to achieve lower costs by attracting low-risk (or avoiding high-risk) enrollees than to pressure providers to be cost-conscious. Thus there are strong incentives to move away from "the best of all worlds" to a situation in which plans actively design benefit packages, provider arrangements, and other schemes to gain favorable risks. A recent article in a periodical for HMO managers, for example, outlines ways "prescription drug benefits can be manipulated to influence selection bias in a health plan" (Curtiss 1991, 9–11). Unlike true cost-containment efforts that reduce expenditures, efforts to attract low-risk enrollees are actually cost-increasing. If successful from a plan's perspective, they ease the pressure to contain costs truly while forcing the higher-risk individuals onto someone else's bill. They also create dead-weight loss through the costs of selective marketing, new enrollee administrative costs, and the like.

A second major problem with biased selection arises from the fact that HMOs have attracted the lower-risk enrollees while the fee-for-service plans have the higher-cost enrollees (Luft and Miller 1988, 97–119; Hellinger 1987, 55–63; Wilensky and Rossiter 1986, 66–80). It is important to note, however, that not all HMOs experience favorable selection. When combined with the general pattern of pegging sponsor contributions to fee-for-service plan premiums, this leads to even more rapid growth in contributions. This pattern of setting the contribution to minimize the pain for fee-for-service enrollees has historical roots in many companies and may also be related to the fact that most managers choose fee-for-service rather than HMO options.

If the higher costs in the fee-for-service plans reflect both their relative inefficiency and an increasing share of high-risk enrollees, then it is politically difficult to force these enrollees to bear the full increase in premiums. Moreover, the more rapidly the fee-for-service premiums rise in such a situation, the more rapidly the relatively lower-risk enrollees in that plan will leave. To keep the fee-for-service plan's net premium in some reasonable range, the employer contribution must often be so high that all the HMOs are free, which creates additional problems around the issue of premium setting, to be discussed below.

Biased selection also creates a problem of perception and political acceptability. Many employers saw the research literature on the costs of medical care for people enrolled in fee-for-service and HMO plans. HMOs marketed themselves as being able to achieve substantial savings, often in the range of 20–40 percent. After years of experience with multiple options, however, many employers say they see no savings.

Some of the reasons for this relate to premium-setting behavior by the HMOs. But another factor is that researchers and businesses focus on different costs. Employers focus on their contributions, while the research studies focus on the total costs of care per enrollee in various plans (Luft 1987; Manning et al. 1984, 1505–10). Total costs include premiums, whether paid by the employee or the employer; out-of-pocket costs for copayments; deductibles; and noncovered services. As fee-for-service costs have risen over the past decade, benefits have become more circumscribed, deductibles have risen, and other costs have shifted to the enrollee (Jensen and Gabel 1988, 328–43).

In spite of this, premiums and the employer contribution have risen rapidly (Savitz 1991, 8 ff.). Thus, from the employer's perspective, costs have increased. If HMO premiums have kept pace with those of fee-for-service, it does not matter to the employer if those premiums include more rather than fewer benefits over time. The fact that those enrolled in the HMOs may have garnered more benefits does not help the firm trying to control its fringe benefit costs. Moreover, if the presence of HMOs has actually led to adverse selection against the fee-for-service plan and to a more rapid increase in fee-for-service premiums, then one could argue that the HMOs have had a net inflationary effect on the employer. Representatives of the fee-for-service plans are quick to argue that their costs are increasing more rapidly because of favorable selection by the HMOs.

Premium Setting. Biased selection would not be a problem if health plans were merely reimbursed for their costs. In fact, most fee-for-service options offered by large employers are fully experience-rated or self-insured by the employer, so their premiums, at least in the long run, reflect expenses. The key aspect of an HMO, however, is that its strong incentives to economize on the provision of services for its enrollees is based on its acceptance of risk. HMOs argue, quite legitimately, that if they were fully experience-rated, then there would be no incentive for them to be efficient.

In the face of biased selection, however, the issue of premium setting becomes a key problem in competition among health plans. The traditional approach used by HMOs is community rating, in which the premiums are based upon the collective costs of everyone enrolled in the HMO. Since the enrollees from a particular firm are usually a very small fraction of an HMO's total enrollee pool, a firm may experience substantially biased selection, with the low-risk people moving to the HMO, but this will have a negligible effect on the HMO's premium. Of course, if the HMO experiences favorable selection from all or most of its enrollee groups, then there will be a noticeable effect on its costs.

Some HMOs are moving toward the use of adjusted community rating, in which the premium is adjusted upward or downward depending on the mixture of the enrollee group relative to the HMO's total enrollment pool. In this manner, a firm with a younger enrollee group would be quoted a lower-than-average HMO premium. Movement toward premiums reflecting the actual experience of the enrollees in that HMO are more problematic, because the number of enrollees from most firms is relatively small. This problem is exacerbated if there are concerns about biased selection.

One may ask why this is more of a problem for the HMOs than for the fee-for-service carriers. One answer is that most HMOs have little expertise with the tracking of costs on an individual enrollee basis and with experience rating. Another answer is that HMOs prefer to maintain the cost-containing incentives of full capitation, but they worry about efforts by benefit managers to dump high-cost cases on them.

The above issues would be problems even in a perfectly operating market. But markets are never quite perfect, and several aspects of the market for employer-based health insurance are important in understanding additional problems related to premium setting (McLaughlin 1988, 207–18). For one, although there may be more than 500 HMOs in the country, most markets have relatively few plans in competition with one another. For example, of the twenty-seven largest market areas served by HMOs, thirteen have fewer than ten HMOs (Palsbo 1990). Even at the metropolitan-area level, the number of competitors is often misleading because many HMOs are available only in limited geographic submarkets. Thus the market is really characterized by monopolistic competition, in which prices are set with careful consideration of responses by local competitors. Second, much of the competition is based upon nonprice characteristics of the various plans. Individual Practice Association (IPA) model plans, for example, often emphasize the wide choice of physician, while group model plans emphasize the identifiable clinic settings and ease of referral.

In this context it appears that two major considerations enter into premium-setting decisions. The first is the level of the premiums for the fee-for-service plan. In general, HMOs have their major marketing advantage when they can offer a lower premium than the fee-for-service plans. But there is really no incentive for the HMOs to offer a premium lower than the employer's contribution. This leads to what is often called "shadow pricing." If, over time, the contribution level roughly parallels the fee-for-service costs, then HMOs have little incentive to force down their premiums. This problem is exacerbated by the long-standing premium cycle for fee-for-service insurance (Gabel et al. 1990, 161–75). At the upswing of the cycle, annual increases are extraordinarily high, so additional pricing leeway is available for the HMOs. The downside of the cycle usually has increases comparable to the cost of living, so there still is little pressure on the HMOs, because few people then switch back to the fee-for-service plan.

In addition to the premium patterns set by the fee-for-service plan, there may be price leadership among HMOs in the local area. That is, if a large HMO sets its premiums at what it feels is a reasonable level, other HMOs may follow, even though they could have accommodated to lower increases. In the past few years in northern California, for example, Kaiser Foundation Health Plan experienced a massive growth in enrollment. Since the nature of the Kaiser plan is fairly capital-intensive, this enrollment growth was followed by substantial premium increases that were explained as an attempt to raise money for capital expansion to serve the new membership better. A slowing in the rate of growth in enrollment for the next year or so would actually have been a benefit in improved service. Not surprisingly, other HMOs in the area also announced relatively large increases in premiums, even though Kaiser's rates both before and after were the lowest.

It is important to note that the implications of premium increases for fee-for-service plans differ from those for HMO plans. Since most of the large employers' FFS plans are experience-rated, the premiums reflect either actual or expected costs of services; the administrative costs for such plans are relatively small. Thus an increase in premium for such plans has little effect on the insurer's bottom line. For the HMOs, however, the marginal premium dollar is often pure profit. Some of the major HMOs are not-for-profit organizations, and such net revenues are recycled as capital investment and additional benefits. Other HMOs are for-profit, however, and employers may be quite distressed at what they see as manipulated pricing that goes not to additional medical care benefits but to transfer profits from their bottom line to that of selected HMOs.

Managing a Multiple-Option Plan. Offering a multiple-option health plan is not a trivial undertaking for an employer, particularly a large one with multiple locations. The annual open enrollment season is often an administrative nightmare, sometimes with a massive number of switchers among plans, each of whom must be disenrolled and enrolled in a new plan, have deductions altered, and be presented with plan descriptions. Perhaps even more difficult are the problems that arise if an employer chooses not to be a passive premium-taker.

First of all, some employers must contract with hundreds of HMOs in order to provide options for their employees across the country. In many cases only a relatively small number of employees will be in most of the HMOs, but a few may have a substantial enrollment. Issues of equity and evenhandedness may require that contracting processes be similar for both the large and the small contracts, meaning either that major opportunities are lost or that the costs of negotiation and monitoring small contracts exceed the potential savings. As a consequence many benefit consultants are recommending that firms pare down the number of HMOs they offer. Regional differences in health care costs, combined with the fact that the fee-for-service plan is usually company-wide, mean that if the contribution is set appropriately relative to the base plan, it is likely to be too high for HMOs in some areas and too low in others. Even within one state, for example, the Kaiser family premium in southern California is 13 percent higher than the premium in northern California, a differential that has existed for at least two decades.

Second, the HMO market is undergoing substantial consolidation, as well as some highly publicized bankruptcies. This means that the employer must be concerned about coverage for enrollees in HMOs that are financially shaky, because should they close, it is not guaranteed that their enrollees will be accepted by other plans. Thus the benefit manager needs to become, at least in part, a financial analyst and an insurance company regulator. This problem is exacerbated by the fact that if a major employer cancels a contract with an HMO because of the fear the HMO may fail, the employer could be accused of "causing a run on the bank" and precipitating a failure that would not otherwise have happened.

Third, if an employer wishes to negotiate rates, develop experience-rated premiums, or devise approaches to offset the biased selection problem, then the level of expertise required increases substantially. These are all new approaches, and there is little experience with them either in the research arena or in the field. Employers may sometimes be correct in seeing negotiated rates as a means to extract concessions from the HMOs. Nevertheless, once the published community rate is jettisoned for negotiated rates, one cannot tell whether a deal is in fact better. The HMO will certainly know more about both its cost structure and the enrollees it has than will the firm. One has only to compare shopping at a supermarket that has posted prices with shopping at an auto dealership that has negotiated prices. Although it is difficult to tell which yields the best prices, few consumers prefer the latter process, where there is always the feeling that the deal was not as good as it should have been. Thus substantial learning about alternative premium setting is required, and there is little confidence that a better approach will be found.

Some firms are taking a different approach. Instead of dealing with thousands of suppliers and always looking for the best price on the items they purchase, they are consciously paring down the number of suppliers and are focusing on those who provide outstanding quality at reasonable cost. Xerox, for example, has reduced the number of its suppliers by 90 percent. Firms pursuing this strategy attempt to develop long-standing relationships with the remaining suppliers and help them better understand the company's needs. This approach can be applied in the health care setting as well. It implies more of a partnership arrangement, however, and less of a classic market solution. Moreover, in the health care setting it may be even more difficult to switch HMOs once long-term relationships are established. While a new supplier of high-quality machine screws can be found fairly easily, enrollees develop attachments to their physicians and may be upset if their HMO is dropped in favor of another one.

Provider Consolidation. In addition to a shrinking number of HMOs in any one local area, the pool of available providers, especially hospitals, is also shrinking. While the number of hospital closures is increasing slowly, in many markets a far more rapid wave of mergers is occurring among local institutions. Many metropolitan areas actually have only half a dozen hospitals, regardless of ownership.

34

In the past decade, for example, only one hospital in San Francisco went out of business, and it was purchased by Kaiser for extra bed capacity. After several mergers, however, three hospital groupings now control 72 percent of the available beds, and the remaining hospitals are generally in areas not very attractive for HMOs (Legnini 1990). One of the three major groupings is Kaiser, and another is the university, so local HMOs have essentially no community hospital alternatives to choose among. This means that free-standing HMOs have little bargaining power in negotiating contracts with local hospitals. Much the same pattern is emerging in Minneapolis-St. Paul (Mayer 1991, 3).

In addition to hospital mergers, there is growing consolidation of physician groups. Large group practices increasingly serve as the focal points for specific HMOs. In other cases, hospitals are purchasing group practices (Grant, Smith, and Lindeke 1990, 16–18). Although this is not the same as the classic staff or group model plan, such as Kaiser, these networks of groups are quite different from the old individual practice associations in which only a small proportion of the physician's practice was prepaid. Now 20–50 percent of the patients may be part of an HMO, enough to develop unique practice styles and referral systems for these patients (Grant 1991, 32–38). The other side is that if one HMO in the area accounts for a substantial share of the groups' prepaid business, it may demand either an exclusive contract or a channeling of its enrollees among the most cost-effective providers. While this is a natural response, the number of viable choices available for HMOs will shrink rapidly, as group practices have to "choose sides."

This type of consolidation is probably a natural outcome of the maturing of the market. It may make it more difficult for HMOs to extract major concessions from the provider population. It also makes it more likely that providers and HMOs will form stable alliances, which then compete on the basis of service but not price. Furthermore, it implies that a strategy based on aggressive price competition among a large number of health plans in a local area is probably feasible in only a handful of localities.

Responses by the Insurance Industry and Health Care Providers. Two additional aspects of multiple-option plans need to be considered. One is the response of the insurance industry through the development of triple-option plans. The other is the effect of increased competition on the health care system and how this has eroded the traditional patterns of cross subsidy.

As indicated earlier, one of the key problems in the multiple-option strategy is the potential for biased selection among plans. In fact, the likelihood of biased selection is so great that if it does not occur, it is

35

worth noting. To date, there have been no examples of effective external means to measure the extent of selection and offset the problems it creates. There is no selection problem, however, if one views the pool of enrollees as a whole. A given pool may be more or less risky than another pool of enrollees, but this is a reflection of the employment mixture, not selection.

One well-known contract negotiated by Allied-Signal with CIGNA was designed to eliminate the selection problem. Allied-Signal offered its employees a choice among traditional fee-for-service, a preferred-provider organization, and an HMO, all underwritten by CIGNA. While there could be substantial biased selection among the three options, it does not matter from the perspective of the employer because the extra costs faced by one of the plans are offset by savings among the others. Furthermore, an important aspect of the initial contract was a premium quotation that was good for three years, thereby guaranteeing savings for Allied-Signal.

The triple-option approach has several major advantages. From the perspective of the employer it vastly simplifies the purchasing of health plan options. It fits in with the notion of paring down the number of suppliers to a select few who can be relied upon. Premium rates can be set in advance, with incentives built in for good performance. One could even imagine rate increases being tied to external factors, such as the consumer price index.

From the carrier's perspective, it eliminates the worry about selection. The triple-option also eliminates other HMOs as competitors. It makes it substantially more difficult for the employer to pit one carrier against another, because there is unlikely to be another carrier with a comparable mix of HMO and PPO options in the relevant geographic areas.

Many of these advantages have a disadvantage. While selection is no longer a problem in setting premiums, it must still be measured in order to provide the appropriate internal signals to the managers of the three options concerning the performance of their divisions. If this is not done, the efficiency of the overall package may be jeopardized. While the linked offering of one HMO, one PPO, and one FFS plan may seem reasonable, not all HMOs are the same. Although many families may prefer to have one small imported car and one large American car, few would be content not being able to choose the brands. Likewise, an employer may prefer the HMO offered by the carrier in one city and a competitor's HMO in another city because of location or quality differences. Finally, while the careful nurturing of supplier-demander relationships may make sense in the long term, it may well be too soon to give up the option of choosing an entirely different set of providers, especially in the context of HMOs. Thus, although the multiple-option approach has much to recommend it, further modifications may well be advised before it is touted as the solution to the problems of multiple-option plans.

It is important to remember that large employers provide coverage only for a small fraction of the population. Much of the current debate about restructuring the U.S. health care system arises from the twin concerns of the large part of the population without any insurance or with only minimal insurance, and the rising costs of insurance for those with coverage. Multiple-option plans are not designed to help the former and seem ineffective in having a major impact on the latter. Moreover, in some ways the growing competitiveness of the health insurance market has worsened the access and cost issues. Until the early 1980s most hospitals were paid on the basis of costs or charges, allowing them to charge the insured patients and their carriers for the unreimbursed costs of those patients unable to pay. Some hospitals had substantially larger pools of uncovered patients, but their costs were buried in the fees for the insured, and payers were not particularly price-sensitive.

With the advent of Medicare's prospective payment system and aggressive price negotiation by private third-party payers and some Medicaid programs, the old system of cross subsidization has fallen apart. In response to competitive pressures by major employers, the large carriers have developed preferred-provider arrangements to contract with selected hospitals at lower-than-list price. Such contracts will cover the hospitals' marginal cost but provide little for the cross subsidy of the uninsured. It is therefore in the hospitals' best interest to avoid patients without insurance, steering them toward the public providers of last resort.

At the same time, small businesses are generally unable to attract the interest of the major insurers and so have less advantageous coverage. In 1989, for example, only 13 percent of firms with fewer than twenty-five employees offered a PPO, in contrast to 25 percent of firms with twenty-five or more employees (Health Insurance Association of America 1990, 49). With hospitals offering discounts to the stronger carriers through their PPOs, costs for the charge-paying insured increase even more rapidly, and are then reflected in rising premiums. Since small employers tend to offer smaller contributions, the rising premiums result in voluntary lack of coverage by employees who are eligible but feel they cannot afford coverage. At the same time many of the small firms are finding themselves canceled by their carriers because of one or two large claims, and they then have to shop around for new coverage at even higher cost.

The development of this multitiered system of coverage is likely to color the policy debate about the health care system. Large employers face problems of biased selection, complex administration, and rising premiums. Small firms find that their costs rise even more rapidly and that they cannot get coverage at reasonable prices. Hospitals find themselves torn between long-term commitments to local populations and the realities of price-based competition, in which aggressive cost cutting may be the only way to survive in a shrinking industry. In this context a multiple-option system as currently structured seems to have little beneficial impact. There may be a role for such an approach, however, in a somewhat restructured environment.

Prospects for a Multiple-Option Solution

The preceding discussion has pointed out several problems in the multiple-option health plan setting. Biased selection is a major problem that requires substantial additional analysis in working out a solution. The administrative problems associated with multiple choices are potentially more soluble. Premium-setting issues involve new adminis-trative approaches and techniques that do not run afoul of antitrust concerns. The latter are also potentially important in addressing the problems of a limited number of choices in most geographic areas. Finally, the growing problem of the uninsured and the falling apart of the small-firm insurance market, in combination with continuing cost increases for all payers, increase the pressure for a solution that works not just for the large-employer segment of the market.

The triple-option solution offered by a single carrier has too many shortcomings to be a solution by itself. It may be possible, however, to build a better model by keeping its strong points and modifying its weaknesses. The principal attraction of the triple-option model is that the employer is offered a bundled premium for all employees, irrespective of the plans they choose, and the carrier accepts the responsibility for efficient management of the system and for providing incentives for enrollees to choose the less costly options. The principal weakness is its locking the employer into a single carrier and that carrier's HMOs in all localities.

One alternative is to develop a "contractor," or intermediary, model (Luft 1986, 566–92; Enthoven and Kronick 1989, 29–37, 94–101). In such an approach, an intermediary would take on the responsibility of negotiating payments to various HMOs, PPOs, and fee-for-service plans. This intermediary would have to develop a method of assessing the extent of biased selection among the plans and would adjust payments accordingly. It could offer the employers a premium that, while possibly reflecting the total composition of its enrollee base, would be indepen-dent of risk selection among the options offered. The employer contri-bution would be allocated among the plans in a way to mimic the risk patterns, and the net employee cost would reflect differences in efficiency, not selection.

The use of an intermediary may entail compromises among employers in the design of their benefit packages, but there need not be uniformity. The level and structure of employer contributions, for example, could vary markedly across firms. Copayments and deductibles could be offered in several packages, and other benefits, such as preventive care options, could also be added.

By pooling the enrollments of many large and small firms in a local area, the intermediary would be far more able to assess risk factors and relative efficiency of plans. Furthermore, it could collect enough information about the quality of care and consumer assessments of the process to provide ratings of the alternatives. Even large employers do not have enough enrollees in most plans to undertake such assessments individually, but collectively they do. Furthermore, because of economies of scale in the collection and analysis of information, assessments impossible to undertake at the firm level may be relatively easy at the level of a local intermediary.

An intermediary could function at one of two levels. The simplest form would be as a broker or benefit consultant, who merely performs the negotiations and provides assessments of plan quality and risk-adjusted premiums. By pooling information from a large number of enrollee groups and negotiating risk-adjustment approaches collectively, the intermediary will have far more power than it would representing each firm individually. When working for individual clients, there is always the fear that a broker may attempt to skew the analysis away from the HMOs. While this incentive is still present for a collective intermediary, it is likely to be blunted by the fact that adjustments that might benefit the fee-for-service plan of one employer could harm that of another. When all employee groups are handled with the same risk-adjustment mechanisms, it is more difficult to "cook" the data. Thus there is strong pressure on the intermediary to collaborate with the various carriers and HMOs to develop a fair approach to assessing risk differences among plans.

The HMOs in an area would have a strong incentive to collaborate with a fair intermediary that would enable them to avoid allegations of favorable selection. The establishment of a generally accepted process of adjusting contributions and assessing plan performance would vastly simplify the negotiation process. Of course, those HMOs that are unfairly benefiting from favorable selection and that could not compete on efficiency and quality would find the intermediary process unattractive. Their decision not to participate would probably not be a major loss.

True managed-care plans and preferred-provider organizations would probably react to the use of an intermediary in much the same fashion as HMOs. To the extent that they are able to improve their relative positions by getting larger shares of the employers' contributions through risk adjustments, it would be to their advantage. The same would probably be true for fee-for-service plans. Most large employers self-insure, using carriers for administrative services only. Thus the intermediary would have to assure all players that any risk adjustments and quality assessments were not biased in favor of the fee-for-service options.

Some carriers may seek to emphasize the captive-triple option—that is, situations in which they bundle the risk and lock the employer into their own provider groups. From the employer's perspective, the use of an intermediary offers the attractive features of such a strategy and removes the unattractive aspects. Thus there is likely to be some carrier opposition to the proposal. Likewise, the role identified is substantially more complex than that usually taken on by benefit consultants, and therefore may be perceived as too risky. In terms of initial implementation of the concept, it may be best attempted where a coalition of major employers strongly favors the idea. If the local area has a wide range of HMOs, including some that are suffering from adverse selection and some that have favorable selection, then provider acceptance is more likely.

A second level of involvement for an intermediary is to take on the risk for a large pool of enrollees. This is less likely to occur among the privately insured unless the intermediary is a carrier, raising questions about its objectivity. But if the intermediary is a semipublic agency it might take on the responsibility for managing Medicaid enrollments in various HMOs and other plans. Several states, including Wisconsin and Arizona, already force their Medicaid eligibles into HMOs and must therefore deal with the problems of biased selection among the plans. Such a semipublic agency could also serve as an intermediary for a health insurance pool for small employers. An analogue is the California Public Employee Retirement System (PERS), which not only provides health insurance options for all state employees but also allows local public agencies such as cities, towns, and school districts to buy into the system. When this is done all the PERS options and management are available to the local agencies, but the agencies are able to set their own contribution levels.

Conclusions

Multiple-option health plans have been less successful than hoped, partly because of problems of competition among health plan options. Some problems arise from the way multiple-option plans have been implemented, particularly the pegging of contributions to increases in the costs of fee-for-service coverage. This apparently irrational policy, however, is probably a reflection of the problems created by adverse selection that increase the costs of the fee-for-service option beyond true efficiency differences. In the absence of reasonable means of addressing the problem of biased selection, it may be impossible to implement a multiple-option system with incentives for people to choose efficient plans and for plans to compete on the basis of efficiency.

In addition, while competition among plans is certainly attractive, most local markets have few hospitals and HMOs. Competition is therefore based more on factors such as style of practice, quality, and marketing than on efficiency. Furthermore, except in a few areas, individual employers represent only a small portion of any HMO's or health plan's business, so direct negotiation and assessment of quality is difficult. If, however, one recognizes the problems of fragmentation on the purchaser side and of concentration on the provider side, and one can devise a mechanism to concentrate purchaser power, then a situation of countervailing power may be established. If this is linked to active attempts to measure and offset the biased-selection problem, a viable solution may be reached.

The attraction of a solution based on intermediaries is that, while focused initially on the market for large-employer plans, it could easily be expanded to the market for small firms and for public sponsors. Furthermore, the intermediary approach is designed to allow the market to work, rather than relying on a bureaucratic or regulatory solution. That is, the intermediary would not be setting insurance or HMO premiums, but only the factors that serve to reallocate employer contributions among plans. Health plans could still set their own premiums and face the market consequences of those decisions. Likewise, labor and management can still negotiate the level of the employer contribution for health insurance versus other forms of compensation. An intermediary may also serve as the focal point for a small-employer pool, which could then provide coverage at rates comparable to those of the large accounts.

Most important, the development of an intermediary model may allow the broad-based assessment of quality of care in various health plans within a local market. This is possible because the agglomeration of enrollees is then large enough to allow statistically reliable estimates of patient outcomes and assessments of the process of care. Using the impartial intermediary to collect and evaluate comparisons across plans and then to publicize the findings would encourage competition to focus on quality and true efficiency differences. With such enhancements the multiple-option model may eventually achieve some of its potential benefits and lead to long-run improvements in the health care system.

References

Berki, Sylvester E., and Marie L. F. Ashcraft. "HMO Enrollment: Who Joins What and Why: A Review of the Literature." *Milbank Quarterly* 58 (Fall 1980): 588–632.

Curtiss, Frederic R. "Drug Benefit Design to Manage Selection Bias." *Drug Benefit Trends* 3 (May–June 1991): 9–11.

Enthoven, Alain. *Health Plan.* Menlo Park, Calif.: Addison-Wesley, 1980.

Enthoven, Alain, and Richard Kronick. "A Consumer-Choice Health Plan for the 1990's: Universal Health Insurance in a System Designed to Promote Quality and Economy." *New England Journal of Medicine* 320 (January 5, 1989): 29–37.

Gabel, Jon, Steven DiCarlo, Cynthia Sullivan, and Thomas Rice. "Employer-Sponsored Health Insurance, 1989." *Health Affairs* 9 (Fall 1990): 161–75.

Grant, Peter N. "Dramatic Developments in IPA, Medical Group Practice, and HMO–Hospital–Medical Group Relations in California." *California Physician* (September 1991): 32–38.

Grant, Peter N., Paul T. Smith, and Jonathan M. Lindeke. "Selling Your Medical Practice: Considering the Role of the Hospital." *Northern California Medicine* (March 1990): 16–18.

Health Insurance Association of America. *Providing Employee Health Benefits: How Firms Differ.* Washington, D.C.: HIAA, Department of Policy Development and Research, 1990, p. 49.

Hellinger, Fredrick J. "Selection Bias in Health Maintenance Organizations: Analysis of Recent Evidence." *Health Care Financing Review* 9 (Winter 1987): 55–63.

Jensen, Gail A., and Jon R. Gabel. "The Erosion of Private Health Insurance." *Inquiry* 25 (Fall 1988): 328–43.

Klinkman, Michael S. "The Process of Choice of Health Care Plan and Provider: Development of an Integrated Analytic Framework." *Medical Care Review* 48 (Fall 1991): 295–330.

Legnini, Mark W. *A Case Study of the Effects of Hospital Competition and Deregulation: San Francisco during the 1980s.* San Francisco: Institute for Health Policy Studies, University of California, 1990.

Lichtenstein, Richard, J. William Thomas, Janet Adams-Watson, James Lepkowski, and Bridget Simone. "Selection Bias in TEFRA At-Risk HMOs." *Medical Care* 29 (April 1991): 318–31.

Luft, Harold S. "Compensating for Biased Selection in Health Insurance." *Milbank Quarterly* 64 (1986): 566–92.

———. *Health Maintenance Organizations: Dimensions of Performance.* 2nd ed. New Brunswick, N.J.: Transaction Books, 1987.

Luft, Harold S., Susan Maerki, and Joan B. Trauner. "The Competitive Effects of Health Maintenance Organizations: Another Look at the Evidence from Hawaii, Rochester, and Minneapolis-St. Paul." *Journal of Health Politics, Policy and Law* 10 (1986): 625–58.

Luft, Harold S., and Robert H. Miller. "Patient Selection in a Competitive Health Care System." *Health Affairs* 7 (Summer 1988): 97–119.

Manning, W. G., A. Liebowitz, G. A. Goldberg, et al. "A Controlled Trial of the Effect of a Prepaid Group Practice on Use of Services." *New England Journal of Medicine* 310 (June 7, 1984): 1505–10.

Mayer, Dean. "In Minneapolis, Talking about Merger Talk." *Health Week* (August 12, 1991): 3.

McLaughlin, Catherine G. "HMO Growth and Hospital Expense and Use: A Simultaneous Equation Approach." *Health Services Research* 22 (1987): 183–205.

———. "Market Responses to HMOs: Price Competition or Rivalry?" *Inquiry* 25 (Summer 1988): 207–18.

National Health Policy Forum. *Where Does Marketplace Competition in Health Care Take Us? Impressions, Issues, and Unanswered Questions from the NHPF Site Visit to Minneapolis-St. Paul.* Washington, D.C.: National Health Policy Forum, January 14–17, 1991, published June 1991.

Palsbo, Susan J. *HMO Market Penetration in the 30 Largest Metropolitan Statistical Areas, 1989.* Group Health Association of America, Research Briefs, number 13, December 1990.

Robinson, James C., Harold S. Luft, Laura B. Gardner, and Ellen M. Morrison. "Method for Risk-Adjusting Employer Contributions to Competing Health Insurance Plans." *Inquiry* 28 (Summer 1991): 107–16.

Savitz, Eric J. "No Miracle Cure: HMOs Are Not the Rx for Spiraling Health-Care Costs." *Barron's* (August 5, 1991): 8 ff.

Wilensky, Gail R., and Louis F. Rossiter. "Patient Self-Selection in HMOs." *Health Affairs* 5 (Spring 1986): 66–80.

3

Managed Competition—
Why We Don't Have It and
How We Can Get It

Richard Kronick

Although enrollment in health maintenance organizations (HMOs) grew substantially during the 1980s, some basic features of the health care economy have not changed:

• Most providers (physicians and hospitals) are still paid on a fee-for-service basis, in which they are paid more for providing more service and in which they are not rewarded for solving medical problems using fewer, rather than more, resources.

• The stock of practicing physicians, particularly specialists, is increasing rapidly.

• Many consumers either have no choice of health plan, or if they have a choice, are not required to pay more for a more expensive plan.

• Even when consumers are cost conscious, competition among health plans is not well managed. As a result, it is much easier for health plans to prosper by figuring out how to select good risks than it is for them to do the hard job of figuring out how to organize the medical care system for quality and economy.

Given these basic features, we should not be surprised that the growth of medical care expenditures accelerated during the 1980s, with scant likelihood that increased expenditures were matched by increased value.

The 1980s were a decade in which the rhetoric of competition in health care was ubiquitous. Some have argued that the dismal performance of the health care economy in the 1980s—accelerating expenditures, increasing numbers of uninsured, and little clear indication of increased value—is evidence that the competitive strategy is fatally flawed. A stronger case can be made, however, that, despite the rhetoric, we as a nation have not seriously tried to create an environment in which providers are systematically rewarded for high-quality, economical care.

Why have we done so little to create an environment that rewards high-quality, economical care when both government and corporate policy makers have given so much rhetorical support to a competitive strategy? The thesis of this chapter is that the primary reason we do not have managed competition is that we have a collective action problem: although it would, arguably, be in every employer's and employee's best interest if the employer were to make its employees cost conscious and actively manage competition among health plans, it is not in the interest of any individual employer and employee group to do so (see Olson 1965 for a discussion of collective action problems).

Converting from historical health benefits practices to a system of managed competition entails both transition costs and continuing administrative costs. If one employer in an area pays these costs, even if it is quite a large employer, providers' incentives will be only slightly affected. If providers are selling to a small number of consumers who reward quality and economy and a large number who do not, why should providers respond to the incentives created by the few rather than those of the many? If only one employer in a community pays the costs to manage competition, provider behavior will not be affected, and health care costs will continue to escalate without being matched by quality increases. Faced with the choice of converting to a system of managed competition and getting nothing for it or not adopting a system of managed competition and avoiding the short-term labor relations difficulties and administrative costs, the choice for most employers will be clear.

If the choice for large employers is clear, small employers are not even given the opportunity to manage competition among health plans. Individual small employers, even more than large employers, are powerless to affect the incentives for providers. Further, even if a small employer were committed to trying to manage competition, it would be unable to implement the strategy—if a health plan wants to prosper by "creaming" those small employers with healthy employees, the small employer cannot counteract this strategy.

This diagnosis points to two reasons we do not have managed competition. First, large employers have little incentive to invest in managing competition, since they will get no return unless a critical mass of other employers in their region makes the same investment. Second, small employers have neither an incentive to manage competition nor (even if they were willing to make the investment) any real ability to create an environment in which high-quality, economical providers would prosper.

If we accept that the reason we do not have managed competition in the health care market is that it is not in the interest of any individual employer to pay the costs of creating the necessary conditions, then solutions that attempt to implement managed competition must focus on ways of overcoming this collective action problem.

For small and medium-sized employers, an attractive solution is to create nonprofit health insurance purchasing corporations (HIPCs) that would pool the purchasing power of small businesses and overcome the collective action problem. Under this proposal, HIPCs would be nonprofit corporations, chartered by state governments. HIPCs would contract with health plans and manage competition among them. Small businesses that wanted to purchase health insurance would arrange this purchase through the HIPC—employees would choose one of the HIPC contracted plans, and some combination of employer and employee premium funding would pay the health plan the contracted price.

The proposed HIPC is similar in concept to multiple employer trusts (METs) and, in the absence of "glue"—that is, some mechanism to induce healthy persons to remain part of the purchasing pool—would face adverse selection problems similar to those that plague METs. One of the problems faced by METs is that there are strong incentives for employers with healthy, younger employers to seek coverage elsewhere, and the MET is caught in an adverse selection spiral—in which it is responsible for progressively sicker enrollees. HIPCs would be subject to these same problems, compounded because of the additional administrative costs involved in managing competition.

Two options for glue should be considered to avoid these problems. First, the availability of tax-free employer contributions for small employers could be conditioned on the purchase of benefits through HIPCs. This change in the Internal Revenue Code would give state governments strong incentives to establish HIPCs and would give small businesses strong incentives to purchase through HIPCs rather than purchasing health benefits independently. Second, a state could require that all insurance sold to a small business in the state be sold through an HIPC: this approach could feasibly be implemented by the states, without any involvement of the federal government.[1]

The remainder of this chapter is organized as follows: the first section reviews the theory of managed competition and the actions that sponsors must take to create an environment in which providers will be rewarded for quality and economy. The second section examines evidence demonstrating how far the current environment is from the one

---

1. ERISA preemptions might well require self-funded businesses to be allowed to fund their own health plans independently of HIPCs. But since few (if any) small employers operate self-funded ERISA plans, this preemption is a theoretical but not a practical problem.

needed if we expect providers to produce the kind of care that consumers want. The third section considers the reasons we do not have such an environment, emphasizing the collective action problem that employers and their employees face. The fourth section proposes solutions to these collective action problems, contrasting the proposed HIPCs to various proposals that have been made for the reform of small group insurance.

The Theory of Managed Competition

Alain Enthoven (1986) has written extensively on the theory of managed competition. His basic premise is that fee-for-service medicine combined with nearly universal third-party reimbursement rewards providers for more service, without regard to whether it is appropriate or beneficial. Especially since so much medical care is art, not science, open-ended payment results in the delivery of much care of doubtful value, with little assurance of quality.

Some have suggested trying to address these problems by imposing copayments and deductibles on the consumer at the point of service. The rationale for doing so is that if consumers are required to pay for services out of pocket, they will question more carefully the need for the services they are receiving and balance considerations of expected benefit with considerations of expected cost. The RAND health insurance experiment demonstrated convincingly that consumers who were required to share the cost of health care used fewer health care services than those receiving free care, with minimal negative effects on health outcomes (Manning et al. 1987).

These results do not imply, however, that if everyone faced modest deductibles and coinsurance that either quality of care would be increased or that growth of expenditure would be moderated. While deductibles and coinsurance would reduce the frequency with which patients sought the care of a physician, once a physician has been contacted the patient has relatively little control over the delivery, or price, of care received. Most physicians would be unwilling to quote a global fee for taking care of a patient who walks in the door with a given presentation of symptoms; at the time of illness, patients are poorly equipped, in any case, to shop for quality and price. Further, given the skewed distribution of health expenditures toward high-cost cases and the strong desire on the part of a risk-averse population for insurance to protect against financial catastrophe in the face of illness, the use of point-of-service copayments and deductibles, at least within the limits that are likely to be acceptable to consumers, would not restrain the growth of health care expenditures.

Others have suggested that insurers should contract with hospitals and physicians on a unit price basis and then review (or micromanage) treatment decisions. This strategy might be successful if medicine were largely a science (that is, if it were clear how best to treat a patient with a given set of symptoms) and if the transaction costs of such review were relatively small. But much of medicine is art, requiring the provider's judgment; given the lack of a scientific basis for much medical practice, adversarial third-party utilization review will not successfully restrain the growth of expenditures if providers earn more by delivering more service. While attempts to identify and select the "good" providers for inclusion in a contracted network can improve quality and economy in the short run, as long as the relationship between providers and insurer remains primarily adversarial, and as long as providers are primarily paid on a fee-for-service basis, even selecting "good" providers will do little, in the long run, to restrain the growth of expenditures.

Some have proposed escaping from the current morass by increasing the scientific basis of medicine. By further supporting health services research and the development of practice guidelines, we will be able to determine what works and what does not work. Armed with this knowledge, physicians can improve the quality of care and limit (either voluntarily or as a result of third-party review) services to those that are known to be effective. Certainly increasing the scientific basis of medicine is to be heartily applauded. We are so far from medicine as science, however, and the transaction costs of adversarial third-party review are so high, that practice guidelines alone are unlikely to be effective in restraining the growth of expenditures.

As argued by Enthoven and others, a potential solution to these problems is to generate competition among groups of providers who have strong financial incentives to manage themselves well—that is, to calculate how many resources are really needed to take care of an enrolled population and to figure out how to move toward higher quality and greater efficiency.

To create such an environment, consumers must be offered a cost-conscious choice among competing health plans and provided information on health plan performance. In a "healthy" competitive market, the prices charged by these health plans will reflect the relative efficiency and quality of care they produce, and consumers will choose the health plans that offer high-quality care at a low price. With this model, consumer choice will reward, and cause to prosper, the health plans that provide cost-effective, high-quality care.

Merely offering competing health plans, however, is not enough to achieve these desirable results. The markets for health plans are not naturally competitive like the markets for transportation and financial services. Left unmanaged, health plans will pursue profits by strategies

48

that destroy competition. The list of profit strategies includes risk selection, market segmentation, product differentiation, biased information regarding coverage and quality, and oligopolistic behavior. As a consequence, efficient plans—that is, health plans in which medical problems are solved using fewer rather than more resources—may not prosper, and inefficient health plans may do quite well.

To create an environment that rewards those providers that organize for quality and economy, a third party, or sponsor, must actively manage the interactions of consumers and health plans. The devices available to sponsors to counteract health plan strategies include managing the enrollment process to prevent health plans from selecting only healthy employees; monitoring the disenrollment process to ensure that health plans are not consistently extruding their sickest members; standardizing the benefits packages offered by competing health plans to keep health plans from segmenting the market and selecting good risks; surveying employee satisfaction with health plan performance and making this information available at the annual open enrollment; gathering and publicizing information on the quality of care in competing health plans; ensuring that each health plan has contracted with centers of excellence for tertiary care; monitoring risk selection among health plans, and, potentially, adjusting the sponsor contribution if a health plan attracts a risk mixture significantly different from the average. In addition, an extremely important strategy for sponsors is to contract with health plans that divide the provider community into competing groups and avoid contracting with health plans that include in their network a large subset of the doctors and hospitals in town.

It will be useful here to consider briefly two types of objections to this theory. First, some (for example, Butler and Haislmaier 1989; and Pauly et al. 1991) would argue that active sponsors are not needed to make a competitive model work. These authors suggest that if individuals are required to purchase insurance, and if a set of rules for fair play governs the behavior of insurers, then no further intervention is needed from the government to create an environment that rewards providers for quality and economy. I think it is unlikely, however, that individuals would be successful in dividing the provider community into competing economic groups or in preventing providers from segmenting the market through product differentiation and other strategies that would reduce competitive pressures. Further, it is unlikely that a set of rules of fair play, enforced by a passive regulator, could prevent insurers and provider groups from profiting through favorable risk selection.

A second critique, made by Stanley B. Jones (1990), is that employers have not been able to manage risk selection problems successfully in multiple choice environments. Jones is certainly correct that few employ-

49

ers have managed these problems very well to date; however, he identifies no reasons these problems could not be managed satisfactorily.

How Close Are We to an Environment of Managed Competition?

Opponents of competitive strategies argue that we tried competition during the 1980s and that it did not work. It is is undeniable that whatever we tried during the 1980s did not work well. What we have tried, however, is far from the model of managed competition outlined above.

Although it is difficult to provide precise estimates, it appears that approximately 40–45 percent of employees who are offered employer-sponsored health insurance can choose between at least one HMO and a fee-for-service plan; most of the other 60 percent are offered only one health plan (see table 3–1). Jon Gabel et al. (1988) report that in 1987, 42 percent of the employers of a nationwide sample were offered an HMO. The sampling frame included all employers with six or more employees. Larger firms were much more likely than smaller firms to offer an HMO option: 13 percent of small employers (fewer than 100 employees) offered an HMO; 31 percent of medium-sized employers (100–999 employees) offered an HMO; and 62 percent of large employers offered an HMO. Subsequent surveys conducted by the Health Insurance Association of America (HIAA) have found similar results—42 percent of employees in the 1989 survey of employers were offered an HMO (and this survey included in the sampling frame employers with five or more employees), and 33 percent of employees in the 1990 survey were offered an HMO (personal communication, Cynthia Sullivan, HIAA).

The suggestion of a decline between 1989 and 1990 in the percentage of employees offered an HMO is concentrated among employees in large firms and is almost certainly a survey artifact of some sort and not an indication of real change. Gail A. Jensen and Michael A. Morrisey (1991) analyzed a 1986 survey of employers conducted by the Bureau of Labor Statistics (BLS) and report that 50 percent of the employees in medium- and large-sized firms were offered an HMO option. Jensen et al. (1987) report that a similar BLS survey conducted in 1985 found that only 25 percent of employees in medium and large firms were offered an HMO. Again, most of the estimated change from 1985 to 1986 must have been due to changes in the questions asked or the sampling frame, not to real change in what employers offered. A 1991 survey sponsored by KPMG Peat Marwick in which the sampling frame was all employers with 200 or more employees found results for these employers that were quite similar to the 1989 HIAA survey results.

Foster-Higgins conducts an annual survey of mostly large employers, disproportionately weighted toward Foster-Higgins clients (and

TABLE 3–1

PERCENTAGE OF EMPLOYEES OFFERED AN HMO, BY SURVEY, 1987–1991

Survey Sponsor	Year	Universe	% of Employees Offered an HMO	Firm Size (%)			
				< 25	25–99	100–999	1000 +
HIAA	1987	6 or more employees	42	13	13	31	62
HIAA	1989	All firms	42	9	21	40	77
HIAA	1990	All firms	33	12	18	36	56
BLS	1987	Medium and large firms	26	n.a.	n.a.	n.a.	n.a.
BLS	1987	Medium and large firms	50	n.a.	n.a.	n.a.	n.a.
KPMG-Peat Marwick	1991	200 employees and more	—	n.a.	n.a.	40[a]	61,[b] 87[c]
Foster-Higgins	1987	Mostly larger; not random sample	—	n.a.	52[d]	76[b]	89[c]
Foster-Higgins	1988	Mostly larger; not random sample	—	n.a.	51[d]	73[b]	92[c]
Foster-Higgins	1989	Mostly larger; not random sample	—	n.a.	50[d]	72[b]	90[c]
Foster-Higgins	1990	Mostly larger; not random sample	—	n.a.	50[d]	72[b]	89[c]

n.a. = not applicable; — = insufficient data.
a. 200–999 employees.
b. 1,000–4,999 employees.
c. 5,000+ employees.
d. <1,000 employees.
SOURCES: HIAA, 1987—Gabel et al. 1988; HIAA, 1989 and 1990—Personal communication, Cynthia Sullivan, HIAA; BLS, 1985—Jensen et al. 1987; BLS, 1986—Jensen and Morrisey 1991; KPMG-Peat Marwick 1991—personal communication, Jon Gabel, KPMG-Peat Marwick; Foster-Higgins, 1987–1990—Foster Higgins Health Care Benefits Survey 1987; Foster-Higgins Health Care Benefits Survey 1988; Foster-Higgins Health Care Benefits Survey 1989/Managed Care; and Foster-Higgins Health Care Benefits Survey 1990/Managed Care.

thus emphatically not a random sample). Survey results from 1987 to 1990 show almost no change in the percentage of employees offered an HMO and are largely consistent with the HIAA survey estimates.[2] The Foster-Higgins surveys find a slightly greater percentage of large firms offering an HMO than in the HIAA survey, a disparity perhaps explainable because of the differences in the sampling frame between the surveys. This hodge-podge of evidence leaves some uncertainty, but it seems likely that most employees in very large firms are offered at least one HMO, few employees in small firms (probably less than 15 percent of employees in firms with twenty-five or fewer employees) are offered an HMO, and, averaging across all firm sizes, 40–45 percent are offered an HMO.

There is even less evidence on the extent to which employees who are offered an HMO are fully cost conscious, but it seems likely that a minority of those offered a choice are required to pay the entire difference between the price of the least costly plan and the price of the plan they choose. Many employees still receive an individual plan without any premium payment, regardless of the plan they choose. Although most employees choosing family coverage are required to make a premium contribution, there are many employers who subsidize part of the difference between the most and the least expensive plan.[3]

In the absence of good data, all estimates are speculative: a reasonable speculative estimate is that 40 percent of employees who are offered a choice of health plan are fully cost conscious when choosing among plans. Combined with the estimate that 40–45 percent of employees covered by group health insurance are offered a choice of plan, a reasonable estimate is that 16–18 percent of employees covered by group health insurance are offered a choice and are required to pay the full amount of the difference in cost between the least expensive plan

---

2. Foster-Higgins reports the percentage of sampled *employers* offering an HMO in the following firm size categories: < 500, 500–999, 1,000–2,499, 2,500–4,999, 5,000–9,999, 10,000–19,999, 20,000–39,999, 40,000 and more. To construct estimates of the percentage of *employees* offered an HMO in firms with fewer than 1,000 employees, I simply averaged the percentage of employes offering a plan in the < 500 and 500–999 category; similarly, I averaged the 1,000–2,499 and 2,500–4,999 categories to construct an estimate of the percentage for 1,000–4,999 employees, and I averaged the estimates for the four larger firm size categories to estimate the percentage for 5,000 employees and over. This simple averaging procedure probably slightly underestimates the percentage of employees in each firm size category who are offered an HMO but has the virtue both of being simple and of producing comparable results across years.

3. My own employer, the University of California, provides a typical example.

available and the price of the plan they chose. Since hospital and physician expenditures for privately insured patients are approximately 50 percent of total expenditures for these types of service, less than 10 percent of all physician and hospital expenditures are accounted for by people subject to a cost-conscious choice of plan.[4]

Further, even among the minority of employees who are cost-conscious consumers, few work for an employer that actively manages competition among health plans. The failings of employers as sponsors are made evident by comparing actual employer practices to the list of strategies enumerated in the previous section. I am not aware of any employers that systematically monitor disenrollment and request corrective actions from health plans that consistently extrude their sickest members. Few employers survey employees on their satisfaction with health plans and make this information available at the time of open enrollment. No employer that I am familiar with routinely publicizes the limited information that is available on quality (for example, rates for Caesarean sections or Medicare mortality rates at health plan hospitals). Few employers risk-adjust the employer contribution to avoid penalizing those health plans that serve sicker enrollees.[5]

In 1990, UC offered three options for coverage—Kaiser, HealthNet, and a self-insured indemnity product administered by Prudential. The monthly prices for family coverage for these three plans were $324, $366, and $561 (for basically similar benefit packages, except that the indemnity plan included copayment and deductibles, and the de facto coverage for mental health in Kaiser and HealthNet were slimmer). The university contributed up to $505 per month, so that the employee need pay "only" $56 per month for Prudential, which can be taken out of pretax earnings. Thus, while most employers require some employee contribution for the purchase of family coverage, many such employees are not fully cost-conscious. Even fewer employees will be cost-conscious when selecting individual coverage.

4. Many Medicare beneficiaries can choose between HMO alternatives and fee-for-service Medicare, and these beneficiaries are cost-conscious when making the choice, but most beneficiaries are not making active choices. For a variety of reasons too complex to cover here, the Medicare HMO program does not pressure fee-for-service providers to search for quality and economy.

5. A few employers, concerned that HMOs are creaming younger, healthier enrollees, do adjust the employer contribution for age and sex. No employer that I am aware of adjusts for factors other than age, sex, and family size.

Although employers often have failings as managers of competition among health plans, the two areas in which many employers are successful should be noted: first, employers manage the enrollment process themselves, correctly depriving health plans of the opportunity to attempt to select favorable risks at time of enrollment. Second, many employers are moving in the direction of standardizing the benefits packages in competing health plans, depriving health

Perhaps most important, few employers engage in systematic efforts to divide the provider community in an area into competing groups. Many employers are content to contract with a number of independent practice association (IPA) model HMOs, each of which may include in its network 80 percent of the doctors and hospitals in town. In such situations, there is little pressure on providers to strive for quality and economy and little economic reward to those providers who are able to increase the value produced by their practice.

Why Don't We Have Managed Competition?

The theory of managed competition suggests that if all purchasers in a market are cost-conscious consumers whose interactions with health plans are actively and intelligently managed by a sponsor, then physicians and hospitals will have strong incentives to try to figure out how to deliver high-quality, economical care. If only one employer makes its employees cost-conscious and manages competition among health plans, however, providers will not respond to the incentives this employer is trying to create, and health care delivery will be unchanged.

Employers and their employees are caught in a classic collective action problem—all would be better off if all paid the costs of managing competition, but any single employer (and its employees) is made worse off if it tries to manage competition and other employers do not. Finding a solution to the collective action problem is made more difficult because the benefits of managed competition have the characteristics of a public good: if some group of employers and employees can create an environment in which providers are rewarded for quality and economy and provider groups respond by organizing for value, then all employers and employees will benefit, regardless of whether they contributed toward creating the desirable environment.

Before considering the ways in which this collective action problem can be solved, we should look at the costs that an employer (and its employees) face in attempting to manage competition. First, employers currently contributing more than the price of the least expensive health plan offered must reduce the employer contribution. While in theory this can be compensated for by an increase in wages, employee dissatisfaction

---

plans of the opportunity to select good risks through benefit design. Non-comparability of mental health and substance abuse benefits remains a problem for many—many employers offer more generous mental health and substance abuse benefits in their fee-for-service product than in their HMO products; this invites those who think they might need such benefits to choose the fee-for-service program.

may still result if employees are not convinced that a particular wage increase is compensating for a benefit reduction, as opposed to simply being a wage increase that would have occurred in any case. Further, even if the wage increase does compensate, on average, for benefit reductions, the employees who choose the more expensive plans will still be worse off than they were at the higher benefit–lower wage combination. Since these employees are likely to be older and more influential within the company, their potential dissatisfaction may be weighted heavily by the benefits managers. For a variety of reasons, the labor relations costs of changing from fully (or largely) employer-paid premiums to making all employees fully cost conscious during annual open enrollment will be particularly large in unionized firms. Especially since a benefits manager cannot promise that moving to cost consciousness will restrain future growth in health care costs, this anticipated labor relations problem undoubtedly discourages some firms from making the transition to cost consciousness.

In addition to the labor relations cost, an employer that wants to manage competition will have higher administrative costs than one that simply offers a choice of health plans without managing competition among them. The employer that is managing competition must monitor disenrollment, survey employees for satisfaction and make this information available to other employees, gather what information is available on quality, put effort into measuring the distribution of risks among health plans, and be willing to calculate risk-adjusted employer contributions. Although it is difficult to estimate the costs of these activities, a very rough guess is that an employer with 1,000 employees might add 4 percent to health benefits costs to do a good job of managing competition and that an employer with 10,000 employees might add 1 percent to these costs. Again, since a benefits manager can provide no assurance (or even likelihood) that such an investment will restrain the growth of costs or produce better quality care—since providers will change their behavior only if many other employers also make such an investment—most employers will decide not to do so.

The problem of dividing the provider community into competing groups is a particularly vexing one in a marketplace with many employers making individual coverage decisions. Consider a hypothetical metropolitan area with three loosely organized groups of hospitals and physicians, each of which produces care of approximately similar quality and efficiency (or inefficiency). Suppose that one insurer comes into town and signs up all three groups for an HMO product, while a second, third, and fourth insurer each enter the market and create an HMO centered around one of the groups. Each group might give some discount to the "pure play" HMO (one that contracted with only one group) compared with the HMO that included all three groups; however, since the cost of care produced by each group is, by assumption, approximately the same, the premium charged by the HMO that includes all three groups should be similar to the premium for each HMO that offers a "pure play."

An employer deciding whether to contract with the single "blended" HMO or the three "pure plays" will be attracted by the blended product. Employees will have the advantage of being able to choose from any of the provider groups in town without changing their health plan; given the assumption of equal premiums, the blended product will be more attractive than any of the "pure plays." But if the blended product is offered and the pure plays are not, then each provider group has little incentive to search for improvements in efficiency and quality in the future. If all employers offered the pure plays rather than the blended product, then, arguably, providers would increase the value of the care they provide in the future. But any individual employer will have happier employees by offering the blended product rather than the pure plays. This logic, combined with the reluctance of providers in many areas to divide into competing groups, creates a situation in many markets in which pure plays are not available and blended products are the only choice.

The arguments made in this section of the chapter apply to both large and small employers but have even more force for small employers. The administrative costs of attempting to manage competition will be larger as a percentage of health benefits costs for small employers than for large employers, and a single small employer has less chance than a large employer of appreciably affecting the providers' incentives. Consider a hypothetical choice faced by a small employer: on the one hand, to pay a broker who does not actively manage competition to choose a selection of health plans for its employees; or, on the other, to pay a broker who does manage competition to choose a selection of plans and to manage competition among them. The second broker would monitor disenrollment, survey employee satisfaction, collect and disseminate information on health plan quality, and provide advice on risk adjustment of the employer contribution. Health plans would presumably charge the small employer the same price whether the employer was advised by the first or by the second broker, but the employer would need to pay more for the second broker's services than for the first broker's services. Why would any small employer pay to buy the managed competition services? No satisfactory answer can be provided.

In addition, since neither the small employer nor the broker can require health plans to guarantee issue or renewability, or prevent health plans from imposing exclusions for preexisting conditions, or prevent health plans from drastically increasing premiums if one member of a small group gets sick, the small employer cannot create an environment that rewards health plans that provide high quality and economical care and punishes those health plans that attempt to prosper by selecting good risks. That is, in the small-group market, health plans have strong incentives to try to figure out how to select good risks; while large employers, if they were motivated to do so, could adopt strategies that would largely prevent health plans from prospering through risk selection, small employers cannot, on their own, bring discipline to the health plan market even if they tried.

How We Can Get Managed Competition

In the second section of this chapter I argued that providers do not currently have strong incentives to improve the quality or economy of care. In the third section I argued that the main reason for the absence of these incentives is a collective action problem: managing competition entails administrative costs for employers, but no single employer can achieve success through its own actions. Further, if that environment can be created, each employer will benefit regardless of whether any one employer contributed to the costs of creating those conditions.

To solve this collective action problem, we must create some incentives for employers to contribute to the public good. That is, we must find some way of rewarding those employers that do make the effort to manage competition. For small employers, there is an additional problem to be solved. Not only must small employers have incentives to invest in managing competition, but also a structure must be created to prevent health plans from prospering through selection of favorable risks.

An attractive solution to both problems is to create a large purchaser that would aggregate the purchasing power of small groups. As discussed earlier, such a purchaser—a health insurance purchasing corporation—would contract with health plans on behalf of small employers and manage competition among those health plans. Small employers purchasing health benefits through the HIPC would make a fixed-dollar contribution toward health benefits that is less than or equal to the price of the least expensive health plan under contract to the HIPC. Employees would choose one of the HIPC contracted plans and pay the difference between the employer's contribution and the price of the plan chosen.[6]

---

6. Under this proposal employers would not be required to offer health benefits—they would be free, just as they are today, to either offer or not offer benefits. Similarly, employees would be free to choose whether to purchase

Just as large employers contracting with health plans almost universally require the plans to accept any employee choosing to enroll, and to do so without imposing exclusions for preexisting conditions, HIPC contracts with health plans should prohibit these exclusions and require acceptance of all groups and individuals wishing to enroll.[7] A health plan would always be free not to renew a HIPC contract but could not selectively do so for some, but not all, of the HIPC membership.

To make this proposal work, "glue" is required for two reasons. First, as discussed in the previous section, if the HIPC is managing competition, the administrative cost of purchasing benefits through an HIPC will be greater than the cost of purchasing through an independent broker. Employers must be given some incentive to pay this administrative fee. Second, and more important, without glue, HIPCs would suffer from the same problem that plagues many multiple employer trusts— namely, that employers with healthy employees will be offered low-price insurance outside the HIPC and employers with sicker employees will purchase through the HIPC, raising the price of coverage for all those purchasing through the HIPC.[8]

Two sources of glue should be considered. First, the Internal

---

benefits; it would make sense, however, to enforce minimum participation requirements just as they are today for many small-group products.

7. When an HIPC is first established, small employers and their employees should be able to purchase benefits with no exclusions for preexisting conditions or underwriting. To discourage opportunistic purchasing decisions, however, businesses that decide not to purchase through the HIPC when the option is first made available but subsequently decide to do so should be subject to underwriting, preexisting condition exclusions, or both.

8. A potential adverse selection spiral must certainly be protected against. It is curious and somewhat comforting, however, that adverse selection spirals do not appear to be endemic to such arrangements. A number of states (including Massachusetts and New Jersey) operate an analogy to an HIPC that is restricted to city and county governments. In these states the state agency that contracts with health plans on behalf of state employees also contracts with these plans on behalf of other public sector employees. Other public sector employers (such as school districts, city governments, or units of county government) can decide whether to purchase health benefits on their own or purchase through the state government purchasing pool (local government employees are rated separately from state government employees). Although this would appear to create an incentive for local government units with healthy employees to purchase benefits on their own and leave the units with sick employees in the state pool, there is no evidence in either Massachusetts or New Jersey that such adverse selection problems have occurred. Research on the number of states with such purchasing arrangements and on their experience with such arrangements would be desirable.

Revenue Code could be changed to require that for the employees of a small business to receive tax-free employer health insurance contributions, the small employer must arrange for the purchase of health benefits through an HIPC. Under this proposal, small employers would be allowed to contract directly with health plans but would lose the ability to provide employees with tax-free employer contributions. Such a change in the Internal Revenue Code would provide states with a strong incentive to establish HIPCs and would provide small employers strong incentives to arrange for the purchase of benefits through them.

A second source of glue, which the states can apply without any changes needed in Washington, would be to amend a state's insurance laws to require that health insurance products could not be sold to small businesses outside the HIPC: that is, to prohibit insurers from selling directly to small businesses. If a state were to change its insurance laws in this way, then a small employer that wanted to provide employer-sponsored health insurance would have no choice except to make a fixed-dollar contribution and allow its employees to choose one of the HIPC contracted health plans.

If either source of glue is used, virtually all small businesses that decide to purchase insurance would purchase through an HIPC. The HIPC would be purchasing on behalf of a large segment of the market—depending on the threshold used to define "small employer," perhaps between 20 percent and 50 percent of the privately insured market would purchase benefits through an HIPC.[9] The HIPC would be large enough to influence providers to respond to financial incentives. Thus, an HIPC that invested in managing competition would be likely to obtain a return from this investment in the form of higher quality, more economical care for its subscribers.

This proposal to establish HIPCs and to provide strong incentives for small employers to purchase benefits through them has some substantive disadvantages and some political liabilities. There are three main substantive concerns. First, because the employees of some small employers would have a more restricted choice of health benefits than they now have, they might be worse off as a result. If a small employer wanted to purchase a policy with a set of coverages different from any

---

9. A sensible approach would be to make HIPCs initially responsible for purchasing benefits for employers with twenty-five or fewer employees. Following a two- to three-year phase-in period, employers with twenty-five to forty-nine employees might be brought in if the HIPC is functioning satisfactorily, followed by a phase in of employers with fifty to ninety-nine employees. Larger employers might be allowed to purchase through HIPCs on terms that were mutually agreeable.

set of coverages under contract to the HIPC, the employer might not be able to, or might be forced to use after-tax dollars to do so. It does not seem likely, however, that the welfare loss would be large. Employees of any large business are restricted to the benefits packages that have been chosen by the corporate benefits manager and do not seem to suffer greatly as a result. Arguably, the employees of many separate small businesses would have more diversity in their preferences than the employees of a single large business and thus suffer a larger welfare loss, but the argument is not persuasive.

Second, some employers with healthy employees might be able to obtain lower prices purchasing on their own than they can when purchasing through the HIPC. This problem could be attenuated if the HIPCs rate the premiums charged to subscribers by age, just as many premiums for small employers are currently age rated. If political considerations do lead HIPCs to charge subscribers community-rated premiums, then some young healthy employees who would have chosen to purchase relatively low-priced, age-rated insurance might choose to be uninsured if their only choice is a community-rated product available through the HIPC.[10]

Third are concerns over how to encourage HIPCs to manage competition well. What dynamic will ensure that the HIPC intelligently selects health plans that divide the provider community into competing groups, standardizes the benefit packages offered by competing plans, makes information available on satisfaction and quality, monitors enrollment and disenrollment, and, potentially, risk adjusts the sponsor contribution? How can the HIPC be held accountable for achieving its goals?

Although there can be no completely satisfactory answer to this question, a variety of mechanisms are available to increase accountability. The HIPC board of directors might be chosen in periodic elections in which the small employers purchasing through the HIPCs each receive one vote. If the HIPC does a poor job—that is, if health plan prices escalate or quality does not improve—the board would likely be replaced. Compensation of HIPC staff might be tied, in part, to the success achieved in reducing cost growth and increasing quality. The federal government might compare and contrast the performances of HIPCs; publicizing this information would put further pressure on HIPCs for good performance.

Regardless of substantive concerns, strong political opposition

---

10. Note that under current arrangements, many young, healthy employees in small businesses who choose to purchase low-priced insurance are not really insured—if they get sick, their policy may be canceled or be subject to a precipitous premium increase. The HIPC proposal would solve this problem.

would be expected from health insurance brokers, who would lose access to a whole line of business. Opposition should be expected from some provider groups, who will oppose any concentration of purchasing power; other provider groups may react neutrally or even positively to the proposal, particularly if the HIPC is structured as a nonprofit agency that is largely independent from government.

The expected reaction to this proposal from small businesses is not clear. Most small businesses that purchase insurance will be favorably affected by the proposal. They will have access to the purchasing power of a large group and avoid the administrative difficulties of arranging to purchase insurance on their own. They will be protected against precipitous premium increases if one or more employees become ill—for the first time, they will really be insured. Further, to the extent that the HIPCs successfully move providers to moderate their growth in costs, small businesses will benefit.

This substantive argument, however, does not necessarily translate into political support. One concern is that many of the trade organizations lobbying on behalf of small businesses also sponsor their own insurance products, and some of these products would be threatened by HIPCs. Further, as mentioned above, some small business may be forced to pay higher premiums, while others may be concerned by restricted choice of insurance products. Some small businesses not currently providing insurance will oppose the proposal, because they expect the other shoe to drop: once HIPCs are in place, if they prove to be an effective method of purchasing for small businesses and if they are able to affect provider behavior and moderate cost growth, the next step might well be to require small businesses to provide insurance (or impose a "play-or-pay" requirement).

Even with these concerns, however, many small businesses should be attracted by the promise of HIPCs. HIPCs would largely solve the problems plaguing the small business market. Further, many small business persons favor entrepreneurial values and should respond positively to the argument that HIPCs will create an environment rewarding providers for quality and economy.

The response of insurers is likely to be pivotal in determining whether state legislation requiring all small-group products to be sold through HIPCs is politically viable. If insurers oppose such legislation, it is doubtful that in many places there would be enough support from the small business community to enact it. Conversely, if insurers strongly support such legislation, their support, along with support from at least some parts of the small business community, would be enough to give the legislation a good chance in many states.

Many insurers are likely to react negatively to the concentration of purchasing power, however. Certainly small insurers without an attractive managed-care product would lose their ability to market to small employers, forcing them out of the small-group market for health insurance. Even larger carriers that believe they have an attractive product to offer would be nervous; if they do not successfully sell a product to the HIPC, they will be shut out of the small-group market. Many insurers, though, may initially be disposed to support the HIPC concept strongly, because it is, I think, in the long-run best interest of both insurers and consumers.

The main alternative to the establishment of HIPCs—small-group market reform as has been proposed by the National Association of Insurance Commissioners, the Health Insurance Association of America, and others—is far from a satisfactory substitute. HIPCs as proposed have two goals: first, to allow small businesses to purchase coverage on terms more like those available to large businesses; and second, to create an environment for providers that rewards quality and economy. Proposals for reforming the small-group market are designed primarily to address the first goal. It is doubtful that many such proposals will, even if enacted, achieve this goal.[11] But even if these reforms successfully made the pricing and products available in the small-group market more similar to those available in the large-group market, they would do very little to solve the collective action problem that has been identified as the main reason for the absence of an environment that rewards providers for quality and economy.

Although traditionally the main functions of health insurance were to spread risk and to process claims efficiently, supporters of private health insurance are now required to argue that the *raison d'être* for maintaining multiple insurers is to foster innovation and quality and efficiency improvements in the delivery of health care. As stated by Jones (1990), among others, to date the existence of multiple private insurers, however, has done little to foster either quality or economy. This situation will persist as long as competition among health plans is unmanaged or poorly managed.

The creation and empowerment of health insurance purchasing corporations to purchase benefits on behalf of small employers would both solve the collective action problems that have inhibited the growth of managed competition and provide a "jump start" for the implementation of managed competition. Without that jump start, it is difficult to foresee the circumstances under which the theory of managed competi-

---

11. It is unlikely that a largely passive regulatory body, like most state-level divisions of insurance, could effectively police a market and punish those carriers practicing favorable risk selection.

tion will receive a fair test.[12] If those constituencies that pay lip service to the notion of a competitive health care marketplace are not willing to support such a jump start (or some similar radical plan), then they will no doubt eventually face a single-payer or all-payer price control system as the only feasible alternative for achieving control of expenditures.

---

12. Adopting a variety of other measures—for example, preempting state-mandated benefit laws, reforming the tort liability system, limiting tax-free employer contributions, and increased effort at developing practice guidelines—will neither solve the collective action problems facing employers nor create, by themselves, an environment in which providers are systematically rewarded for quality and economy.

References

A. Foster Higgins & Company, Inc. *Health Care Benefits Survey*. Princeton, N.J.: 1987, 1988, 1989, 1990.

Butler, Stuart, and Edward Haislmaier, eds. *A National Health System for America*. Washington, D.C.: The Heritage Foundation, 1989.

Enthoven, Alain. "Managed Competition in Health Care and the Unfinished Agenda." *Health Care Financing Review*, Annual Supplement, 1986: 105–19.

Gabel, Jon, et al. "The Changing World of Group Health Insurance." *Health Affairs* 7(1988): 48–65.

Jensen, Gail A., and Michael A. Morrisey. "Employer Sponsored Post Retirement Health Benefits: Not Your Mother's Medigap Plan." Wayne State University, September, 1991. Unpublished manuscript.

Jensen, Gail A., Michael A. Morrisey, and John A. Marcus. "Cost Sharing and the Changing Pattern of Employer-Sponsored Health Benefits." *Milbank Quarterly* 65 (1987): 521–50.

Jones, Stanley B. "Multiple Choice Insurance: The Lessons and Challenges to Private Insurers." *Inquiry* 27 (1990): 161–66.

Manning, Willard G., J.P. Newhouse, N. Duan, E.B. Keebler, A. Leibowitz, and M.S. Marquis. "Health Insurance and the Demand for Medical Care: Evidence from a Randomized Experiment." *American Economic Review* 77 (1987): 251–77.

Olson, Mancur. *The Logic of Collective Action; Public Goods and the Theory of Groups*. Cambridge: Harvard University Press, 1965.

Pauly, Mark, et al. "A Plan for Responsible National Health Insurance." *Health Affairs* 10 (1991): 5–25.

4

Biased Selection—
Fairness and Efficiency in
Health Insurance Markets

Roger Feldman and Bryan E. Dowd

Whenever multiple health plans are offered to a group of individuals, risks are unlikely to be distributed equally among plans. Health risks also are unlikely to be distributed equally between groups who buy health insurance through their place of employment and individuals who purchase health insurance directly. Last, the average health risk of people with insurance may differ systematically from the risk of the uninsured. A crucial question for health plan reform concerns the effect of nonrandom or "biased" selection on the fairness and efficiency of health insurance markets. The analysis of biased selection depends crucially upon whether insurers can identify high and low risks prior to enrollment and the extent to which insurers can risk-adjust their premiums. We will explain the consequences of biased selection under four possible scenarios: when insurers can or cannot identify high risks prior to enrollment; and when they are or are not permitted to risk-adjust their premiums.

Most proposals for national or state-sponsored health insurance explicitly prohibit risk-adjustment of premiums, even if losses differ widely and systematically among risk types. When insurance is made available to certain groups of buyers at rates below cost, the other buyers of insurance can be viewed as providing a subsidy to the favored group. Thus we will be particularly interested in the analysis of biased selection when insurers can identify different risk types but are prevented from charging different rates. Will the resulting subsidy of high risks be efficient and equitable?

Efficiency and Equity Principles in Economics

Our theoretical framework is taken from welfare economics and the microeconomic theory of consumer behavior under risk. Welfare economics is the source of several definitions of "efficiency." An efficient *allocation* of a given amount of consumer goods is reached when no one can improve his position without causing someone else to leave a preferred position. The usual description of allocative efficiency in economics relies on Vilfredo Pareto's preference function or indifference map. Each person is assumed to be able to compare the utility or satisfaction derived from consuming different combinations of goods. Subject to his or her initial allocation of goods and the opportunities to buy and sell, each person will choose a final allocation that maximizes his or her satisfaction. This can be accomplished by exchanging any two goods until his or her willingness to substitute these goods in consumption is just equal to the market rate of exchange. The willingness to substitute two goods is called the rate of commodity substitution (RCS). If all consumers face the same market rate of exchange, then the resulting final allocation of goods will be efficient. If goods X and Y can be exchanged at the rate of one-to-one, for example, then everyone would exchange X and Y until their willingness to trade is exactly one-for-one.

Efficiency in *production* is achieved when the output of each good is maximized, given the output levels of all other goods. To do this, the rate at which inputs can be substituted in production must be equal for all goods. The rate of substitution in production is called the rate of technical substitution (RTS). For example, the RTS for plastic and aluminum should be equal in the production of all goods that use these two inputs. If this condition is met, then these two inputs cannot be rearranged to increase the production of one good without decreasing the production of another good.

Both conditions for efficiency are met when the utility of each consumer is maximized—given the utilities of all other consumers, the technology of production, and the constraints that supply equals demand for every input and for every good. This general condition for efficiency requires that consumers' RCS for any pair of goods equals the rate at which these goods can be transformed in production, which is called the rate of product transformation (RPT).

Competitive markets provide a means to achieve efficient allocation and production of goods. Since all consumers face the same prices in competitive markets, they will voluntarily exchange goods until their willingness to trade (the RCS) is equal to the ratio of competitive prices of those goods. Likewise, all producers in competitive markets face the same prices for factors of production and goods. The threat of being undersold by competitors will drive each producer to use resources efficiently. This means that the rate of technical substitution for any two factors of production will be set equal to their common price ratio.

Finally, the consumers' RCS will equal the rate of product transformation. To see why this is true, we use an example taken from an economics textbook (Henderson and Quandt 1971). Imagine there is only one input that produces two commodities, Q_j and Q_k. Consumers will exchange these commodities until RCS $= p_j/p_k$. If there is perfect competition among entrepreneurs in product and factor markets, then $p_j = r/MP_j$ and $p_k = r/MP_k$, where r stands for the price of the factor of production and MP_j and MP_k are its marginal products in each good. Since all consumers and producers face the same prices under perfect competition, RCS $= p_j/p_k = (r/MP_j)/(r/MP_k) = (1/MP_j)/(1/MP_k) =$ (marginal cost of good j in terms of input)/(marginal cost of good k in terms of input) = RPT.

To summarize, the economist's contribution to the problem of allocating goods and factors of production is to show how improvements can be made that make at least one individual better off without making anyone else worse off. Once these efficiency-based improvements are exhausted, the economist has no more to offer than has any other member of society. Further changes require value judgments regarding the initial distribution of resources and the prices at which these resources can be exchanged. For example, the competitive allocation of resources might seem unfair to those who start off with little to sell. Equally troublesome is the situation where some people's initial resources have a very low price or the things they want to buy have a very high price. Equity criteria are usually considered by the economist to arise through a process, such as the political process, which is distinct from the economic exchange of goods and services. This process places values on the initial distribution of resources and on the final allocation of goods among consumers.

Nevertheless, economists can play an important role in evaluating alternative policies designed to achieve equity or fairness among consumers. For example, society may judge that some sellers of labor cannot earn enough, at the going wage rate, to afford a "minimum" standard of living. One solution to this problem is to raise the wage rate for unskilled labor above the competitive level through legislation. This policy has the drawback that users of unskilled labor will attempt to substitute skilled labor and capital in production. A subsidy designed to reduce the price of a consumption good has the drawback that consumers will use more of the subsidized good and fewer of the nonsubsidized goods. The resulting allocation of goods will be inefficient, because it does not meet the condition that consumers' RCS equals the rate of product transformation. Consumers will act as though the subsidized good is relatively cheaper than other goods, although the marginal cost of the good in relation to other goods is unchanged by the subsidy. Economists generally favor subsidies that increase consumers' purchasing power without altering the relative prices of goods. Competitive markets then will allocate consumers' purchasing power efficiently, leaving the subsidy to address perceived inequities in the initial distribution of resources.

Application of Efficiency and Equity to Health Insurance Markets

By its very nature, insurance is a way of sharing losses (Long 1972). The price of insurance in a given time period is necessarily set so that relatively many people pay more in premiums than they collect in claims, and relatively few collect more in claims than they pay in premiums. But identification of the "many" and the "few" within a particular class of insured individuals is fortuitous. A subsidy is introduced by lowering the price of insurance for a particular class below what is believed to be the expected cost for that class. Most proposals for national health insurance and for state-sponsored health insurance in those states that have proposed such programs feature pricing techniques that make insurance available to certain classes of buyers at rates below their expected costs. The rates are altered so that other classes of buyers pay rates above their expected costs. Because each group equates its marginal willingness to buy insurance with a different price, this subsidy causes the allocation of health insurance among consumers to be inefficient. Consumers in the group receiving the subsidy will demand too much health insurance because the price has been reduced to them, whereas those in the group paying the subsidy will demand less insurance than they would purchase in a competitive market.

As we said earlier, it is normal for risks to be distributed unequally among health insurance plans. In a competitive market, members of the same risk class face the same price of insurance, but the price of insurance differs among risk classes. High risks will pay more than low risks for the same amount of coverage. Many policy makers view this outcome as unfair to the high risks and propose that premiums should be the same for all risk classes. Subsidizing high risks, however, is inefficient. Therefore we appear to have reached an impasse, in which the cost of achieving equity among risk classes is the inefficient allocation of resources in health insurance markets. The subsidized class would like to buy too much insurance, whereas those who pay the subsidy demand too little coverage. Analysis of this apparent conflict between equity and efficiency is the central topic of our chapter.

We focus explicitly on the analysis of price subsidies in the market for insurance. Other causes of market failure may be equally important but are outside the scope of our chapter. For example, the health insurance industry as a whole enjoys a partial exemption from federal antitrust laws. This exemption has allowed the industry to maintain anticompetitive practices, such as setting prices through collective action and excluding firms that offer lower-cost products from the market (Goldberg and Greenberg 1991). As a result of higher insurance prices, the rate of product transformation will not be equal to consumers' RCS between health insurance and other goods. Consequently the allocation of resources between health insurance and other goods in the economy will be inefficient. Another form of distortion, probably less common in health insurance than in medical care service markets, results from monopoly power over inputs. When the medical profession excludes other providers of inputs and fixes the price of its own labor above the competitive level, then both the production of medical services and the allocation of medical care versus other goods will be inefficient.

Economic Model of Consumer Behavior under Risk

How will biased selection affect market outcomes? The answer depends crucially on the information available to insurers and whether insurers are allowed to charge different premiums to individuals with different levels of risk. This suggests that we must analyze four possible situations: whether insurers can or cannot identify members of different risk classes; and whether they are or are not allowed to vary premiums by risk class.

Our basic model assumes that consumers have equal initial resources, denoted Y, but they differ in their health risk. For simplicity, only two risk classes and one type of medical care with a fixed expenditure are considered. "High risks" have probability ρ_h of being sick and spending X dollars on medical care, and $(1-\rho_h)$ probability of being well and having no medical care expenses. "Low risks" have ρ_l probability of spending X dollars and $(1-\rho_l)$ probability of no expenses.

The two commodities that consumers exchange in this model are net income in the sick and well states of the world. Net income means income left over for other goods after paying medical care premiums if they are well and receiving reimbursement if they are sick. Expected utility is therefore defined as $\rho U(Y - X + R) + (1 - \rho)U(Y - P)$, where P stands for the insurance premium and R is the amount reimbursed by the insurance company. We have omitted the subscripts on ρ, but each group is understood to have its own value for ρ. The rate of commodity substitution is found by differentiating this function with respect to well and sick income, holding expected utility constant. This defines Pareto's indifference curve for a given level of consumer welfare as $-dY_s/dY_w = [(1 - \rho)/\rho]U'_w/U'_s = 1/RCS$. The subscripts in this expression stand for well and sick states of the world.

The consumer's welfare is maximized when the RCS is set equal to the price of insurance, which we define as "dollars paid when well per dollars received when sick." If insurers can enter and leave the market freely and they do not collude to fix prices, then the expected premium per person in a given risk class will be driven down to the point where it is just equal to the expected insurance payout per member of that class, or $(1 - \rho)P = \rho R$. Therefore, the price of insurance is $-P/R = \rho/(1 - \rho)$ under conditions of free entry and price-taking by insurers. We will refer to this price as the "competitive price" of insurance.

Setting the reciprocal of the competitive price equal to 1/RCS, we get $(1 - \rho)/\rho = [(1 - \rho)/\rho]U'_w/U'_s$, or $U'_w = U'_s$. The consumer's welfare is maximized when marginal utility is equal in both health states. Since utility depends only on net income in our model, this implies that net income must be equal in both health states. This model can be represented by a two-dimensional graph (figure 4–1) with axes that measure Y_s vertically and Y_w horizontally. A line with a 45 degree slope from the origin indicates all points where net incomes in both states of the world are equal. The consumer's preinsurance endowment (point E) must lie below the 45 degree line because he or she has Y income if well and $(Y - X)$ if sick. From the endowment point, a straight line drawn upward and to the left represents the reciprocal of the competitive price of insurance; for simplicity call this the "competitive price line." In equilibrium, the consumer's Pareto indifference curve must be tangent to the competitive price line. This occurs along the 45 degree line, where incomes in both states of the world are equal.

We can introduce the two risk types into the graph by drawing two competitive price lines from the endowment point: Eh for high risks and El for low risks. Line Eh is relatively flat, indicating that high risks have to pay a higher price for insurance than do low risks. One might say that the premium-to-payout ratio is higher for high risks; premiums are measured by moving to the left along the horizontal axis of figure 4–1, and payouts are measured by moving up the vertical axis. Also shown in figure 4–1 is a competitive price line Ef for all consumers if they were charged one price for insurance. The slope of Ef is $-(1 - \pi)/\pi$, where $\pi = \lambda\rho_h + (1 - \lambda) p_l$ and λ is the proportion of high risks in the total pool. We can now use this graph to analyze the four cases that were mentioned above.

Insurers Can Identify Risks and Charge Different Premiums. This case represents economically efficient allocation of insurance. Each risk type purchases insurance until its risk-adjusted competitive price is equal to its RCS. This occurs at contracts L^* and H^* for low and high risks, respectively. These contracts equalize net income in both states of the world, an outcome known as "full insurance" for both risk types. As shown in figure 4–1, however, full insurance for high risks involves a

FIGURE 4–1

CONSUMER BEHAVIOR WHEN INSURERS CAN IDENTIFY RISKS AND
CHARGE DIFFERENT PREMIUMS

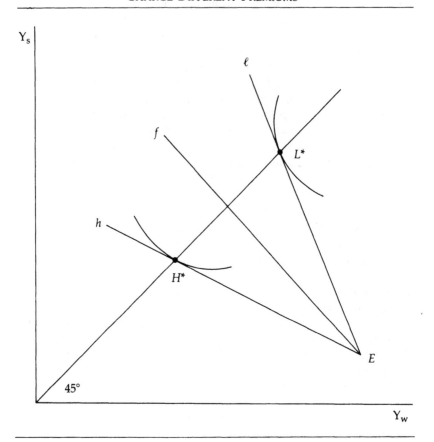

SOURCE: Authors.

large premium and a small payout. Low risks pay much less for each dollar of reimbursement under their full insurance policy.

Economically efficient allocation of insurance will occur if insurers can freely enter and leave the market and do not collude to fix the price of insurance. The threat of being undersold by competitors drives each insurer to price its policies at the lowest possible rate for each risk type. Because it can identify risk types prior to enrollment, high risks are not allowed to purchase policies intended for low risks. Obviously they would like to do so, and unless they could be identified and excluded from the low-risk policy, the market could not reach the equilibrium shown in figure 4–1.

This case points to a sharp contrast between the economist's notion of efficiency, which basically means that each consumer does the best possible job of allocating his or her given resources subject to competitive prices, and the policy maker's concept of fairness. The latter concept views the higher premium, the higher ratio of premium-to-benefits, and the lower payout for high risks as being grossly unfair. These views drive the policy maker to recommend a single premium for all risk types. It noteworthy that the policy maker's interpretation of fairness results in the subsidy of premiums for wealthy, high-risk individuals by poorer, low-risk individuals.

Insurers Can Identify Risks but Cannot Charge Different Premiums. Suppose that a single premium for all risk groups is required by law or regulation. The result will be active recruitment and retention of low risks by insurers, and active discrimination or disenrollment of high risks, to the extent that this is legally and technically possible. The phrase "cream-skimming" has been used to denote this type of behavior by insurers. Mark Pauly (1984) notes that cream-skimming should not occur in competitive insurance markets in which premiums can be adjusted for risk. The expected outcome in such markets is that high risks will be allowed to join or to remain in a health insurance plan, but they will pay a higher premium. Forcing insurers to charge the same premium for everyone will cause cream-skimming.

Alain Enthoven (1988) refers to health plans' incentive to cream-skim within uniform premium categories as "perverse," but it is no more so than other forms of profit seeking. Profit-maximizing insurers facing a single premium for all risks will cream-skim to the point where the marginal benefits and marginal costs of cream-skimming are equal, regardless of the level of the single premium. Even if allowances are made for some observable risk factors—for example, premium discounts for nonsmokers—the insurer will cream-skim within premium categories if it possesses additional information about health risks in those categories.

In order to attenuate the incentive to cream-skim, Enthoven (1978) proposed that premiums for private health plans should be regulated by actuarial categories based on age, sex, and location. Gradually these would be replaced by more precise and refined systems of predicting medical costs. All individuals within a risk class would pay the same premium. To the extent that these rating variables do not capture everything that is explainable about the variance of risk within a class, health insurance plans could be expected to cream-skim within Enthoven's actuarial risk categories. Newhouse and colleagues (1989) found that the rating factors proposed by Enthoven—age, sex, and location—plus aid-to-families-with-dependent-children (AFDC) status explained only about 11 percent of the total explainable variance in health care spending in a nonaged population. These rating factors explained 17 percent of the variance that could be accounted for by observable variables, such as health status and prior year's use of services, other than knowing the identity of the individual. Thus even without individual risk rating, insurers could be expected to cream-skim within Enthoven's risk categories.

Enthoven (1988) recommends that actuarial risk categories be supplemented by additional payments for certain high-cost diagnoses and elevated capitation payments following high-cost episodes, to reflect the additional costs usually associated with such patients. There are two problems with this type of after-the-fact adjustment. First, the medical conditions that trigger extra payments may be endogenous to some extent. Providing extra payments for such conditions will reduce the health plan's incentive to utilize preventive medical care. Second, even if the incidence of high-cost conditions is exogenous, the cost of treating an illness, once it occurs, has a large discretionary component. Thus the proposed system of adjustments would require a definition of the cost of an efficient treatment pattern. The health plan's sponsor would have to determine the cost of treating a stroke in the most efficient setting, for example. The most efficient setting may differ for each patient. Research on identifying predictable differences in cost and medical outcomes is still in its infancy, even for high-cost conditions.

Cream-skimming is especially likely to occur in the Medicare program, where health maintenance organizations (HMOs) can enroll beneficiaries for a capitation payment based on age, sex, location, welfare status, and institutionalization. These factors explain only a fraction of the variance in health care spending that could be explained by prior knowledge of enrollee health status (Manton 1990). Although risk-contracting Medicare HMOs are prohibited from screening potential enrollees and they must hold at least one open-enrollment period each year when anyone can join the HMO, empirical studies indicate that HMOs enjoy favorable risk selection within Medicare's actuarial rating categories (Eggers 1980; Eggers and Prihoda 1982; Brown 1988). Pauly (1985) has suggested that at least some of this favorable risk selection may occur because low-risk enrollees are attracted to the conservative practice style of HMO physicians. Alternatively, many people must switch their physician to join a group or staff model HMO, and low risks may be more willing to switch than high risks. Our assessment is that favorable selection is caused by characteristics of both the patient and the HMO.

Medicare HMOs also might encourage high-cost enrollees to convert to fee-for-service (FFS) Medicare. The HMO's physicians may support this strategy, since in many cases the physicians can continue to treat these patients under FFS Medicare. The HMO might even sell an FFS Medicare supplement (Medigap) policy, so that patients would see little difference between enrollment in the HMO and enrollment in FFS Medicare with a Medigap policy sold by the HMO. Brown (1988) found that high risks are indeed more likely than low risks to disenroll from Medicare HMOs. Thus it may not be reasonable to expect that Medicare HMO risks will resemble Medicare FFS risks as the HMO population ages. One can expect to find favorable risk selection in Medicare HMOs over the long run.

What can we say about the long-run consequences of biased selection for efficiency and equity when insurers cannot adjust premiums for known risk differences? We know that cream-skimming has the potential to subvert the intended subsidy from low to high risks. This is not quite the whole story, however. We need to describe how cream-skimming insurers will compete in equilibrium. Mark Pauly (1985) has provided this analysis for us. He assumes that HMOs can identify the low risks and will compete to enroll them. To succeed in this competition, HMOs will have to offer more amenities or higher quality to low risks and correspondingly lower quality or fewer services to high risks. Eventually HMOs will competitively drive away all the profits from enrolling low risks. Equilibrium in this regulated market may entail a small loss in efficiency, since healthy people might prefer to receive benefits in cash rather than in extra services. But the market is functioning as well as it can, given that premiums cannot be adjusted and cash rebates are not allowed.

We would like to extend Pauly's argument, because we believe that the efficiency loss from forcing insurers to ignore risk differences may be somewhat worse than he imagined. In particular he overlooks the effect of this policy on the welfare of high-risk individuals. Enforcing equal premiums may in fact make both risk groups worse off, compared with the competitive equilibrium. Our analysis is shown in figure 4–2, where Ef is the competitive price line for an insurance policy that ignores risk differences. Any policy with the same premium and payout for both groups will break even if it is located along Ef.

One such policy might be represented by point C, with premium P_C and payout R_C. The zero-profit payout for this premium, however, would be much larger if the policy could be offered only to low risks. As we have drawn figure 4–2, the zero-profit payout to low risks would lie at point L^*, which is exactly the policy that low risks would choose if offered insurance at a competitive price. Under Pauly's assumption that insurers

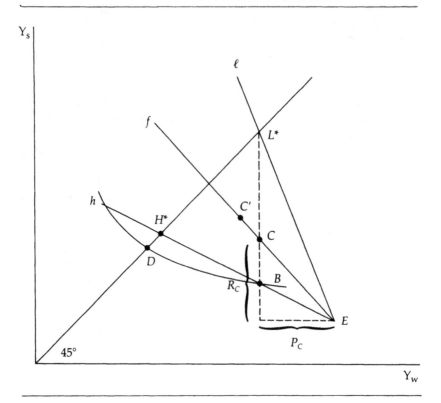

SOURCE: Authors.

compete for low risks, they will eventually offer them the payout of policy L^*. Since L^* is the competitive contract for low risks, they are no better or worse off than they would be under competitive pricing.

But high risks are worse off than they would be under competitive pricing. They will lose services until they are offered the payout at point B. Competitive pricing would allow them to choose contact H^*. Therefore the unsuccessful attempt to create cross subsidies between groups is economically inefficient, because one group's satisfaction is unchanged and the other group is made worse off by this policy. The monetary value of this efficiency loss can be found by extending the high risk's indifference curve that passes through point B until it cuts the 45 degree

74

line at point D. Distance DH^* along the 45 degree line is the amount of money that would have to be given to high risks to compensate them for the lost opportunity to buy policy H^*. A corollary to this argument is that a common policy that holds the high risks harmless cannot be offered without making low risks worse off. Such a common policy would have to contain much more insurance than low risks would willingly buy at competitive prices.

Finally, we can show that both groups may be worse off under the common policy. Simply imagine that the common policy is C' with a slightly larger premium and payout than C. This new policy still leaves high risks worse off than they were with the competitive policy H^*, and it also leaves low risks worse off than with competitive policy L^*. The attempt to be fair to high risks may hurt everyone.

Insurers Cannot Identify Risks or Charge Different Premiums. This case might be called "successful community rating." Because the same contract is offered to all risks and the insurer cannot cream-skim, the low risks subsidize high risks at a rate below the high risks' true actuarial cost. We will analyze the consequences of successful community rating for efficiency and equity.

First we should point out that successful community rating is not guaranteed when insurers do not have enough information to skim the good risks prior to enrollment. Passive selection by enrollees who prefer managed care and selective disenrollment might still defeat community rating. Nevertheless, if only one insurer is permitted to enter the market and that insurer offers only one contract, then passive selection and disenrollment are not possible. This situation might correspond to a geographic market served exclusively by a single-contract insurer. Blue Cross plans practiced this type of community rating before they were challenged by commercial health insurers. An employer that allows only one single-contract health plan to enter the firm can also enforce successful community rating.

We will concentrate less on the causes of successful community rating and more on its consequences. Mark Pauly (1970) has argued that community rating is similar to a tax on healthy policy holders, with the amount of the tax proportionate to the quantity of insurance they buy. To reduce their tax burden, healthy policy holders will reduce the quantity of insurance they purchase. If they could pay the same tax in a lump sum and buy insurance at the competitive price, they would choose to insure fully against risk. Since full insurance against risk is better than incomplete insurance, it follows that community rating is an inefficient method to subsidize high risks.

We can use our graphic model to present this argument. Contracts

FIGURE 4–3
CONSUMER BEHAVIOR WHEN INSURERS CANNOT IDENTIFY RISKS
OR CHARGE DIFFERENT PREMIUMS

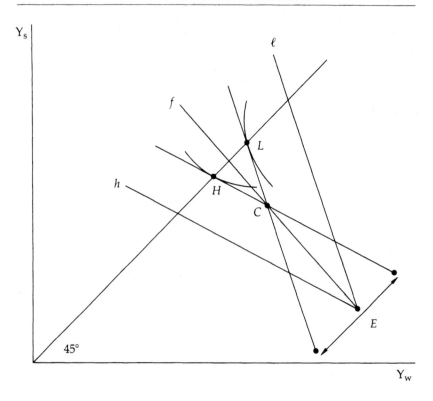

SOURCE: Authors.

along line Ef in figure 4–3 will break even, provided that they are bought by both high and low risks. Point C represents one such contract. Contract C would be picked apart by insurers if they had enough information to cream-skim, but we now assume that insurers do not have this information or, more likely, that only one plan is offered. Contract C causes low risks to subsidize high risks. If this tax were converted into an income transfer, payable in both states of the world, it would move the high risks' endowment point up and to the right at a 45 degree angle. The low risks' endowment would move down and to the left at a 45 degree angle. An income transfer of equal value to the subsidy would allow both groups to buy contract C if they wished and if it were offered

76

to each group at the competitive price for that group. The opportunity to buy contract C is represented by lines parallel to *Eh* and *El*, originating from the post-tax endowments. Consumers facing competitive prices, however, would not want to buy contract C. High risks facing competitive prices would purchase *H* and low risks would purchase *L*. The utility value of these contracts is greater than the value of C for *both* risk groups.

The literature on community rating is silent regarding the location of contract C. We have drawn the community-rated contract so that it represents incomplete insurance. By pure luck contract C might involve full insurance—that is, it might lie exactly on the 45 degree line that denotes equal income in both states of the world. In this case, which we emphasize would happen only by luck, the community-rated contract is efficient. Nevertheless, there are plausible political reasons to expect that contract C will involve more-than-complete insurance—that is, it will lie above and to the left of the 45 degree line. High-risk groups will lobby the political process to push C in this direction. They will be joined by provider-interest groups, whose incomes would be increased by having both groups purchase more-than-complete insurance coverage.

Since the implicit tax is off-budget, there is presumably no reason why it would have to compete against other public spending programs. Thus the only people who might resist more-than-complete insurance are those who pay the tax. Who are these people? Table 4–1 shows how family expenditures for personal health care services in the United States in 1977 were related to age of the family head (NCHSR 1987). Families headed by persons aged nineteen–twenty-four spent $582, on average, for personal health care in 1977. Using the May 1991 medical care component of the consumer price index (CPI) to convert 1977 medical care spending into current dollars, this represents $1,789 per young family in current dollars. Families headed by persons aged twenty-five–fifty-four spent $3,747 in current dollars, and those headed by persons between ages fifty-five and sixty-four spent $5,115. Average 1977 medical care spending by all families headed by persons aged nineteen–sixty-four was $3,753 in current dollars.

Table 4–1 also shows the total annual 1987 money income of families in each age interval (Bureau of the Census 1989). Because of a slight difference in reporting, the youngest census age category is eighteen–twenty-four years. In 1987 the total annual money income of the youngest families was $18,830, on average. This represents $22,477 in current dollars, using the May 1991 CPI.

Assuming that the level and distribution of expenses would not be affected by insurance, a community-rated medical care premium for the entire population in table 4–1 would cost $3,753. Young families, who

TABLE 4–1

FAMILY MEDICAL CARE SPENDING AND FAMILY INCOME, BY AGE, 1977

Age of Family Head (years)	Number of Families (1,000s)	Medical Spending (1977$)	Medical Spending (1991$)	Total Income (1987$)	Total Income (1991$)
19-24	8,418	582	1,789	18,830	22,477
25-54	43,137	1,219	3,747	41,085	49,042
55-64	12,345	1,664	5,115	40,088	47,852

SOURCE: NCHSR 1987; Bureau of the Census 1989.

earn less than half as much as the other two groups, would receive a payout ratio of 48 percent on this policy. In other words they would collect only 48 cents for every dollar paid in premiums. The large group of families headed by persons aged twenty-five–fifty-four would break even on this policy, collecting almost as much as they paid in premiums. Older families would receive $1.36 for every dollar paid in premiums. Therefore the income distribution consequence of community rating is that young (aged eighteen–twenty-four) families would subsidize older (aged fifty-five–sixty-four) families. This subsidy flows from a group that earns $22,477 per year to a group that earns $47,852 per year.

This is a very rough comparison, limited by the availability of data to the broad income classes and the years cited above. It does not adjust for family size or other measures of need, nor does it account for other measures of ability to pay. Inclusion of the latter would show that families in the fifty-five–sixty-four age group have the highest median net worth of all families (Bureau of the Census 1986). Community rating also subsidizes activities of dubious social value, such as smoking and excessive consumption of alcohol. One study (Pupp 1981) estimated that the annual cross subsidy per smoker in a community-rated health insurance plan was $38.10 in 1974. The author calculated that the total annual cross subsidy in a universal national health insurance plan would have been $2.04 billion in 1974. The current cost of this cross subsidy would be $8.43 billion.

Community rating also has implications for equity between the insured and uninsured populations. According to one estimate (Moyer 1989), 31.1 million Americans lacked health insurance during 1987. Thirty percent of the uninsured lived in impoverished families, and another 18 percent lived in families above the poverty line but with less than 149 percent of poverty income. The uninsured were also disproportionately found in the eighteen–twenty-four age group. Thus it appears that the people who would have to pay the community rating tax are also likely to be uninsured. Viewed from this perspective, community rating would increase the number of uninsured because it would raise the price of health insurance for many people in this group.

Insurers Can Charge Different Premiums but Cannot Identify Risks. Consumers in insurance markets may have information that is not known to the insurer. For example, a person may know that he or she has a history of cancer in the family. The seller of insurance cannot discover this information easily, and the consumer's incentive is to conceal it. Nevertheless, insurers can tailor their benefit packages to get consumers to signal what kind of risk they are. This case has received a great deal of attention in the theoretical literature on insurance (Rothschild and Stiglitz 1976; Wilson 1977). These theoretical analyses have shown that insurance markets will work poorly, if at all, when unequal information is present. A likely scenario is that the insurer quotes a competitive price for full coverage of low risks. Needless to say, this policy will be very attractive to high risks who will flock to it. Since the insurer cannot exclude high risks, the policy will lose money and it must be withdrawn from the market. It is replaced with a competitively-priced policy for low risks that features limits on coverage. High risks will choose not to buy this policy because it does not offer the protection they desire. Low risks will buy it because some insurance is better than no insurance. A full-coverage policy competitively priced for high risks can also be offered, and it will be chosen by high risks. As Rothschild and Stiglitz (1976) note:

> One of the interesting properties of the equilibrium is that the presence of high risk individuals exerts a negative externality on low risk individuals. The externality is completely dissipative; there are losses to the low risk individuals, but the high risk individuals are no better off than they would be in isolation.

In our opinion, the main flaw with this argument is that the theory's predictions do not describe how health insurance markets really work. We know of no example where low risks are prevented from buying as much health insurance as they want. Although many Americans lack any health insurance and most have incomplete coverage for some risks, such as nursing home care, these gaps in coverage can be explained without using the adverse selection theory. About one-fifth of all uninsured Americans are under age fifteen. Half of uninsured adults do not work full-time for any part of the year (Moyer 1989). Thus they are unlikely to be eligible for the tax subsidy for employer-paid health insurance. The employed uninsured usually work for small firms that do not offer health insurance, even at the subsidized price (Swartz and

Bovbjerg 1985). State laws requiring coverage of expensive "add-ons" make it even more difficult for low-income people to afford basic health insurance.

The lack of adequate long-term care insurance can also be explained by more prosaic factors. A competitively-priced, long-term care insurance policy would be very expensive. Many beneficiaries die in nursing homes and therefore would not want insurance except to protect their estates. Thus the demand for long-term care insurance is not adequate to support a market for this type of protection (Pauly 1990).

Some health policy analysts tell a story that resembles the adverse selection theory but turns out on closer inspection to be quite different. In this story, a low coverage policy—for example, one with deductibles and coinsurance—is offered by an employer. This policy attracts low-risk employees and sells for a low premium. Those employees who are more likely to use health services would prefer a different policy that covers the first dollar of expenses. Such a policy is offered, but it costs so much that the relatively good risks switch back to the low-coverage policy. The premium for first-dollar coverage rises as the risk pool worsens. Finally, the high-coverage policy becomes so expensive that it must be withdrawn from the market.

We have argued elsewhere (Feldman and Dowd 1991) that market segmentation of this type is limited by two factors: the preferences of high risks for their favored coverage, and the fact that the low-risk premium must rise as it attracts people from the other policy. But even if health insurance markets tend to unravel into segments composed of low and high risks, this is not evidence of market failure. Instead it shows that a competitive market will not subsidize the first-dollar coverage that is desired by high risks. When the fair premium for first-dollar coverage is revealed to them, they discover that it is too high. This outcome may not be fair to these people, but competition does not promise outcomes that are fair. It only promises outcomes that are efficient.

In Rothschild's and Stiglitz's (1976) model, varying the level of coverage offered is the only means the insurer has of identifying low and high risks. This unrealistic assumption can be avoided if the low-risk plan can devise some way of excluding high-risk individuals other than by offering less coverage than they wish to buy. It is not necessary that the health plan be able to identify high-risk individuals, a priori. All that is needed is for the low-risk plan to introduce some feature to which low-risk individuals are at least indifferent and that high-risk individuals abhor. As noted earlier (Pauly 1985), healthy individuals may be attracted to the conservative practice style of HMO physicians. The opposite may be true for high-risk individuals, who may find the tightly monitored resource use of HMOs so objectionable that this feature presents enough of a barrier to maintain a quasi-competitive equilib-rium. In this equilibrium, high-risk individuals would pay higher premiums and have less coverage than low-risk individuals, since managed-care plans would bid up the benefits in competition for low-risk individuals. Enrollees in the managed-care plan would be subjected to tightly controlled resource use.

A quasi-competitive equilibrium has two objectionable features. First, just as in the case of a priori risk identification, this equilibrium may be inequitable, since high-risk individuals have to pay higher premiums and receive fewer benefits than do low-risk individuals. Second, the wrong individuals may be in the managed-care plan. There seems to be little value in having persistently healthy people enrolled in tightly managed health plans. The latter objection might involve both inequity and inefficiency. Having the unhealthy elderly enrolled in unmanaged fee-for-service Medicare, for example, is inequitable to nonelderly taxpayers who provide a substantial subsidy of Medicare's costs. It also is inefficient, since the government's contribution to Medicare HMOs is based on costs in the unmanaged FFS sector. Medicare costs could be reduced by transferring these unhealthy enrollees to managed-care plans.

Some enrollees may prefer unmanaged care, however, and their preferences could be accommodated without loss of efficiency if all beneficiaries choosing unmanaged FFS Medicare had to pay the full marginal cost of this alternative. Some high-risk individuals, whose preference for unmanaged care exceeds the extra cost, would stay in that system; others would transfer to managed-care plans. The resulting distribution of enrollees would be efficient. In addition, loss of enrollees to managed-care plans might encourage less efficient insurers to adopt proven managed-care techniques, especially those that are acceptable to high risks.

Critical Issues for Reform

We have analyzed four possible markets for health insurance: where insurers can or cannot identify low and high risks prior to enrollment; and where insurers are or are not allowed to risk-adjust their premiums. What can be said about which of these markets is most efficient or equitable? How can we enter the most favored market? A diagram of the four possible insurance markets is shown in figure 4–4.

It seems clear to us that the least desirable situation is the one in which insurers can identify risks but are not allowed to risk-adjust their premiums. This is an invitation for insurers to cream-skim to the extent that they are technically and legally able. The result of cream-skimming

81

FIGURE 4–4

A DIAGRAM OF FOUR POSSIBLE INSURANCE MARKETS

Can insurers identify risks?

		No	Yes
Can insurers risk-adjust premiums?	No	Successful community rating	Cream-skimming
	Yes	Rationing coverage for low risks Quasi-competitive equilibrium	Competitive equilibrium

SOURCE: Authors.

will be a welfare loss for one or both risk groups, not to mention the resources that insurers spend on skimming. Unless society is willing to spend a great deal of money to provide benefits of little marginal value to low risks, the cream-skimming equilibrium will make high risks worse off than they would be under perfectly competitive markets with a priori risk identification. Since cream-skimming is inefficient and is likely to be unfair to high risks, it would therefore seem reasonable to allow insurers to adjust their rates to reflect risk differences.

Can we be sure, however, that insurers will not default to the lower left box, in which they can adjust their rates but cannot identify risks? First, as we argued above, the empirical evidence simply does not persuade us that coverage for low risks is rationed in real-world insurance markets. Even if this box were realistic, market segmentation of low and high risks could be maintained by less objectionable methods than rationing. One of these methods is managed care. If low risks are attracted to managed-care plans and high risks are repelled by them, then consumers could signal their risk type by their preference for managed care. We might prefer to have high risks enrolled in the managed-care plan, but if they are determined not to join it, then society has little justification other than paternalism for forcing them to do so.

What can we say about successful community rating versus rationing coverage to low risks? Clearly the subsidized community-rated policy is preferred by high-risk individuals to the policies that would be offered in a Rothschild-Stiglitz rationing equilibrium. Low risks, on the other hand, might prefer buying a rationed policy rather than paying a large tax through community rates. Thus the choice of these two boxes is likely to be viewed differently by the two risk groups. For the theoretically inclined, there is one situation in which both groups would prefer community rating: enforced community rating will make both groups better off when the Rothschild-Stiglitz equilibrium does not exist. We regard this case as a theoretical curiosity.

The comparison of most importance for health policy is between successful community rating and competition. Community rating improves the welfare of high risks and reduces that of low risks, compared with the competitive equilibrium. Except in one special case—where the community-rated policy involves full insurance for both groups—we showed that this method of subsidizing high risks is inefficient. It could be replaced by an income transfer of equal value that, coupled with the opportunity to buy insurance at competitive prices, could make both groups better off. We also strongly question whether the subsidy of high health risks by low risks is fair. The problem is that low-risk families also have low incomes and few household assets. Although our opinion carries no special moral authority, we think that low-income families should not subsidize high-income families. The subsidy of unhealthy personal habits is also questionable.

What can the sponsor of a public or private health benefit plan do in order to enter the box in figure 4–2 labeled "competitive equilibrium"? We have analyzed this question in detail elsewhere with special reference to the Medicare program (Dowd et al. 1990), so that only a summary is needed here. First we recommend that competition be used to determine the correct price of health insurance benefits. Finding the right price is probably the most important contribution that competition can make in health insurance markets. Unless the health plan's sponsor can find the right price, it is likely to pay too much for health insurance; then, unless it has an unlimited budget, it will purchase too little health insurance for its beneficiaries. Competition can ensure that health insurance is purchased for the lowest possible price. Specifically, the government's premium contribution for Medicare should be set equal to the lowest price submitted by a qualified health plan for Medicare Part A and Part B benefits, or some other basic benefit package specified by the federal government, in a predefined market area.

The basic benefit package should not be more generous than the amount of coverage that high risks would be willing to purchase in competitive equilibrium. Benefits more generous than the level denoted by R^* in figure 4–5 would result in overinsurance of high risks. A health plan bidding to supply this level of coverage would submit a bid that reflected both efficiency in producing the benefits and any selection

83

FIGURE 4–5
GOVERNMENT AND BENEFICIARY
CONTRIBUTIONS FOR MEDICARE

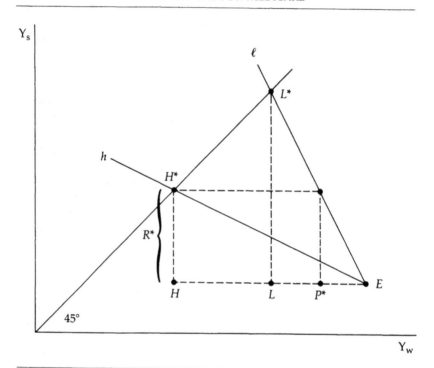

SOURCE: Authors.

advantages that the plan may have in recruiting low-risk enrollees. For example, if HMOs are more successful in recruiting low-risk enrollees because of the conservative practice style of HMO physicians, then this advantage would be reflected in a low bid—distance EP^*—by HMOs for basic coverage.

Next we recommend that the government should pay the low bid on behalf of any enrollee in any health plan. Both low- and high-risk enrollees would wish to supplement the government's contribution with an additional out-of-pocket payment in order to purchase their desired levels of coverage. Low risks would pay P^*L to purchase additional benefits represented by policy L^*, and high risks would pay P^*H to purchase basic Medicare benefits. While it may seem unfair to require an out-of-pocket premium contribution by high risks for basic coverage, we question whether the government's contribution should be adjusted

84

for risk. The available methods for determining actuarial risk categories may be too crude, relative to the opportunities for health plans to cream-skim within categories. Finally, we question whether government subsidies should be based on how much people spend for medical care. Income and, possibly, asset holdings seem to be a more equitable basis for determining ability to pay for health insurance.

References

Brown, Randall S. "Biased Selection in Medicare HMOs." Paper presented at the Fifth Annual Meeting of the Association for Health Services Research (San Francisco, Calif., June 26–28, 1988).

Bureau of the Census, U.S. Department of Commerce. "Household Wealth and Asset Ownership: 1984." *Current Population Reports*, Series P–70, Household Economic Studies, no. 7 (July 1986).

———. "Money Income of Households, Families, and Persons in the United States: 1987." *Current Population Reports*, Series P–60, Consumer Income, no. 162 (February 1989).

Dowd, Bryan, Jon Christianson, Roger Feldman, and Catherine Wisner. *Issues Regarding Health Plan Payment under Medicare and Recommendations for Reform*. Report prepared under Cooperative Agreement no. 99-C-99169/5 for the Health Care Financing Administration (March 22, 1990).

Eggers, Paul W. "Risk Differential Between Medicare Beneficiaries Enrolled and Not Enrolled in an HMO." *Health Care Financing Review* 1 (Winter 1980): 91–99.

Eggers, Paul W., and Ronald Prihoda. "Pre-Enrollment Reimbursement Patterns of Medicare Beneficiaries Enrolled in 'At-Risk' HMOs." *Health Care Financing Review* 4 (September 1982): 55–73.

Enthoven, Alain C. "Consumer-Choice Health Plan." *New England Journal of Medicine* 298 (March 23 and 30, 1978); 650–58 (Part 1), 709–20 (Part 2).

———. *Theory and Practice of Managed Competition in Health Care Finance.* Amsterdam: North-Holland, 1988.

Feldman, Roger, and Bryan Dowd. "Must Adverse Selection Cause Premium Spirals?" *Journal of Health Economics* 10 (October 1991): 350–57.

Goldberg, Lawrence G., and Warren Greenberg. "Health Insurance Industry Shouldn't Be Exempt from Antitrust Laws." *HealthSpan* 8 (May 1991): 3–9.

Henderson, James M., and Richard E. Quandt. *Microeconomic Theory: A Mathematical Approach.* Second Edition, New York: McGraw-Hill Book Company, 1971.

Long, John D. "Insurance Subsidies and Welfare Economics." *Journal of Risk and Insurance* 39 (September 1972): 341–50.

Manton, Kenneth G. "Patterns of Health and Functioning in the Enrollment of Social Health Maintenance Organizations." Health Care

Financing Administration, Contract no. 500-85-0042, 1990.

Moyer, M. Eugene. "A Revised Look at the Number of Uninsured Americans." *Health Affairs* 8 (Summer 1989): 102–110.

National Center for Health Services Research and Health Care Technology Assessment, U.S. Department of Health and Human Services. "A Summary of Expenditures and Sources of Payment for Personal Health Services from the National Medical Care Expenditure Survey." *National Health Care Expenditures Study*. Data Preview 24 (May 1987).

Newhouse, Joseph P., Willard G. Manning, Emmett B. Keeler, and Elizabeth Sloss. "Adjusting Capitation Rates Using Objective Health Status Measures and Prior Utilization." *Health Care Financing Review* 10 (Spring 1989): 41–54.

Pauly, Mark V. "The Welfare Economics of Community Rating." *Journal of Risk and Insurance* 37 (September 1970): 407–18.

————. "Is Cream-Skimming a Problem for the Competitive Medical Market?" *Journal of Health Economics* 3 (April 1984): 88–95.

————. "What Is Adverse about Adverse Selection?" *Advances in Health Economics and Health Services Research*, vol. 6. Eds. Richard M. Scheffler and Louis F. Rossiter. Greenwich, Conn.: JAI Press Inc., 1985.

————. "The Rational Nonpurchase of Long-Term-Care Insurance." *Journal of Political Economy* 98 (February 1990): 153–68.

Pupp, Roger L. "Community Rating and Cross Subsidies in Health Insurance." *Journal of Risk and Insurance* 48 (December 1981): 610–27.

Rothschild, Michael, and Joseph Stiglitz. "Equilibrium in Competitive Insurance Markets: An Essay in the Economics of Imperfect Information." *Quarterly Journal of Economics* 90 (November 1976): 629–49.

Swartz, Katherine, and Randall R. Bovbjerg. *Summary Report: Project on the Uninsured and Private Sector Initiatives to Broaden Health Insurance Coverage*. Washington, D.C.: The Urban Institute, December 1985.

Wilson, Charles. "A Model of Insurance Markets with Incomplete Information." *Journal of Economic Theory* 16 (December 1977): 167–207.

5

Why Preserve
Private Health Care Financing?

Clark C. Havighurst

As it is taking shape, the national health policy debate of the 1990s poses no great threat to the existing system of private health care financing. Although some serious proposals would shift to a single-payer system like Canada's, the proposals with the best political prospects all reflect Senator George Mitchell's view that "we must build upon the existing public/private mix in our health care system" (House 1991, 21). Congressman Henry Waxman, another political leader eager for major reform, has opined that "it is politically nonviable to talk about scrapping the existing system" (House, 1991, 6). Thus, those in the business of privately financing health care can probably rest easy in the knowledge that Americans prefer incremental over radical change and are likely to settle for regulatory reforms that do no more than keep private coverage viable and make it more accessible to working Americans.[1]

But as a policy matter, precisely why should private financing be preserved? In this chapter, I question whether private coverage has a raison d'être. To some extent I am using my prerogative as a Duke

---

1. The so-called play-or-pay mandate, which appears in both the Mitchell and the Waxman bills (S. 1227 and H.R. 2535, the Pepper Commission Health Care Access and Reform Act of 1991, respectively) and which ostensibly preserves private financing, may prove, however, to be a wolf in sheep's clothing. The play-or-pay strategy is popular in Congress because it transforms a politically objectionable new payroll tax into more palatable regulation—by allowing employers to escape the tax simply by insuring their workers. Some play-or-pay proponents probably hope, however, that either now or in the future the employer tax can be made low enough by supplementation from general revenues that employers will increasingly elect public coverage, causing the public payer to triumph in the end. Setting the tax rate in a play-or-pay system would be a politically sensitive undertaking, pitting defenders of private health insurance against both small business and supporters of a government-dominated system.

University law professor to act as a (Blue) Devil's advocate—to devil, as it were, the Blues and other private health insurers. But I am quite sincere in my skepticism about both the ability and the willingness of private entities, including the whole range of alternative delivery and financing systems with which we are familiar, to address effectively the vital issue of health care spending. Although a single-payer system might be only a second-best solution to our cost problems, a strong argument can be made for preferring it over the current regime of private intermediaries that lack—and do not appear even to want—the tools that are needed to tackle the cost problem at its root. If we are nearing a critical decision about the future of our health care system, let us use the occasion to ask explicitly whether private financing is worth preserving as the principal mechanism by which the cost of health care is made bearable in the United States.

Although I am sincere in questioning private health care financing as we know it, my main goal here is to demonstrate that private financing could perform a unique and useful function in the health care enterprise. A prerequisite, however, is the resurrection of private contracts as effective vehicles for specifying precise, enforceable rules to govern medical care in particular circumstances. Unless contracts can be made viable instruments for expressing and implementing meaningful, econ-omizing choices by consumers, we should stop pretending that privately financed medical care is a product of a free market.[2] Instead, we should acknowledge that the most important decisions about health care are ultimately under the control of central authorities and that these authorities—essentially, the courts and the medical profession acting in tandem—are accountable to neither consumers in the marketplace nor voters in the political process. A national health policy that leaves vital decisions in such hands is an invitation to runaway costs. Unless private financing plans can somehow employ private contracts to transmit clear, enforceable signals from cost-conscious consumers on the demand side of the market to providers on the supply side, a single-payer health policy

---

2. For the observation that the moral hazard associated with private health insurance—that is, the propensity of insureds to incur excessive risks or costs—does not alone prevent the market from allocating resources efficiently in the health care sector (since moral hazard may be an acceptable cost of any program providing desirable financial protection), see P. Joskow (1981, 22). Joskow's observation holds, however, only if private insurers are doing all that is efficient to limit the impact of moral hazard. If either regulatory restrictions or their customers' incentives (resulting from poorly designed tax subsidies, for example) cause them not to control costs optimally, then a serious misallocation of resources can occur—possibly involving, in this case, whole percentage points of GDP.

may be the only reasonable one. If the private financing industry is a barrier to—instead of a vehicle for—democratizing the market for health services, it may deserve to be consigned to what Karl Marx called "the dustbin of history."[3]

A Raison d'Être for Private Financing?

There is a presumption in favor of private arrangements for financing health care not only in the current political climate but also among economics-trained policy analysts. Nevertheless, the private financing of health care has few enough followers around the globe and has revealed enough shortcomings in the United States that the burden of proof in objective policy discussions should probably be on those who believe that private financing should be preserved. In any event, wherever the burden of proof belongs, one can fairly expect the private health insurance industry to put its best foot forward in policy discus-

---

3. The reference to Marx is ironic at more levels than initially meet the eye. The case I will make against the private financing industry lies largely in its complicity in the medical profession's collective domination of crucial decisions about medical care; although less obviously the "lackeys" and "running dogs" of the medical profession than in earlier days, private health plans still kowtow to professional authority on many issues, as will be shown. Perhaps the greatest irony, however, is the similarity between the medical profession's one-party rule of the world of medicine and the powers formerly exercised by communist elites in Eastern Europe and the former Soviet Union. Consider the following (Havighurst 1990b, 429):

> With no intention to push the analogy too far, it can be observed that communism, too, was based on a paradigm under which a single elite group set itself up as the ultimate authority on what was good for the people. In the name of the people whose interests it purported to serve, that elite group monopolized the flow of information and opinion. Transactions between willing buyers and willing sellers were not allowed, and freedom of choice was sacrificed to an ideology of equality.
> [Like the recent overthrow of communist regimes,] the decentralization strategy in American health care is also an attempt to empower people by giving them choices they have previously been denied. The suggestions I have offered for carrying the decentralization strategy forward to its logical conclusion would foster *glasnost*, would invite market-driven *perestroika*, and would further weaken the medical profession's one-party rule. Fortunately, however, there is no reason to think that the medical profession would suffer the same fate as old communist parties. Instead, precisely because the profession has a legitimate claim to the people's continued respect, it would continue in its vital role as an advocate for important patient interests—even in a fully decentralized, fully democratic health care system.

sions and not to rely principally on political inertia to ensure its survival.

The Industry's Stance on Access and Cost Issues. If proponents of private financing are to establish its net advantage over a single-payer system, they must demonstrate its ability to address two distinct policy challenges: (1) ensuring access and (2) controlling cost. Unfortunately, the private financing industry itself recognizes shortcomings only in access.

Private health insurers have not been able to ignore the failure of the private market to make health care accessible to all working Americans. The number of Americans lacking health coverage of any kind rose significantly in the 1980s, reversing a trend that had encouraged the nation to assume that private insurance and public measures would eventually converge to ensure everyone's access to health services. Now, well over 30 million Americans, most of them working persons, lack any financial protection against the cost of health care, and the coverage of many more persons is insecure, dependent on continued employment or continued insurability. Similar shortcomings of private insurance in protecting the elderly led to the creation of the Medicare program in the 1960s. A comparable single-payer program for the nonelderly may be enacted in the 1990s if private insurers cannot demonstrate a greater ability and willingness to cover all employed persons.

In recognition of the new questions being raised concerning private health insurance, the Health Insurance Association of America and the Blue Cross and Blue Shield Association have acknowledged the difficulty of keeping private coverage available on reasonable terms and have suggested some specific remedies. Thus, the industry has endorsed some regulation of underwriting practices that would make voluntary health insurance more effective in serving both private and social objectives.[4] In

---

4. Although private insurance is socially beneficial, it exists to serve only private ends. Indeed, private insurance is nothing more than a vehicle by which individuals facing similar risks can agree to pool them. One problem in the current market is that not everyone wishing health insurance can find a pool of comparable risks that will accept them, especially because insurers, increasingly fearful of the staggering cost of unknowingly accepting a single bad risk, have each erected increasingly arbitrary underwriting barriers. This failure of the private market may be correctable to some degree by regulation (see, for example, HIAA 1991).

Other perceived deficiencies in private insurance relate to its failure to meet the redistributive objectives of social insurance. The objective of social insurance that sets it apart from private insurance is to pool *dissimilar* risks, so that those with less exposure or more wealth will subsidize those who are less fortunate. As regulation is used to force private insurers to serve more and more social objectives, the freedom of individual insurers to innovate, to offer alternatives, and to serve the interests of homogeneous insured groups is impaired. Beyond

addition, the HIAA and the Blues, hypothesizing that many of the uninsured have been simply priced out of the health insurance market, have made some constructive proposals to facilitate the offering of new, low-cost insurance options (for example, HIAA 1991). The industry's political strategy is apparently to offer policy makers ways of expanding the number of persons who can be insured privately so that fewer persons will require public coverage financed by explicit taxes.

Health insurers have been less willing to confront the failure of the private market to ensure the efficiency of health care spending. Yet the incrementalist policy of tinkering with private insurance and public programs to close the gap between them is justified only if private intermediaries can address cost issues more effectively, sensitively, and fairly than could a single public payer.[5] Indeed, a privately financed system must possess more than just a marginal advantage in achieving

some point, there is no reason to maintain, at high administrative cost, the fiction that insurance is a private undertaking. This chapter raises the question whether private health insurance is serving, or even aspiring to serve, its private purposes well enough to be preserved.

5. As demonstrated by the Medicare and Medicaid programs, a dominant public payer can seek to lower costs by exercising monopsony power against providers, demanding lower unit prices for the services provided. A public program is somewhat more limited in its ability to control the volume and type of services provided, however, because, although it can set general policies, it is bound to meet constitutional and administrative law standards of due process in resolving specific disputes with beneficiaries and providers. See generally Kinney (1986) and Blumstein (1976). Although private payers are not similarly bound by law to incur large administrative costs in resolving every dispute, later discussion observes that, under current conditions, they must fear potentially devastating lawsuits over their decisions to deny coverage for desirable care. This chapter advocates improving the legal environment for cost-containment efforts by private payers, thus giving them a comparative advantage over a single governmental payer in the American scheme.

The monopsony feature of the single-payer model should make it unattractive to a neutral policy analyst, who should object to its potential for exploiting producers, misallocating resources, and reducing the quality of care. Many policy makers, however, are attracted to the single-payer model precisely because of its ability to drive hard price bargains with providers; providers obviously resist it for the same reason and hope to preserve a system of relatively passive private financing. Like private payers, providers will support the more extensive market and legal reforms advocated in this chapter only if they feel truly threatened by the prospect of a single public payer. Indeed, arguments comparable to those addressed to the proponents of private financing in this chapter might be addressed to a provider audience in the same spirit in the hope that they too can be induced to give up their support for the dysfunctional status quo and seek to preserve private financing on the only principled basis that is available.

efficiency over a single-payer system because the latter is clearly superior for solving access problems. Thus, the incrementalist strategy would require new taxes to finance expanded health coverage for the uninsured; tax-shy legislatures are unlikely to provide such funds.[6] Conversely, a single-payer strategy would be self-financing to the extent that it would yield administrative savings[7] and allow ineffective or marginally bene-

6. All the while that many have believed that enactment of a public guarantee of universal health coverage was only a matter of time, the target (as some would define it) has been receding, rather than getting easier to hit. Thus, the cost of state-of-the-art health care has risen significantly faster each year than the nation's ability to pay, as measured, for example, by GDP. And the incremental public cost of giving everyone an entitlement to mainstream medical care increases each year it is not done. By the same token, creating an entitlement today commits government and society to coming up with new money each year to cover its increasing cost—unless a method of limiting the entitlement can be devised. See note 8 below.

7. The policy debate has recently directed attention to the allegedly high administrative costs of the current system of private health care financing. See, for example, U.S. General Accounting Office (1991) (concluding that a Canadian-style system, eliminating private insurance and run by federal and state governments, would result in savings of $67 billion a year, largely through scaled-back administration) and Woolhandler & Himmelstein (1991) (estimating up to $100 billion in savings from introducing a single-payer system). Among the many possible reasons why these savings may be overestimated is the fact that government must bear a heavy burden of due process in implementing its policies (see note 5).

Administrative costs of private health plans have grown in the 1980s as insurers have adopted managed-care techniques and other cost-containment measures to control for the moral hazard that necessarily accompanies any kind of insurance but is particularly troublesome in health insurance (see note 2). Notably, however, Americans already have the option of buying, through staff-model and group-practice health maintenance organizations, private protection that does not entail all the administrative costs of insured fee-for-service medicine. It is a fair question whether the availability of such options to consumers obviates concern about administrative costs in the rest of the system. (In other words, should we not assume that if consumers choose costlier fee-for-service insurance, they have reason, after allowing for tax subsidies, to spend their money that way?)

Without addressing the difficult question of the relative magnitude of government's and insurers' administrative costs, one can see how such costs might shift the burden of proof to the private sector. Although the operation of free markets always entails special costs in marketing, searching, and duplication of effort, those costs are usually justified by the countervailing benefits that flow to consumers from the diversity of products, from continual innovation, and from the incentives that result from making sellers accountable for the

ficial care to be redirected to more productive uses in caring for those who previously lacked health insurance.[8] Unless private financing has some distinct advantages over public financing, there is no convincing reason to preserve it.[9]

In these circumstances, private health care plans should be required to make a better case for their own survival than they have made so far. In so doing, one would expect them to demonstrate their success, or at least a promising potential, in the one area where a private, competitive system might have something special to offer: the decentralization of decision making on the myriad of difficult trade-offs with which modern medicine confronts us. As the following discussion reveals, however, the private sector has not shown that it can help consumers address the crucial dilemmas that must be resolved if health care costs are to be optimally controlled. On the contrary, private health care plans appear to be bent on avoiding such responsibilities, justifying questions concerning their future.

---

quality and cost of their products in the democratic marketplace. Given the apparently high cost of maintaining an array of private health care plans all carrying out essentially the same functions, it is reasonable to ask whether public monopoly might be more efficient. The health insurance industry is responsible for showing us specifically what we are getting in return for the additional costs we are asked to bear.

8. Savings achieved by a single payer by rationing care can be used directly for unmet needs, thus avoiding the necessity for a new explicit tax. Thus, the plan can generate resources by, in effect, "taxing" away from heavily insured patients that care which is worth less than it costs and can then redistribute that care to those who are needier. This is a fairly efficient tax-and-spend program because the exchanges it forces are Pareto-appropriate. Thus, the cost to the deprived patient is, by hypothesis, less than the cash generated, and the benefit to the newly treated patient may exceed, by some measure, the amount spent to obtain it. Although the differing marginal utility of income is a shaky basis for defending redistributions of cash, perhaps people can be persuaded to accept in-kind redistribution of medical care on the ground that it has differing marginal utilities.

9. Precisely because redistributive goals in medicine would be easier to achieve through a single-payer system than through welfare-medicine programs funded by explicit taxes, there is a danger that private health care financing will survive only because the taxpaying majority wishes to preserve its own health care while limiting assistance to those who are in need. Indeed, realism compels the conclusion that private financing is most likely to prevail, not on its own merits, but as a bulwark against egalitarian medicine, whether of the leveling-down or the leveling-up variety (see note 8). It is possible to imagine, however, single-payer systems in which individuals could supplement the public payment to obtain more or better services, thus yielding administrative efficiencies without forced homogenization of care.

Do They Give Us Any Choice? The raison d'être of a competitive market for health care financing is, or should be, to promote pluralism and to offer consumers meaningful choices so that they can seek good value for the money they have to spend. Private firms engaged in administering privately financed health care could most effectively carry their burden of proof on the question of their long-term utility by showing that they are both able and willing to offer consumers these benefits. Unfortunately, however, neither traditional health insurers nor modern alternative financing and delivery systems have ever demonstrated that they are eager to facilitate the exercise of meaningful choice by consumers. Institutions that are not true to their raison d'être deserve to face an uncertain future.

Even though most health care in the United States has been privately financed from the beginning, the marketplace does not yet offer consumers a full range of options. Specifically, they are denied the chance to make many economizing choices that would be both rational and responsible in light of the extraordinary cost and often limited benefit of state-of-the-art medical care. The reasons why consumers' options are restricted are not all immediately apparent. (The most critical of them will be discussed later.) Certainly, however, the fault does not lie entirely with private financing plans themselves.[10] Although private health plans might have been more courageous and creative in addressing their customers' needs, their failure to offer a full range of choices does not necessarily mean that private financing could never be a vehicle for responsible pluralism. Failures can be forgotten to the extent that (1) they were the consequence of exogenous factors; (2) those exogenous obstacles to innovation have been or can now be effectively removed; (3) the industry is committed to removing them;[11] and (4)

---

10. But see Havighurst (1988, 254–55):

> [M]any of the theories offered [to explain why commercial carriers were for a long time nearly useless in combating the influence of moral hazard on the cost of insured health services] absolve commercial insurers from blame for neglecting cost containment. There are, however, several points at which industry members might have opted to compete but chose instead to adhere to traditional patterns. Despite the plausibility of some of the industry's excuses for behaving as it did, its overall performance can be fairly criticized.

11. Although private insurers have fought, in court and in legislatures, many kinds of regulatory, legal, and other constraints on their ability to control costs, some forms of regulation have gone largely unchallenged. Indeed, challenges were likely only when the particular regulation or other constraint (including those imposed on the industry by organized medicine) put the commercial

individual health plans are eager and able to assume the new responsibilities that would then devolve upon them.

The performance and prospects of private health care financing may look different depending upon whether one focuses on traditional health insurance, both commercial and nonprofit (for example, the Blues), or on alternative mechanisms, such as group-practice and staff-model HMOs, that more closely integrate the delivery of medical care with its financing. One serious barrier to consumer choice in traditional health insurance has been state regulatory legislation prescribing the content of health insurance policies—so-called mandated-benefit laws. The health insurance industry is actively campaigning against such laws in attempting to serve the small-employer market more effectively (HIAA 1990, 1991). It has also accepted the preemption of the Employment Retirement Income Security Act that frees self-insured employers from such state mandates, while seeking a more general preemption of such laws to improve its ability to serve employers that are too small to self-insure. In this area there is little to fault in the industry's public position.[12] Insurers have convincingly demonstrated that poor public policy, not any inherent failing on their part, has prevented them from performing one of their essential functions in designing efficient coverage.

Mandated-benefit laws do not, however, explain all the failures of traditional health insurers to serve as useful vehicles for discovering and executing consumers' precise wishes about their medical care. Instead of competing to define and to enforce standards of medical practice to meet the tastes and pocketbooks of particular insured groups, insurers have viewed their task as limited to underwriting the cost of state-of-the-art medical care; the content of such care is, in their view, the responsibility of someone else, such as the medical profession, the U.S.

---

insurers at a competitive disadvantage vis-a-vis HMOs, the Blues, or employer self-insurance. "On the record, it appears that, for whatever reason, the insurance companies have been content to live with legal constraints on their own competitive behavior except where those constraints did not bind their competitors as well" (Havighurst 1988, 242, giving examples). The point is helpful in explaining insurers' disinterest in pursuing the competitive and law reform strategies recommended in this chapter. It also reveals why I have tried here to impress upon the industry that instead of pursuing short-term self-interest, it should justify its existence on policy grounds or face extinction.

12. The insurers' resistance to regulation of this kind bears out, however, the observation in note 11 that the insurance industry objects strenuously to regulation when it places insurers at a competitive or political disadvantage, but generally acquiesces in constraints whose only effect is to interfere with the ability of all forms of private health care financing to serve consumer interests.

Food and Drug Administration, or some other authoritative decision maker. Insurers have yet to present themselves as definers and executors of the wishes of insured groups. Yet the members of such groups, having contributed to a common fund, need precise rules to govern one another's use of the fund and to minimize the fund's exposure to abuse—that is, moral hazard. Although insurers have rarely entertained the possibility that a particular insured group might wish to establish its own rules, the costs of standard medical care are so high and its benefits so often problematic that consumers badly need some alternatives. They can reasonably expect private insurers to provide them.

Health insurers might respond to the foregoing observations by pointing to their extensive efforts in utilization management. To be sure, managed-care programs have achieved some success in preventing expenditures for inappropriate services. For the most part, however, such programs are unilateral efforts by insurers and do not offer opportunities for consumer choice, in the sense that insured groups can select the particular standards to be used in policing their own care. Indeed, payers generally do not even disclose their screening criteria either to their insureds or to providers. The apparent rationale for nondisclosure is that the criteria are designed only to ensure that care is economically provided within the range of professionally accepted standards, which alone define patient entitlements. Thus, utilization management has been designed to fit within the professional paradigm that treats the medical profession as the ultimate arbiter of the appropriateness of care.[13] Consistent with this paradigm, insurers economize only around the fringes and do not purport to customize the care of particular insured groups to match their members' resources and preferences.

Other managed-care programs, particularly group-practice and staff-model health maintenance organizations, appear to have given consumers some true options, not just different versions of the same largely standardized product. These private plans have somewhat more freedom—de facto, if not de jure—to depart from professional standards of care in the interest of efficiency. Because they promote economizing

---

13. Although the degree to which individual plans "hassle" physicians probably influences the extent to which the latter voluntarily omit marginal services, insurers, holding to the paradigm, do not concede that reducing the intensity of care could have adverse consequences for patients or that they are assuming any of the physician's responsibility for the care provided. Legally, the insurer and the utilization manager are bound by professional standards in their substantive determinations of coverage; contracts govern only the procedures followed in making such determinations. See, for example, Wilson v. Blue Cross (1990).

by altering physician incentives and not by second-guessing treatment decisions, such plans are less likely than third-party payers to find themselves in an open dispute with a patient backed by a treating physician. Although the legal system does not clearly authorize HMO physicians to depart from professional norms and standards (Bovbjerg 1975), there is some room for group-practice and staff-model HMOs to implement such departures sub rosa without undue legal risks. Well-run plans have thus been able to evolve distinctive styles of practice, respecting, for example, the frequency of hospitalization. Nevertheless, the substantive differences between plans, if any, are never made explicit, nor are they negotiable or subject to variation in response to the requirements of a particular group. An alternative delivery system is just that: a self-contained, self-governing entity that, like the dominant system, determines unilaterally, without negotiation or disclosure, what the consumer will get. Although group-practice and staff-model HMOs do offer consumers new options, they have felt no competitive need to press the limits of their freedom to innovate and to economize, leaving the range of choice still closely circumscribed.

In response to criticism of their failure to offer consumers an optimal range of choices, private health plans might say that there is no way that they can do all that I suggest. They could observe, among other things, that they are ultimately required by law to accept and to defer to the standards of the medical profession in deciding what services to provide or to pay for. This response has a great deal of truth, as later discussion will show (see also Havighurst 1983). Nevertheless, the legal compulsions under which insurers and other private health plans operate do not entirely explain their individual and collective failure to use to the maximum effect all the available economizing tools, to develop new tools, to test the limits of the law by innovative contracting, and to advocate legal reform wherever it is necessary to untie their hands. Moreover, if what the industry says is true, then private health plans serve hardly any purpose other than to execute decisions that are made by central authorities. If private plans have no appreciable room for maneuver and are unlikely to get such room—that is, they cannot legally or practically offer consumers meaningful choice—then it is hard to see why, as a policy matter, we need them at all.

To the extent that private financing plans lack (or are barred by law from using) the tools they need to offer a full range of reasonable choices to consumers, they should be aggressively developing new tools and advocating creation of a legal regime in which to use them. But one does not hear the private insurance industry expressing any interest in assuming new responsibilities. On the contrary, health insurers expressly advocate the creation of a single authoritative point of reference on each question arising in medical practice so that all can underwrite precisely the same services—instead of competing to design coverage attractive to differently situated groups. Thus, the HIAA has expressed a desire for "a mechanism . . . to grant certification of medical efficacy and cost-effectiveness to newly developed procedures, technologies and equipment before they become part of common medical practice" (HIAA 1990, xiv). Similarly, health insurers are eager for authoritative practice guidelines developed "with the participation of the physician community . . . by nongovernmental agencies" (HIAA 1990, xiii-xiv). Far from seeking to assist consumers in deciding precisely what services to buy (and not to buy) from the health care industry, health insurers strongly prefer that someone else provide definitive prescriptions. Private health insurers thus appear to be straying from, rather than living up to, their raison d'être. Likewise, the HMO component of the private financing industry, although perhaps offering some de facto relief from central control, is not advertising a willingness to depart from authoritative standards promulgated by higher authority.

The Debatable Wisdom of Joining What One Cannot Fight. In defining themselves only as executors of clinical policies set by others, private health plans may have been making a virtue of necessity. There is little doubt that taking any other stance would violate the dominant paradigm of medical decision making and invite criticism, misunderstanding, and perhaps litigation challenging the insurer's right to make "medical" judgments. Yet precisely this paradigm of medical care must be challenged if runaway health care costs are to be brought under appropriate control, whether by the private sector or by government.

The medical profession's preferred paradigm of the medical care enterprise originates in a deep-seated belief that medical care is not a commodity like other consumer goods and services. Under the paradigm the characteristics of medical care are a scientific and professional matter, to be determined with no more than cursory regard to cost considerations (Havighurst 1990b). Accordingly, all important decisions concerning medical care are entrusted exclusively to professionals who are accountable only to the medical profession itself or to standards of its making. This paradigm implies a distinctly passive role for health insurers. Historically, this passivity was reflected in the practices of the original provider-sponsored insurance plans (the Blues) and enforced by professional hostility to any independent cost-containment initiatives by insurers (Goldberg and Greenberg 1977; Havighurst 1978). It was also embodied in regulatory limits on the freedom of health insurers to act as consumer agents in selecting providers or to assume what were deemed to be professional functions. Because the paradigm implies that a payer's role is only to ensure that professional norms are followed, a payer has little room to resist paying for care unless it is demonstrably useless or harmful. Under the paradigm any independent health plan or other consumer agent that seeks to fight the cost-containment battle in the treacherous no man's land of quality/cost trade-offs runs grave legal and business risks.[14]

The professional paradigm of medical care derives strength from both the scientific pretensions of medicine and the ethical and egalitarian belief that the standard of medical care ought not to vary according to ability to pay. These twin pillars of the paradigm make it relatively easy for the medical profession to assert its authority over the definition of standards and to block actions premised on the alternative view that medical care can be treated as a consumer good and purchased in greater or lesser quantities according to the preferences of purchasers and the availability of resources. Even though government reduces the potential for inequality to some extent by subsidizing the purchasing power of lower-income persons (and could do more), the idea that health care might safely be made an appropriate object of consumer economizing has simply not taken hold. Because of the way the paradigm works, people can be ostensibly free to purchase coverage in a competitive market while lacking real freedom because of constraints operating on their purchasing agents.

Private health insurers, finding it too difficult to fight the professional-scientific-egalitarian paradigm of medical care, have apparently elected to go along with it. Indeed, nothing indicates that they aspire to survive as anything other than cogs in an essentially monolithic health care system—executors of decisions made, not by the customers whom they serve, but by whatever powers may be. To be sure, HMOs have challenged the paradigm to the extent of offering alternative delivery and financing arrangements and, in some cases, alternative styles of medical practice. But HMOs have generally positioned themselves close to their more traditional competitors both in price and otherwise. Certainly, they have not undertaken to define contractually any substitute for their legal obligation to adhere to professional norms and standards in medical practice.

In disavowing any creative independence and offering the public only variations on themes originated by the medical profession, private health plans are undercutting the policy justification for their own survival. Indeed, instead of offering the public the benefit of decentral-

---

14. For a graphic illustration of the no man's land in which the benefit curve still slopes upward but at a lesser rate than the cost curve, see Havighurst and Blumstein (1975, 16–20).

ized decision making and choice regarding medical care, they are giving the nation the worst of both worlds: mostly centralized decisions implemented at unnecessarily high administrative cost (see note 7). If private health plans serve little purpose in preserving meaningful pluralism and facilitating consumer choice, it may be wiser simply to acknowledge that centralized decision making is here to stay and to appoint a single payer to make and administer decisions for us all. It would be a pity if private health care financing were to survive only because of political factors and not because of its ability to offer consumers responsible alternatives to the professional paradigm of medical care.

Putting a Better Foot Forward

Let me now suggest how proponents of private health care financing could most convincingly justify its continued prominence in the U.S. health care system. Because the historical record is not reassuring about the ability of private health plans to fight cost battles where cost curves slope upward faster than benefit curves, the policy argument for their survival must emphasize, not their past accomplishments, but their long-range potential as implementers of consumers' economizing choices.[15] The prospect that private health plans will eventually engage the real enemies of consumer-inspired cost containment is brightened somewhat by the progress they have already made toward assuming independent functions and responsibilities in organizing health care and in bargaining with providers. Beginning their innovative efforts only in the 1980s,[16] private financing intermediaries have pioneered in the area

---

15. For an article raising serious questions about the ability of government to control costs in the crucial area where the benefits curve is not flat and suggesting that the private sector might have a comparative advantage, see Havighurst and Blumstein (1975). This chapter explores what the private sector has yet to do to realize its potential in this regard. If the private sector refuses to pick up the ball and a single-payer strategy is adopted, the earlier article shows why it may be wiser not to create an open-ended entitlement program, such as Medicare, but to assign the government purchaser a fixed budget within which to live. Only if government must make either-or rather than yes-no choices will it be able to economize in the face of powerful claims that beneficial services are being unfairly or inappropriately denied to individuals.

16. Before 1980 the private sector tended to rely on government to control the cost of health care through various regulatory measures, existing or prospective. Only when Congress rejected the Carter administration's ambitious hospital cost-control bill in 1979 did responsibility for private health care costs shift decisively to private purchasers. As the Reagan administration concerned itself exclusively with the cost for federal programs in the early 1980s, the private

of managed care and have been increasingly able, as bulk purchasers, to obtain lower prices from some providers. If private payers can demonstrate that they have exhausted neither their energies nor the possibilities for innovation in responsible cost containment, they may reasonably expect to survive in a reformed health care system.

Private health plans have been inhibited in performing their essential function of offering consumers a full range of benefit/cost options by some circumstances that are not of their own making. Certain of the most substantial constraints operating on them have rarely been identified as critical problems, however, either in the industry itself or in national health policy. Nevertheless, once they are identified, these constraints could be effectively contested in practice, in the courts, and in the legislatures. Private health plans, instead of seeking merely to secure their place in the monolithic health care system of the future, should be actively advocating pluralism, testing the limits of their competitive freedom, and, where necessary, seeking legal reforms to maximize their effectiveness as consumers' agents in freely purchasing health services. Indeed, if they refuse to adopt this agenda for completing the market-oriented reforms of the 1980s, there is every reason why their future should be placed in jeopardy.

The Limited Utility of Private Contract. The primary barrier preventing consumers from being offered a full range of health care options is the limited utility of private contracts as instruments for legitimizing innovation and for specifying rules to govern particular consumer-provider-payer relationships. As things stand in the health care sector, vital terms of such relationships are prescribed, not by the parties themselves, but by the courts, borrowing standards wherever necessary from the medical profession. Such as they are, the contracts that cover the financing and delivery of health services uniformly embody, implicitly or explicitly, the premise that professional norms and standards must be consulted to resolve any disputes. Rarely, if ever, do such contracts attempt to define any alternative standards. The reasons why contracts take this form are complex but need to be understood in assessing the full potential of private financing. If private contracts are incapable of carrying the load of private reform, then public reforms carried out by a single government-sponsored payer may be the only plausible alternative for American health care.

The limited role of private contracts in defining the appropriateness and scope of medical services is explainable in part by the professional

---

sector took an impressive series of initiatives—stopping short, however, of the even more radical measures recommended in this chapter.

paradigm of medical decision making. Historically, the paradigm dictated noninterference with the doctor-patient relationship and the patient's free choice of provider, foreclosing any role for payers in influencing treatment choices or in bargaining with providers on the consumer's behalf. Financing plans that threatened to act as the consumer's agent in selecting or controlling physicians—undertaking, that is, to replace what Charles Weller (1984) has called "guild free choice" with "market free choice"—faced severe repercussions in the form of provider boycotts (Goldberg and Greenberg 1977). In addition, the professional paradigm was embodied in legal rules proscribing the corporate practice of medicine and other forms of intermediation and in ethical prohibitions against physicians' engaging in contract practice or otherwise submitting to lay interference. Under the paradigm a deep-seated tradition of entrusting all medical decisions to professionals grew up. This tradition was embodied in a range of conventional expectations and assumptions that, with or without statutory recognition, permeated legal doctrine. Because of the legal and other risks created for those who might attempt to write their own rules, innovation in the procurement of medical services was directed into narrow, legally authorized channels, particularly the development of HMOs, in which more efficient styles of medical practice could evolve to a limited extent without explicit contractual authority.

Although private health plans clearly would not have progressed much in contractually specifying alternative standards of medical practice in the face of the medical paradigm, an even more fundamental problem prevented medical standards from being established contractually. As a purely practical matter, writing an insurance policy or health plan that effectively specifies the services that the plan will pay for (and that participating providers will be minimally obligated to provide) is an extraordinarily difficult undertaking. Each contract would have to be the equivalent of a medical textbook with rules to govern virtually every medical exigency. Moreover, its specifications would have to be adapted specially to reflect the wishes and resources of the particular group of consumers being served. In light of the high transaction costs of developing and implementing such contractual specifications, it was both logical and efficient for draftsmen to adopt the professional standard of care as the explicit or implicit touchstone for determining obligations.[17]

Because adopting professional norms and standards as the point of reference in private contracts may have been a rational and efficient response to the high transaction costs of doing otherwise, the convention

---

17. For the view that contract failure accounts for widespread reliance on professional standards, see Epstein (1986, 207) and Havighurst (1986a, 266–72).

of relying exclusively on professional standards might have emerged even if the professional paradigm had not been embodied in law and enforced by a physician cartel. But partly because no one saw fit to challenge professional standards, significant legal obstacles to the private specification of standards of care did develop and now impede any effort to retract the earlier delegation of decision-making authority and to reassert consumer sovereignty and freedom of contract. Indeed, the powers that originally devolved upon the legal system and the medical profession by default are now so firmly entrenched in legal thinking that most people cannot imagine a return to a contractual regime. Yet, as a result of the unconstrained growth of medical technology and the dramatically increased cost of state-of-the-art medical care, the cost of adhering to the old convention is much higher than ever before, and private health plans might reasonably wish to rethink their original policy of going along with medical standards instead of writing their own. It is highly regrettable that the legal system has so thoroughly internalized the professional paradigm and assumed such far-reaching prescriptive powers that the option of returning to a contract-oriented regime is widely discounted as a practical possibility.

Possessing both de facto and de jure authority to define, in the last analysis, the scope of the most crucial provider and payer obligations, the legal system now constitutes a significant, though generally unrecognized, regulatory regime governing the provision of health services. Even though this regulatory regime is not statutory and is administered by judges and juries, it does not differ from other forms of regulation in restricting consumer choice. Under it, private financing plans find themselves effectively bound to underwrite any care that meets the law's requirements and barred from specifying a different set of payment obligations by contract. Likewise, because providers of care must measure up to the law's standards, they do not have the option of agreeing with their patients to be bound by a different set of expectations. Because deviations from professional standards are so effectively precluded by law and circumstance, Americans are forced either to purchase first-class, state-of-the-art, Cadillac-style medical care or to forgo health coverage altogether. With such regulation in place, it should be no surprise that so many persons have had to forgo coverage. By the same token, if health plans were free to specify alternative rights and obligations, many more Americans would be able (especially with new public subsidies to enhance their purchasing power) to purchase acceptable coverage.[18]

---

18. The idea that all citizens must have equal access to all medical care was rejected as an ethical proposition (in favor of a societal obligation to ensure at

Judicial overregulation of health care is most apparent in medical malpractice litigation. In malpractice cases the legal system regularly gives professional norms and standards—even ill-defined and poorly conceived ones—the force of public regulations. One objection to such norms and standards is that because they are rarely written down, they provide a poor guide for physician practice. This vagueness of professional standards in turn induces the widespread practice of defensive medicine, as physicians, in an effort to avoid entanglement with a seemingly arbitrary legal system, err consistently on the side of spending too much rather than too little. Moreover, judicial enforcement of customary standards of medical practice inevitably fosters inappropriate spending because the market in which such standards emerge is severely distorted by defensive medicine and third-party payment. In various ways, therefore, malpractice law compels or induces a style of medical practice that is far costlier than many Americans would purchase if they had a choice.[19]

Judicial regulation of the health care industry under the medical profession's norms and standards also occurs in lawsuits brought by patients or providers to challenge refusals by health insurers to pay for questionable services. Judges can frequently find a legal warrant for prescribing private obligations in contract language that commits a payer to cover all care that is "medically necessary" (or the equivalent). Health insurance policies also typically exclude "experimental" treatments, causing frequent disputes over whether costly new technologies have achieved professional acceptance. Such contract provisions obviously reflect the difficulty that payers have in specifying more precise limitations. Yet courts, ignoring the draftsman's problem, typically construe such contracts liberally (that is, against the insurer), thus overriding payers' attempts to limit their obligations so that they can charge lower premiums. Moreover, just as they do in judging medical malpractice, courts naturally look to professional standards to determine what must be paid for. Because cases of this kind pit a sick patient against a corporate deep pocket, payers have good reason to fear an adverse outcome, possibly accompanied by punitive damages. As a result, they

---

least adequate care for everyone) by a presidential commission in the early 1980s (President's Commission 1983).

19. It is ironic that physicians have come to hate the tort system so much. After all, in drawing its standards from customary medical practice, the law embodies, at least in principle, the medical profession's own paradigmatic belief about where legal standards should be found. In addition, physicians benefit from the paradigm-linked presumption that payers must pay for any measure, however costly, that the law arguably requires practitioners to take.

are unable to be aggressive in implementing, ex post, any economizing provisions in contracts that were in the general interest, ex ante, of the insured group and perhaps also of the plaintiff.

Although the idea of letting providers or payers depart from professional standards will strike many as unthinkable, such standards are rarely satisfactory as regulatory rules governing all medical care. Not only are most professional standards imprecise, being implicit in variable medical practice (Wennberg 1984) and discernible only after the fact through the testimony of partisan medical experts, but many common professional practices have shaky scientific foundations (Eddy and Billings 1988). Under a legal regime dedicated to enforcing such standards, even responsible economizing is hazardous to both the plan and the provider. Moreover, the law gives physicians good excuses for practicing defensively and for incurring high costs, perhaps far beyond what courts would actually require. If an insurer's challenge to a questionable physician practice might end up being evaluated in court under ill-defined or dubious professional norms, the legal risk and cost of pursuing the effort to economize might easily be too great.

One possible solution to these defects in the dominant regulatory regime might be to improve the quality of professional standards and to make them clearer and more accessible to physicians, to payers, and to courts. Responding in part to the lack of clear, validated standards of medical practice, professional organizations of physicians have recently launched a promising movement to create "practice guidelines" (Havighurst 1990a). By spelling out appropriate measures for diagnosing and treating various conditions, such guidelines could greatly improve the quality of regulation of medical practice by malpractice courts (Havighurst 1991). Health insurers and government have high hopes that practice guidelines will soon provide them with objective, uniform standards for making payment decisions.

But making professional standards clearer and more scientific will not necessarily make them suitable for every purchaser. Just as customary practice rarely reflects anyone's careful comparison of benefits and costs, professional organizations engaged in setting explicit practice standards have no reason to give cost considerations appreciable weight. Indeed, physicians regularly assert ethical reasons for not taking costs into account in either treatment decisions or standard setting. A real danger, therefore, is the further standardization of medical care by practice guidelines developed by professional organizations when greater flexibility and contractual freedom are necessary to permit responsible economizing. At best, the profession's guidelines may not actively foreclose economizing measures that physicians and health plans might take independently. Although professional groups will prefer guidelines that preserve practitioners' clinical freedom, such guidelines will be of little affirmative use to insurers and will effectively block any economizing measures that physicians do not collectively find acceptable.

Normally, a purchaser specifies by contract the characteristics of goods or services being purchased. In the health care sector at the moment, however, the legal system, operating in conjunction with the medical profession, bears the primary responsibility for defining the scope and quality of the services that must be provided, with contracts performing only limited functions. With the legal system defining most patient entitlements, consumers and their agents lack effective means to authorize providers to omit any services, however doubtful their value, that professional standards seem to mandate. Most lawyers would doubt the receptiveness of courts to any contract that purported either to alter the legal standard applicable to providers or to relieve an insurer of the obligation to pay for all care that a physician reasonably prescribes. Thus, careful and responsible efforts to customize provider and payer obligations are deterred by the risk that courts would not respect them. Payers can accept this state of affairs as a *fait accompli,* or they can protest against it in the hope of giving the private financing industry, at long last, a chance to live up to its raison d'être. Change is unlikely, however, if private health plans will not take up the cause as their last best hope for ensuring their own survival.

Although this chapter focuses on private arrangements, the legal system also dictates many of the payment obligations of public financing programs, such as Medicaid. Again, the payer's general obligation is to cover everything falling within the bounds of accepted medical practice. If the private sector, using innovative private contracts, can make headway against such professional norms and standards despite the professional paradigm, perhaps the public sector can follow its lead. In a more likely scenario, however, private payers will have to learn from public initiatives such as one under way in Oregon that is seeking to prioritize medical care, to put intelligent limits on what will be paid for, and to extend legal protection to providers who abide by the new rules (Fox and Leichter 1991). More than anything else on the horizon, the Oregon experiment represents a serious effort to set alternative standards to guide provider performance and to put scarce resources to their most beneficial uses. It is time for private health plans to begin to respond to that challenge as a service to their customers—or face extinction.

New Ways of Specifying Patient Entitlements. Despite the legal system's current hostility to economizing that departs in any way from standards developed or espoused by physicians, private health plans might still avoid having the courts finally specify their participating providers' obligations to patients. If explicit language articulating alternative rights could be incorporated in a series of contracts binding patients, the payer, and providers of covered services, courts would have to take those contracts seriously. Despite questions concerning the enforceability of clauses that seem to deny patients the benefit of state-of-the-art medical care, care in drafting, marketing, and administration would improve the prospect that a court could be persuaded to accept the parties' economizing choice. The court would probably have to be satisfied that the economizing move was initiated in the interest of the consumers and was carefully explained at the outset. But if the economizing initiative were well conceived and implemented, courts might well approve it. The legal barrier, therefore, may not be insurmountable.

Private health plans still have far to go, however, in discovering practical and effective ways to specify in advance precisely what their customers want to purchase from health care providers. Indeed, innovation of this kind has only just begun. One type of contractual reform that has been pursued involves authorizing utilization managers to second-guess physician judgments during pretreatment review. As noted, however, contracts providing for utilization management apparently have not articulated any alternative to the professional standard of care that presumably governs the actions of case managers and any dispute that may arise. The conservatism reflected in these generally beneficial reforms effectively proves the limitations of the private contract as a vehicle for widening consumer choice.

Another area of only limited innovation is the modification of legal rights of plan subscribers in the event of medical malpractice. Numerous private health plans maintain a contractual requirement that subscribers submit any malpractice claims to arbitration; few, if any, however, have adopted suggestions by academics that they consider contractual changes also in the substantive tort rights of their subscribers in order to attract physicians to the plan on favorable terms and to reduce the pressure on physicians to practice defensively.[20] Accepting a cutback in their tort rights could well be in the financial interest of plan subscribers, given the high cost of the limited financial protection that tort law gives consumers. Although lawyers tend to doubt that tort doctrine can or should be altered by private agreement, in the right circumstances a court

---

20. See generally "Medical Malpractice" (1986, 143–320). The basic idea is simply that health plans might implement voluntarily, by contract, some of the reforms that some states have implemented by mandatory legislation. See Havighurst (1986b).

might be persuaded to relax its regulatory grip and to enforce a contract affecting tort rights as written. Just as the medical profession should not be the final arbiter of the standards of medical care, the legal system's prescriptions of patients' legal rights should yield to consumer choice, reasonably exercised.

Even further from payers' thinking than these reforms at the moment is the idea of rewriting the substantive standard of care applicable to physicians treating plan subscribers. How this might be done is not obvious. A few years ago, however, I proposed the following contract clause for possible use by HMOs concerned about being held to inefficient standards of care in future malpractice suits:

The Duty of the Plan's Physicians to You
The Plan warrants that each of its physicians possesses at least the skill and knowledge of a reasonably competent medical practitioner in his or her specialty and undertakes to you that its physicians will exercise that skill and knowledge in a reasonable and prudent manner in your case. In so doing, a Plan physician may sometimes depart from practices customary among other physicians. Such departures shall not be deemed to breach the foregoing undertaking, however, unless they are expressly found to have been unreasonable and imprudent; evidence to support such a finding shall include the testimony of experts knowledgeable about practices customary among physicians in other organized health plans in which physicians are not compensated on a fee-for-service basis. In instances where the Plan has consulted with the Members' Advisory Panel concerning a particular practice or method of diagnosis or treatment and obtained the Panel's approval of a particular clinical policy, adherence by the Plan's physicians to that policy shall not be deemed unreasonable and imprudent unless such approval was obtained by misrepresentation or unless changes in medical knowledge between the time such approval was obtained and the time you were treated indicate that continued adherence to such policy was unreasonable and imprudent. You agree that the undertaking in this paragraph fully defines the duties of the Plan and its physicians to you. (Havighurst 1986a, 271–72)

Although several lawyers expressed interest in this contract language, no health plan has attempted anything comparable.

Other contractual reforms of the substantive standard governing physician liability are potentially available. A particularly radical proposal, which is more defensible than it might seem, would bar malpractice claims against plan providers for anything short of gross negligence, suitably defined (Havighurst 1986a, 272–75). An altogether different approach would be provision, as a contractual substitute for subscribers' tort rights, of automatic compensation on a no-fault basis for designated injuries, thus ensuring that more of the funds dedicated to redressing patient injuries would in fact go for that purpose and not into fault finding and litigation (see, for example, Tancredi and Bovbjerg 1991). Although each of the private reforms of tort doctrine proposed here might seem to benefit physicians more than plan subscribers, something of the sort is necessary to allow economizing to proceed on any legal basis other than strict liability. Any effort to reduce health plan premiums that entails possible departures from accepted medical practice must include some legal protection, through contractual modifications of ordinary tort rights, for cooperating providers.

A more direct contractual cost-containment strategy for private health plans would involve specifying not just a different general standard of care for tort law purposes but the actual services that the payer undertakes to pay for and that providers undertake to provide to plan subscribers in particular medical circumstances. Although this strategy has theoretical appeal as the way to give consumers the greatest collective discretion in purchasing health services, the problem of transaction costs would remain. A dramatic—indeed a revolutionary—breakthrough may emerge from the recent movement to develop practice guidelines, however. Depending upon how it evolves, this movement could yield a new technology that allows consumers to exercise critical control over how their health care dollars are spent. Practice guidelines could thus prove—if payers seize the opportunity presented—to be the salvation of private health care financing in the United States. Indeed, the private financing industry could make the strongest case for its own survival by advocating and actively participating in the development of practice guidelines as new tools for consumers and health plans in choosing health services.

The chief obstacle to realizing the promise of practice guidelines in making and implementing consumer choices is, once again, the professional paradigm of medical decision making. The developing guidelines movement is widely expected to yield only a single set of professionally approved new standards. Such authoritative guidelines would then be employed as regulatory standards in administering malpractice law and in determining the legal obligations of private and public financing plans. The health insurance industry itself, in keeping with its acceptance of the medical paradigm, has welcomed the development of guidelines in just this spirit—as new rules that will provide an objective point of reference for utilization management. Regrettably, health insurers have yet to identify the potential value of practice guidelines as new contractual tools with which to modify consumer-provider-payer relationships in accordance with consumer preferences. Once again, the industry has eschewed any meaningful role in helping consumers write their own tickets in purchasing medical care, leaving them still at the mercy of regulatory standards developed by the medical profession. If private payers refuse to accept the challenge of customizing coverage to suit the pocketbooks of their customers, their utility in the health care system of the future should be questioned.

An alternative scenario, however, is quite plausible. The guidelines movement might easily fail to yield definitive sets of authoritative rules and produce instead overlapping, alternative guidelines emanating from a variety of sources, not all of them authoritative professional bodies speaking for medical interests alone. Some guidelines might be produced by private health plans themselves, particularly HMOs—perhaps by making relatively modest modifications of guidelines produced by professional organizations. Whereas professional bodies seem inclined to write guidelines that set only upper and lower boundaries—"parameters" is the American Medical Association's preferred name for practice guidelines—of acceptable care, guidelines produced by individual health plans or other expert bodies might be, not general standards suitable for governing all care, but relatively precise prescriptions suitable for defining the entitlements of particular insured groups. If such alternative, competing guidelines materialize, consumers and their agents will have for the first time a practical means of specifying in advance the services that they do and do not wish to purchase from providers on a prepaid basis. And the private financing industry will have a whole new raison d'être—something it badly needs if it is to claim a legitimate role in the future health care system.

If practice guidelines develop pluralistically, the parties to particular private health plans will find it increasingly feasible to escape regulation under professional norms and to create their own legal environment by incorporating selected practice guidelines in their contracts. To minimize confusion and to assist consumers and their agents in relying on guidelines generated from a variety of unofficial sources, government and private organizations could establish certification programs to identify those guidelines that meet minimum standards—for objectivity, scientific grounding, disclosure of their underlying rationales, and so forth.[21] With such certification conferring legitimacy on economizing moves reflected in the guidelines, courts would be more likely to enforce

---

21. See Havighurst (1990a, 804–19) (arguing that the federal Agency for Health Care Policy and Research should assume such a certifying function under existing legislation).

the agreed limits when disputes arose. An innovative malpractice reform bill pending in Congress (S. 1232, the Medical Injury Compensation Fairness Act of 1991, introduced by Senator Pete V. Domenici) already contemplates that private health plans might adopt practice guidelines, selected from those certified by the federal government, as contractual standards governing provider liability (Havighurst and Metzloff 1991).

Certainly, many difficulties must be overcome before health care choices can be effectively decentralized and deregulated. Nevertheless, private contracts incorporating practice guidelines should ultimately be able to structure health plans that economize sensitively and according to patients' essential needs. Whereas many current economizing efforts merely shift costs to insured patients or exclude certain services categorically, practice guidelines incorporated in health care plans could make such plans efficiently selective in the many gray areas of medical practice. Indeed, once guidelines are developed with appropriate care and in appropriate detail, they could implement a relatively consistent plan policy toward risk and cost across the entire range of beneficiaries' medical needs. They could thus provide not only well-conceived specific standards but also reference points for interpolating standards to govern in situations that the guidelines did not fully anticipate. Contracts also should spell out a process for utilization managers, in cooperation with physicians, to apply the guidelines in particular cases. Well-designed procedures would go far toward legitimizing economizing decisions affecting the treatment of individual patients.

The suggestion that all future medical exigencies could be antici-pated and provided for in practice guidelines incorporated in binding patient contracts may strike some people as unrealistic. And certainly, as a practical matter, guidelines could never provide for every eventu-ality and should not be relied upon slavishly in the face of inevitable uncertainty and technological change. But real-world relationships should be amenable to explicit restructuring through new, administrable mechanisms for coping with cost issues. Contracts of the kind known in law and economics as relational contracts, instead of rigidly defining and anticipating every detail of the parties' future relationship, supply a basic structure that can accommodate unpredictable events and facilitate adaptations that further the parties' mutual long-term purposes. Private efforts must be made, with government support, to design contractual relationships of this character, acknowledging that medical progress and other exigencies can never be fully anticipated by contractual language. I hope that representatives of the private financing industry, instead of merely calling impractical and unrealistic the strategies I have proposed for private health plans, will work toward making private contracts truly useful vehicles for implementing a full range of consumer choices. If private payers are unwilling to challenge the legal and practical obstacles that prevent them from realizing their raison d'être, the question remains: Who needs them?

Conclusion

At an AEI conference in January 1983, I warned of the dangers of pursuing a market-oriented national health policy without addressing the limitations of private contract:

> One way in which market advocates could go wrong . . . is by assuming too readily that interacting private parties and institutions would be free and uninhibited in their competitive efforts to translate consumer cost concerns into economizing behavior by providers. In fact, many efficiency-dictated reductions in the quantity, quality, and cost of inputs, in utilization levels, and in insurance coverage for marginally beneficial services are quite possibly now inhibited by much more than just the system's weak cost-consciousness. . . .
>
> . . . The specific concern is the flexibility of private contract and its utility as a vehicle for introducing new standards in the health care industry. Doctrines of private law—the law of torts and contracts—may impose on private parties duties that are inconsistent with both efficiency and the parties' contractually specified obligations. . . . [T]here is . . . a serious question whether enough freedom of contract prevails to allow competition to bring about in fact all of the reforms in health care financing and delivery that competition theorists expect it to yield. (Havighurst 1983, 22–23)

As I feared, health policy in the 1980s proceeded with an inadequate awareness of the degree to which the courts, in administering the law of medical malpractice and interpreting insurance and other contracts, effectively regulate the delivery of medical care according to rules supplied, one way or another, by practicing physicians.

This regulatory regime, which effectively forecloses consumers from writing their own specifications of what they wish to purchase from health care providers, should be ignored no longer. As long as private health plans lack the freedom to record and to execute their customers' collective wishes and to enter into binding agreements on their behalf with health care providers, they may serve too little useful purpose to justify preserving them in their present role—in view of the high administrative costs they necessarily entail and the impediments they necessarily present to efforts to ensure access to care for all citizens. The practical limitations of private contracts in the health care sector thus bear on the fundamental choice that the nation must make between a market-oriented and a government-dominated health care system. At issue, ultimately, is the freedom of individuals, acting through insured groups, to decide for themselves how much of their resources to invest (perhaps with matching government subsidies) in extraordinarily expensive medical services of sometimes debatable benefit. If these intensely personal, sometimes life-and-death decisions are to be made by a central authority and not by citizens making their own choices, then it may be better to put representative government explicitly in charge and not to rely any longer on undemocratic institutions—the courts and the medical profession—to act on our behalf.

I have argued in this chapter that firms engaged in the business of privately financing health care can make a plausible case for their own survival only by challenging—both in the policy debate and in their day-to-day business of writing and administering contracts to finance health services—the practical and legal obstacles that impede the use of private contracts to express consumer choices in purchasing health care.[22] The challenge I have issued to private health insurers and other health plans is primarily calculated to inspire them to identify and to live up to their raison d'être. But if they fail to respond to this challenge, there is little reason not to let them pass from the health care scene.

References

Blumstein, J. "Constitutional Perspectives on Government Decisions Affecting Human Life and Health." *Law and Contemporary Problems* 40 (Autumn 1976): 233–301.
Bovbjerg, R. "The Medical Malpractice Standard of Care: HMOs and Customary Practice." *Duke Law Journal* 1975: 1375–1414.
Eddy, D., and J. Billings. "The Quality of Medical Evidence: Implications for the Quality of Care." *Health Affairs* 7 (Spring 1988): 19–32.
Epstein, R. "Medical Malpractice, Imperfect Information, and the Con-

---

22. I might also have argued that the private financing industry should be expected to lobby actively on behalf of a major limitation of the federal tax subsidy for employer-purchased health coverage to ensure that consumers will not overinsure but will instead seek an optimal mix of financial protection, self-insurance, and cost-containment services. This might, however, be asking too much of the industry. After all, we allow the residential housing industry to operate on a competitive basis even though the allocation of resources to that sector is heavily subsidized through the tax system. In any event, I have focused instead on obstacles to consumer choice that the industry could reasonably hope to overcome if it tried and that no one else is likely to challenge.

tractual Foundation of Medical Services." *Law and Contemporary Problems* 49 (Spring 1986): 201–12.

Fox, D., and H. Leichter. "Rationing Health Care in Oregon: The New Accountability." *Health Affairs* 10 (Summer 1991): 7–27.

Goldberg, L., and W. Greenberg. "The Effects of Physician-Controlled Health Insurance: U.S. v. Oregon State Medical Society." *Journal of Health Politics, Policy and Law* 2 (1977): 48–78.

Havighurst, C. "Professional Restraints on Innovation in Health Care Financing." *Duke Law Journal* 1978: 303–87.

———. 1983. "Decentralizing Decision Making: Private Contract versus Professional Norms." In *Market Reforms in Health Care*, edited by J. Meyer, 22–45. Washington, D.C.: AEI Press, 1983.

———. "Altering the Applicable Standard of Care." *Law and Contemporary Problems* 49 (Spring 1986a): 265–76.

———. "Private Reform of Tort-Law Dogma: Market Opportunities and Legal Obstacles." *Law and Contemporary Problems* 49 (Spring 1986b): 143–72.

———. "The Questionable Cost-Containment Record of Commercial Health Insurers." In *Health Care in America: The Political Economy of Hospitals and Health Insurance*, edited by H. Frech, 221–58. San Francisco: Pacific Research Institute for Public Policy, 1988.

———. "Practice Guidelines for Medical Care: The Policy Rationale." *St. Louis Law Journal* 34 (1990a): 777–819.

———. "The Professional Paradigm of Medical Care: Obstacle to Decentralization." *Jurimetrics Journal* 30 (1990b): 415–29.

———. "Practice Guidelines as Legal Standards Governing Physician Liability." *Law and Contemporary Problems* 54 (Spring 1991): 87–118.

———, and J. Blumstein. "Coping with Quality/Cost Trade-offs in Medical Care: The Case of Professional Standards Review Organizations." *Northwestern University Law Review* 70 (1975): 6–68.

———, and T. Metzloff. "S.1232—A Late Entry in the Race for Malpractice Reform." *Law and Contemporary Problems* 54 (Spring 1991): 179–98.

Health Insurance Association of America. *The Health Insurance Industry Strategy for Containing Health Care Costs*. Report of the Board of Directors. Washington, D.C.: HIAA, 1990.

———. *Health Care Financing for all Americans: Private Market Reform and Public Responsibility*. Washington, D.C.: HIAA, 1991.

Joskow, P. *Controlling Hospital Costs: The Role of Government Regulation*. Cambridge: MIT Press, 1981.

Kinney, E. "The Medicare Appeals System for Coverage and Payment Disputes." In *1986 Recommendations and Reports*, ed. by Administrative Conference of the United States. Washington, D.C.: Government Printing Office, 1986.

"Medical Malpractice: Can the Private Sector Find Relief?" *Law and Contemporary Problems* 49 (Spring 1986): 1–348.

President's Commission for the Study of Ethical Problems in Medicine and Biomedical and Behavioral Research. *Securing Access to Health Care*. Washington, D.C.: Government Printing Office, 1983.

Tancredi, L., and R. Bovbjerg. "Rethinking Responsibility for Patient Injury: Accelerated-compensation Events, a Malpractice and Quality Reform Ripe for a Test." *Law and Contemporary Problems* 54 (Spring 1991): 147–78.

U.S. Congress, House. *Health Care Cost and Access: Hearing before the House Committee on the Budget*. 102d Congress, 1st session, June 19, 1991.

U.S. General Accounting Office. *Canadian Health Insurance: Lessons for the United States*. Washington, D.C.: Government Printing Office, 1991.

Weller, C. "'Free Choice' as a Restraint of Trade in American Health Care Delivery and Insurance." *Iowa Law Review* 69 (1984): 1351–92.

Wennberg, J. "Dealing with Medical Practice Variation: A Proposal for Action." *Health Affairs* 3 (Summer 1984): 6–32.

Wilson v. Blue Cross of Southern California. 271 Cal. Rptr. 876 (Cal. App. 2d Dist.), 1990.

Woolhandler, S., and D. Himmelstein. "The Deteriorating Administrative Efficiency of the U.S. Health Care System." *New England Journal of Medicine* 324 (1991): 1253–58.

Commentary on Part One

Stanley B. Jones

Recently I watched a CNN special documentary on East Germany that focused on that nation's automobile, the Trabi. Except for some additional plastic in place of steel, this automobile is the same as it was thirty-two years ago. The engine and chassis have not changed. When the reporter asked Trabi management representatives why, they replied, "There are plenty of people who want to buy it as it is, so why change it?" The CNN commentator observed that this shows a basically mismanaged and distorted marketplace.

My thoughts went to the U.S. health insurance industry. I do not think the engine and chassis have changed for thirty years or so. It has remained a transaction-based industry.

What do I mean by that? In the industry, we process pieces of paper that bill us for health care services to individuals. We process billions of individual transactions. It is essentially the same process as in decades past.

Pressures on insurers from the market and from policy makers to influence how doctors and hospitals organize and provide health care have led the industry to develop "managed care." This is important. Insurers now concede that care and its costs need to be managed, and that the insurers have a major role.

In today's managed care, however, the vast majority of the effort involves processing pieces of paper, paper billing for individual transactions. What has been added is the questioning of these papers as they go by, to see whether they fit our rule-book definitions. We have become fancier and fancier in our computer capability to review these transactions, but it remains nevertheless a review of transactions as they go by.

Unfortunately we have not noticeably changed the way doctors and hospitals organize and provide care. Richard Kronick correctly observes that in most areas of the country the various insurers have formed Independent Practice Associations that sign up most of the same doctors, and then rely on review of their bills to "manage care"—the same old transaction-based approach. In fact we have succeeded more in annoying

116

and angering the hospitals and doctors than we have in bringing about any changes in organization or delivery of care.

It is not as if we do not know how to do better. When we started talking about marketplaces, multiple choice, and competition fifteen or twenty years ago we had one proven, successful model. It is not necessarily the only model, but it is one model: the staff- or group-model HMO. During the past several decades we have developed painfully few new staff- and group-model HMOs. Instead we have created managed-care activities that are more consistent with our transaction-based chassis and engine.

What is unusual and important about staff- and group-model HMOs is that they join the provider in mutual-risk situations and shared ventures, requiring them to work together to manage care. The industry has been slow to do this because it is a transaction-based industry, and it is difficult to change the engine and chassis.

How could this happen in America, with our free markets? It is one thing in East Germany to see a Trabi, but in America? Why are employers letting this happen? We hear a lot about employers' "buying smart" and "buying right" in health care, but in truth it is not happening. The chapters by Luft, Kronick, and Havighurst all acknowledge as much.

Recently I wrote a paper lamenting that employers are throwing out the HMO baby with the multiple-choice bathwater, as they get frustrated with the difficulties and complexity of managing multiple choice. I have heard many examples of how it could be worse. They could throw out the baby and keep the bathwater. Many employers are eliminating their staff- and group-model HMOs and returning to just one indemnity plan. Indemnity carriers are pushing employers to do this by threatening to refuse to offer traditional coverage unless the employer thins out the competition by getting rid of some of the HMOs.

I do not understand why employers are not smarter about this. There must be a profound economic reason. It may have something to do with markets other than insurance—such as labor markets, where the employer has to attract the employees he needs in order to do business successfully. This concern always comes out ahead of his concerns about health care and insurance. Health insurance seems to be number three on his priority list.

In any case, the employer's failure to buy smart propels policy makers to look for a better buyer—one that can change the insurance industry, push it off its transaction base, and make it a stronger manager of care. Intermediaries, as Harold Luft calls them, and purchasing corporations, as Richard Kronick calls them, make some sense in that regard. But there are some big questions, such as how to motivate insurers and employers.

117

If they are not motivated by billion-dollar-a-year price tags for health insurance, then what will motivate them to make the investment in staff and resources to do the job?

I have always thought motivation comes from money, power, or sex. Sex is out. Power? Perhaps power, if we make the purchaser a public agency and we elect the folks who oversee it. Money? If we make the purchaser private and put profits on the line, maybe we can motivate them that way. But it will take a lot of motivating—a lot of change.

G. Robert O'Brien

I feel somewhat like the hen in the henhouse with the foxes all around—so much to say and so little time to say it.

I believe the United States has the best medical system in the world, evidenced by our procedural outcomes and by the number of foreign people that come here for procedures for themselves or their families. I agree that the system needs to be changed. Things are different today from the way they were a decade ago, but the system does not have to be scrapped. The delivery system in the United States today is large and complex, and no one—even here in Washington—knows exactly what to do to correct and improve it. From the chapters in part one it is clear why it has been difficult to reach a consensus on what should be done. We all agree we have two fundamental issues to grapple with: cost and access.

On access, one hears people talking—especially in the insurance industry—about the need for small-case reform. It is more than words. Some fundamental changes have to be made so that we aggressively pursue that business. The government has to finance more of the poor who are or should be entitled to Medicaid. We need to work through a public-private partnership, to handle individuals covered neither through Medicaid nor through employer-provided insurance.

On the cost side many things have to be done. Basically we have to change behavior. We have to override or eliminate many of the state-mandated benefits that add 15 to 20 percent of the cost to these programs across the country. Individuals need to be better consumers and better decision makers with regard to health. We should not rely entirely on the medical delivery system to make our choices.

We must establish high-risk pools for individuals with severe medical problems. They should not fall through the cracks of the system. A safety net should catch them. As Clark Havighurst indicates in chapter five, we have to do something with medical malpractice reform. It is becoming too expensive for the system.

We have to take aggressive action to prevent the enactment of anti–managed-care legislation on the part of various states. They are chipping away at some of the progress that has been made on managed care over the years.

We hear a lot about managed care, and many people wonder what it is and whether it is working. Managed care focuses on the two major issues of quality and cost. Does it work in just the staff models, as Stan Jones suggests, or does it work in other forms?

Quality is primary. If any carrier is perceived as lacking in quality, it goes out of business. Managed care establishes the credential standards by which it selects its providers. It uses knowledgeable individuals to select physicians who will be in networks. Many patients on their own continue to select physicians based on convenient location rather than medical competency.

Managed care monitors physician-practice patterns. It gives the physicians data on the practice of medicine in their communities to facilitate their decision making. There are few truly bad practicing physicians in the United States, but rapidly changing technology necessitates providing good ones with data so they can make correct decisions.

The role of the primary-care physician is to assist the patient in making decisions in the health care delivery system. Because managed care aggressively pursues contracts with high quality care institutions, primary care physicians enable patients to select those institutions where they will pay a reasonable price and will get an excellent outcome from their procedures.

Unquestionably, managed care holds down costs while preserving quality. Most major employers are moving in the direction of incorporating managed care in their employee benefit programs. Recently we lost a contract for which the difference in price was only two-tenths of 1 percent. Clearly there is competition on price where quality among different carriers is equal.

With regard to the charge that triple-option plans do not have or encourage quality, note that the triple-option plans are bid in the marketplace every year. Normally every plan in the insurance industry is competitively bid, and so the individual employer has a choice. Most large employers are not dealing with 100 HMOs nationwide but rather are narrowing their selection to one, two, or three HMOs because of the complexity.

I would be the first to say that we have an imperfect system. We have to make changes. If I believed the dollar outlay would be lower were the federal government to take over, or that it would be more efficient, or would deliver better quality care, or would not have the same bureaucracy, then I would be in favor of moving in that direction. But I think we do have an efficient delivery system. CIGNA's administrative expenses are lower than 5 percent, we bring quality of care, and we assist the individual and the family member in making the right decisions for what they need in the delivery system.

Carl J. Schramm

My commentary might be entitled, "the limits of economic analysis"—or, more whimsically, Lenin's question—What is to be done?

Economists have a reason for liking to captivate the imagination with discussions of oligopoly, and monopoly, and observations about subsidies and free riders. It is because these are provocative notions in classical economics, concepts that stimulate the imagination. We economists talk this way because, candidly, when it comes to economic analysis, our imaginations usually remain unfulfilled. There simply are realities out there that cannot yet be captured either by our systems of thought or by the functional systems we have in place. That is the case with our complex scheme of health care financing.

First, health care is by no means a classical market. Yes, there is ample evidence of day-to-day competitive outcomes, but there remain institutional forces that are going largely unobserved and undiscussed. Nevertheless, two chapters in part one are, by implication, attempts to address and restructure these institutional forces. Certainly Clark Havighurst's approach, which examines quintessential institutional forces, would turn those forces upside down and yet make them work to an economically satisfactory result.

The major economic forces in the health care equation that have not been addressed are doctors and hospitals. From 1983 to 1991 our country produced 40 percent more doctors, despite the fact that the Institute of Medicine declared the physician market glutted in 1979. And since not one medical school has closed, we may have another 40 percent practicing in another few years. This "overproduction" has occurred, and continues to occur, despite a glutted marketplace.

Overproduction of physicians—all the economists and all the economic theories notwithstanding—turned out to be extremely profitable for the medical community. In fact, 1990 showed us the all-time record high in the level of physician income. The same is true of hospitals: some are operating at 40 percent excess and are not shutting down; and for-profit hospitals compare favorably with the Fortune 500.

Those of us who wear insurance company hats wrestle every day with what were once thought to be the laws of economics. Take mandated benefits, for example. A physician with a new technology—in vitro fertilization, for example—can easily find the path to his state legislature. At the point where this new technology becomes a mandated benefit that insurers must pay, the natural law has failed; the political power of the physician, or whoever is pushing the new technology, has in effect created a distortion in the marketplace. This is not physician-bashing; this is empirical observation of how behavior and certain social structures operate to distort the classical rules of economics.

The medical institutions—doctors and hopsitals—are characterized by confused price-taker identities. Many such institutions were once eleemosynary—not so far back in their history, they were charitable. We did not change them overnight in 1980 by bathing them in the waters of Reaganesque ideology. Go into a hospital and you will be washed in a shower of eleemosynary talk. But even though some of these institutions may be taking part in a competitive market and perhaps even plundering that market, the institutions themselves are confused as to *what* they are, *who* they are, and *how* they are to act.

Most of these institutions—despite paper after paper by economists—do not at all resemble price takers. They are not worried about market competition. Go look at the recession and ask the architects, and the engineers, and the construction crews, where are the buildings still going up? They will point to one sector—hospitals.

The bizarre economic reality created by doctors and hospitals, in tandem with our legal and political institutions, illustrates that we have not yet discovered the economic axioms of insurance—either social insurance or private insurance. The axiom is that the price of insurance is equal to the aggregated level of risk that is insured. That means that health insurance simply will not be cheap as long as it insures for the health care delivery done in this environment.

We operate with other institutional problems. Government ranks highest among the institutions we no longer trust, and government is powerless to conduct even the debate on reform. We no longer trust universities; we no longer trust banks; we no longer trust the savings and loans, unless we come from the Midwest, where S&Ls don't fail. As people ran out of things to distrust, they decided in 1991 to distrust the insurance companies.

This is the environment we live in. And while our economic analysis might be very interesting and captivating, and a nice way to spend a rainy morning in this complicated environment, it will not help us to answer Lenin's question: What is to be done?

We must focus on several areas. First, we must come to grips with the axiom of insurance: the cost of insurance is the collective cost of the risk insured. That by itself should put to death the quick fix. It is simply not the case that if we socialize the risk, the system will all be vastly more efficient.

How do we know this? You will hear from some people that Medicare does what private insurers do at a fraction of the cost. But no one seriously believes that government is efficient, at least not in the way government runs Medicare and Medicaid. What is the single most frequently heard complaint to members of Congress from constituents? "I call and call Medicare, and no one answers the phone."

Government cannot do it. A number of other suggestions are equally inefficient. Roger Feldman has examined community rating and found inequities there that would affect efficiency profoundly—and for the worse. We must also grapple with health insurance from the perspective of administrative costs. We have to look at the choices America faces—including the choices that are part of cost-containment, where private insurance in fact can do better than the government.

A radical departure in the world of commercial health insurance, and one that can help us to tame costs, is managed care. Here we play a different role from that of the past; insurers must become the disciplinarians of the system. In the wake of the indemnity model of insurance, where insurers were a passive payer, we have now assumed an aggressive role and are disciplining the system on behalf of our customers.

Yet another step we must take is simply to "get real" about the market disability of the poor. No one yet speaks of the failure of the government to keep faith with its insured, but the evidence of Medicaid is abundantly clear and well understood.

Finally, we must understand what we face. We cannot go further in the national debate without focusing on the supply side. What are we going to do about America's insatiable appetite for medicine? What will we do about this country's inclination to buy it all through the public purse without assuming the tax responsibility? And about our readiness to enrich ourselves through a vastly expanding physician population? What about those structural problems within the hospital industry, an industry that seems to lack a means of discipline?

Collectively we must work toward some mechanism to help modulate and control the debate. One theme we hear often is that of paternalism: Big Daddy may be central government or, although not as clearly articulated, the "pure" market forces at work. Others end up talking about an intermediate zone, where we are really looking toward managed competition.

We do need a role for government. It must begin to set statutory limits on the behaviors of various actors; and, as government sets about doing this, it also has to go about the business of reestablishing a credible and efficient role for itself. Yet the irony exists that government cannot yet speak clearly about the health care financing problem; so far, the private insurance industry happens to be the interest that speaks most clearly.

We may sound as if we are throwing down the gauntlet to many other interests—economists, the medical community, government. And perhaps that is a salutary role for us to play. We want those interests to look at America's health care financing problems with the sense of realism that we in the insurance industry bring to them. We want the other players to have an awareness of the complexity of the issues, as well as a sense of their own responsibility. Seeing things as they are, and broadening the debate, is something we need to do to answer with any measure of success the question, What is to be done?

The Nature of the Problem

Discussion of Part One

HEATHER J. GRADISON, American Enterprise Institute: Mr. Havighurst, I am surprised by what you have said about a single-payer system. Do you advocate having a single-payer system for the United States?

CLARK C. HAVIGHURST, Duke University: I made the case for a single-payer system to afford the health insurance industry the opportunity to tell us why it is superior, and it has not yet done so to my satisfaction. Two of its representatives who are contributors to this volume are in a position to do so. Carl Schramm says his managed care is better than the government's managed care. Although I approve of most managed-care efforts, I see all private managed care as managing always to the same objective—the same professional standard—just as a government single payer would do, and that does not impress me.

My chapter is intended as a tour de force to persuade the private sector to do its job of offering consumers a market full of choices, which it is not doing. If Mr. Schramm is correct in claiming that we do not have a market in any classic sense, then why do we pretend to have one? Can we make it work? If not, then we are wasting time.

MS. GRADISON: But Robert O'Brien writes of losing a contract over a small percentage of a competitive bid. Other issues have been raised, too, about informed as opposed to uninformed employer purchasing. Clearly we have a market at work here.

DAVID DRANOVE, Kellogg Graduate School of Management, Northwestern University: This discussion suggests that the performance of the health care system hinges critically on the performance of the insurance sector. But the performance of the industry hinges most critically on the performance of providers. And when I look at providers, I see a very competitive marketplace. For example, count the number of hospitals that have seminars and spend a lot of money learning continuous quality improvement methods. Or look at the number of antitrust cases being litigated and the evidence emerging from them suggesting that prices really do respond to market competition, a number of previous studies notwithstanding. We may not like the outcome of that competition, but we should examine how insurers guide the performance of providers, not the nature of competition between insurers.

DONALD W. MORAN, Lewin/ICF: It is noteworthy that both Mr. Luft and Mr. Feldman and the subsequent discussion focused on observed price behavior as an indicator of whether competition exists in these markets. I am especially struck by Mr. Dranove's last comment. One difference between government and private industry is that between issues associated with price and those associated with the volume and character of services delivered. A substantial degree of product differentiation and volume growth in the health care system is independent of considerations of price. There has been a big difference between the respective ways government and the private sector have gone about these things. The government used whatever force was at its disposal to singlemindedly attack the price side of the equation. It spent the past fifteen or twenty years hammering away at unit prices of various services, while attempting to reconfigure the product a little bit; the private managed care industry concentrated primarily on the volume of services. Obviously, that is a far more complicated task.

HAROLD S. LUFT, University of California, San Francisco: I will give a minor example of price competition and encourage everybody to remember that all the players are in this game for the long run.

The University of California is a very large employer. A few years ago we decided to put our fee-for-service contract on dental insurance out to bid. We took the low bidder and went to a new carrier. There was a substantial difference in the new rates, probably a 15 percent differential. A few years later we sought health insurance bids and got about half the number we anticipated. It was a very attractive contract—80,000 lives—but nobody was willing to play because we had walked away from a high-bid carrier in the dental insurance situation. Consequently the university no longer puts contracts out to bid.

Price competition works when people make many, frequent, small purchases. But major players with major contracts have to think about the long-term consequences of playing tough. It may be that one cannot play any more after walking away from a bid.

WARREN GREENBERG, George Washington University: In view of Mr. Havighurst's comments, we should compare the competitiveness of the health insurance industry with that of other industries—the detergent

125

industry, the tie industry, the apparel industry, the petroleum industry, or even our system of higher education. What has competition brought to these industries? No one says we ought to have a single seller of gasoline, or detergent, or ties or apparel, or any number of the goods we buy. Even considering the administrative costs of running a market and making such consumer choices as choosing a university, no one says that to reduce administrative costs we ought to have only one university or one apparel shop in the country.

We ought to ask why health care should be different. Is bias selection in health insurance the real reason why health markets are different from other markets?

RICHARD KRONICK, University of California, San Diego: Certainly one big difference is that most people are insured, so that price is not a factor at the point of purchase. That ties in with an observation Carl Schramm made: the cost of insurance is the collective cost of the risk of the insureds, as if that were somehow an exogenous factor.

The real question is, How many resources are providers going to require to keep us well? There is little science here, but there is much judgment for providers to exercise. How do we create a system that gets providers to exercise that judgment the way we as purchasers wish? Mr. Jones is correct in saying that the transaction-oriented approach insurers have taken to managed care is doomed to failure. With so much art and so little science, we cannot write down a set of rules and discipline the market through adversarial, third-party review. To get real change we must change the way hospitals and doctors are organized. The transaction-oriented approach to managed care is not going to do that.

MR. DRANOVE: The approach that is not transaction-oriented is the staff-model HMO. When I was a graduate student of Alain Enthoven's in the late 1970s and early 1980s, there was a rush of excitement that there might be proposals to make the staff-model HMO the model for the United States. Why has this not occurred?

Throughout the 1980s I have seen no regulatory entry barriers, other than through the tax system. And I have seen few institutional entry barriers. Yet I do not see many staff-model HMOs. Other than Kaiser, which has made inroads in some markets outside California, there has been almost no growth of staff-model HMOs. Why has the American public not taken to them, if they are so good at reducing the bad transaction cost associated with other types of insurance?

H. E. FRECH III, University of California, Santa Barbara: I am surprised by this discussion, which implies that managed care is not working. That implication seems odd, given the tremendous improvement in the number of instruments being used in managed care and the great growth of preferred provider organizations (PPOs). Research shows that even the loosest managed care saves a substantial amount of money. This is a new development, an innovation in the market.

I see an optimistic picture when I look at the growth of managed care and the increase in coinsurance and copayment in the market. Managed care requires management, but coinsurance and copayments are guaranteed to work. The private health care sector looks promising, and I do not understand the pessimism I am hearing.

C. EUGENE STEUERLE, Urban Institute: I have a question for Mr. Feldman. He made a strong case for preventing certain types of discrimination in insurance policies—in particular, community-rating. He pointed out that if we force community-rating, we may require a common set of prices that are not age-adjusted in appropriate ways. But insurance by its very nature is designed to discriminate by certain patterns. That is, insurance defines certain groups, for whom it charges a common price. How far along this continuum toward community-rating might he want to go? Would he regulate nondiscrimination by race, by sex, by size of family, by the riskiness of the job, if we decided that had certain effects we wanted to correct?

ROGER FELDMAN, University of Minnesota: I have my own value judgment, and I am unwilling to go more than an inch. How far would one go in allowing the sponsor to risk-adjust the premium that is paid on behalf of individuals?

At one point in the president's economic report, I thought that would be a good idea. Since then I have zig-zagged on the question. Mr. Luft believes that sponsor risk-rating would be a good idea, up to the point where it is not worthwhile for the health care plan to attempt either further adjustment or cream-skimming.

RITA RICARDO-CAMPBELL, Hoover Institution: Payment of health insurance premiums by the businessman is a form of compensation paid to employees. It evolved during World War II, when there was a freeze on wages. The only thing an employer could do was to add fringe benefits, so health insurance premiums grew because they were a business expense and were excluded from employee income.

Therefore, why should we expect employers to take the risk of discriminating among their employees in the form of how much health insurance premiums they will pay for each? Under the present system employers have the incentive to hire younger people rather than older people, single people rather than married people, and so forth, because the health insurance premiums of those groups would be much lower. We should address the problem of how to phase out the employer's payment of compensation in the form of after-tax health insurance premiums and get it into the hands of the consumer—the employee.

MR. LUFT: For large employers who are essentially experience-rated, the employment pool determines the premium. In other words, if we hire older workers, we pay more. It does not matter what the premium is. The young ones go to the HMOs, and the older ones stay in fee-for-service plans. With risk-adjusted contributions the employer contributes less money to the HMO and more money to fee-for-service plans, but the total amount is based on the composition of the employment pool. There are enormous incentives not to hire older workers because the employer must pay for pensions as well as health insurance.

G. ROBERT O'BRIEN, CIGNA Corporation: The reason staff-model HMOs have not grown faster is that the capital required to start up a staff model is extensive. The data for cost control and quality for an individual practice association (IPA) are close to those for a staff-model HMO.

MARK V. PAULY, Wharton School, University of Pennsylvania: Much of the discouragement heard in evaluation of performance comes from people on a unicorn hunt, saying that any carrier not identified as highest quality is out of business. People are searching for high quality at lower cost, and perhaps that unicorn does not exist. Perhaps we need to give up a little bit of quality. Maybe we have to call the nurse at Hartford before having a biopsy.

I am incredulous that Stan Jones is incredulous at learning that employers may not be interested in cutting health costs, because it may hurt their chance to recruit good employees. Employees may in effect be saying, "I do not like your insurance policy, which restricts my behavior, and you do not offer me enough of a cash wage to make up the difference." That is their way of saying they are still not serious about saving health care costs if they have to give up something. Sooner or later that will happen, but Americans may not be ready for health care reform just yet.

STANLEY B. JONES, private consultant: Employee resistance is the fundamental proof that our reliance on the purchasing practices of employers to restructure and discipline the provider market is poorly placed and ill-founded.

On a technical note, I have seen no good studies to show that we are realizing major savings or even documentable savings on managed-care systems that are less drastic than staff and group models. Nor have I seen studies that show IPAs can do as well.

MR. FRECH: It is not my research, but two solid studies, one by Feldstein, Wickizer, and Wheeler (1988) and the other by Khandker and Manning (1992), show substantial savings from preadmission utilization review alone. That is why I say that even the loosest managed care gives substantial savings. The lowest number either of them found for preadmission screening was 6 percent savings on the hospital side—and that for something just started. That is a powerful and encouraging result.

MR. JONES: The problem from the payer's perspective is that over the years the insurer comes to believe that the savings from most managed care, except for staff and group models, is lost in other expenses, and so he cannot find the net savings. Therefore, he is unable to quote a favorable premium, using all those devices. We can find little pieces of savings, but we cannot document a total impact on premiums to keep them down and constrain their growth. Perhaps Mr. Moran can.

MR. MORAN: I can agree with both Mr. Jones and Mr. Frech. It is very difficult to rate generic medical and surgical benefit plans at the group level. What is not tough to rate at the group level is the growing body of specialized managed-care carve-outs. The clearest example is the type of psychiatric carve-out of the type done by Preferred Health Care, APM, or other such firms. In those plans utilization differentials are dramatic. Even if the actuaries are conservative, these employers are essentially taking out explicit capitation contracts. They are willing to bank on these specialized managed-care designs, performing in a predictable way. So in that segment of the market, I disagree with Mr. Jones that insurance carriers cannot define areas for managed-care savings.

MR. HAVIGHURST: The basic problem is this. The insurer is a purchasing agent for the consumer and in purchasing health services from the health industry, the consumer ought to have the means of saying explicitly what he or she wants or does not want to buy. The managed-care system does not do that. It puts everything in a black box, giving very little disclosure of what the standards are. The consumer has little choice, except whether to take managed care or not.

I like the idea of contracting and having more opportunities for the consumer to make those choices explicitly in their contracts. The legal system resists the idea that consumer contrasts could authorize deviations from what seems to be accepted medical practice, however costly it may be. We need finally to break away from the notion that the medical profession tells us what we must buy. It is time to seek ways of specifying what we want to buy. The insurance industry has to perform that function for us. Otherwise it is not a useful institution.

References

Feldstein, Paul J., T.M. Wickizer, and J.R. Wheeler. "The Effects of Utilization Review Programs on Health Care Use and Expenditures." *New England Review of Medicine* 318 (May 19, 1988): 1310–40.

Khandker, Rezaul K., and Willard G. Manning. "The Impact of Utilization Review on Costs and Utilization." In Peter Zweifel and H.E. Frech III, eds. *Health Economics Worldwide.* Dordrecht: Kluwer Academic Publishers, 1992, pp. 47–62.

PART TWO

What Should Be the Role for the Private Sector in Improving Access to Health Care?

6
Mandated Benefits and Compensating Differentials— Taxing the Uninsured

Michael A. Morrisey

Robert J. Blendon and Jennifer N. Edwards (1991) have categorized the growing number of U.S. health care proposals into four categories: (1) those that mandate employer health insurance coverage together with an expansion of government coverage for the nonworking and the poor; (2) those that require employers either to provide coverage or to pay a tax, together with an expansion of government coverage for the nonworking and the poor; (3) tax credit plans; and (4) all-government plans. Since their enumeration in 1991, several more proposals have entered the market. The majority of these proposals fall into the first two categories—expanding the role of employers.

Because of this interest in mandating employer-sponsored coverage, it is important to understand the workings of the labor market and the effects of such mandates on the employment relationship. That is the purpose of this chapter. The results are disconcerting. Mandates are expensive. Lots of people are affected besides those who are currently uninsured. There is a significant trade-off between exemption of small business and coverage of the uninsured. Mandates imply some shifting of employment across firms. Most important, however, mandated coverage will be predominately paid for by uninsured workers themselves.

The argument, in a nutshell, is that workers are paid what they are worth. Compensation takes many forms: wages, benefits, and working conditions. When a law requires that a labor contract include a specified level of health insurance, then wages, other benefits, and working conditions will adjust downward until the value of the goods and services produced by the worker is again equal to compensation. These compensating differentials paid by the currently uninsured workers are the principal means by which mandated health insurance coverage will

133

be financed. Not unlike the Medicare Catastrophic Coverage Act, the mandated benefit proposals tax the recipients of the benefits. Like the Medicare beneficiaries also, many of the beneficiaries will perceive themselves as worse off after they have coverage.

The second section of this chapter proceeds with a brief description of the salient features of mandated benefit programs and a review of the estimated effects of mandates on health insurance coverage and costs. The third section analyzes the effects of mandates in the labor market. The fourth section reviews the empirical evidence of compensating differentials. The final section summarizes the chapter and draws some conclusions.

Description of Programs

The best-known employer mandate proposal is the Minimum Health Benefits for All Workers Act, introduced by Senator Edward Kennedy. The American Medical Association's Health Access America and the Pepper Commission recommendations also make employer mandates key features of their programs for reform.

Although the plans differ in detail, they all involve certain key features. Employers are required as a matter of federal law to provide health insurance coverage to their workers. The government will define both a bundle of minimum services that must be included in the benefit packages and the extent of any deductibles, copayments, or stop losses. Eligible workers are generally defined as those working at least ten, seventeen and one-half, or twenty hours per week. Each spouse is to be covered by his or her own employer, if both are employed; dependents are to be covered and are allocated across parents' plans. The plan is to be paid for by an allocation of the premium to both the employer and the worker, usually specified as an eighty-twenty split. Other features may include a provision to subsidize the purchase of insurance by small employers. This subsidy is often financed from general tax revenues.

Other proposals fall into the so-called play-or-pay category. Employers are mandated to provide health insurance in accordance with the provisions just described. But if an employer chooses, it may pay a tax instead. The tax is generally specified as a percentage of payroll. Senate bill 1227, the HealthAmerica: Portable Health Care of All Americans Act, would set the pay option at 8 percent of payroll.

The proposals also generally call for an expansion of Medicaid or some new government program to cover those unattached to the labor market. The joint provision of mandates and Medicaid (or other government program) is essential for two reasons: it draws most of the uninsured into some form of coverage, and it keeps on-budget government expenses to a minimum.

Estimates of Access and Cost

Because employer mandate proposals have been under consideration for several years, many efforts have been made to estimate the number of persons affected and the cost of providing this coverage. The efforts have disagreed because of different operational definitions of the uninsured and because of the assumptions about the extent to which the currently insured change insurance plans or find their existing plans expanded. Nonetheless, they are in the same ballpark.

Estimates of the number of uninsured using 1987 data reported about 37 million uninsured (Swartz 1988; Chollet 1987). These estimates, however, were too large as a result of some imprecise questionnaire design in the Current Population Survey used by most analysts.[1] Estimates in 1988 put the number at about 30 million people. The 1989 data have now been analyzed. The Employee Benefit Research Institute (EBRI) reports that some 34.4 million people below age sixty-five are without health insurance (Foley 1991). The Congressional Budget Office (CBO 1991) estimates put the number at 33.1 million. Thus 34 million uninsured—about 15 percent of the population—is our best guess.

EBRI and CBO are reasonably consistent in finding that 85 and 81 percent, respectively, of the below-age-sixty-five uninsured are in a family affiliated with the labor force. The differences in these estimates appear to be due to differences in the treatment of part-time, part-year workers and those not in the labor force.

Estimates of the number of uninsured affected by a mandate are quite consistent, at least using the 1988 CPS data. Approximately 24.4 million uninsured would be covered by an employer mandate.[2] More recent CBO estimates are lower. For a mandate covering all firms with ten or more workers working more than twenty-five hours, 17.6 million previously uninsured would get coverage. This is approximately 52 percent of the uninsured.

This lower estimate is, in part, a reflection of the policy parameters in an employer mandate. By placing the firm size and hours worked limits at ten workers and twenty-five hours, respectively, small firms and part-time workers are less affected. This means there will be less labor market disruption but also less employer-sponsored coverage. EBRI reports, for example, that 39 percent of the uninsured are affiliated with a firm of fewer than twenty-five employees (Foley 1991). If the

---

1. For a careful discussion of the changes in the Current Population Survey and an estimate of 31.1 million uninsured, see Moyer (1989). Similar conclusions are drawn by Needleman et al. (1990) and Holahan and Zedlewski (1989).
2. For a detailed review of alternative estimates, see Morrisey (1991).

mandated program is to make a bigger dent in the uninsured, it must extend into smaller firms.

The 17.6 million uninsured, however, are not the only people affected. If the employer plan is mandated, some people with nonemployment-related coverage will be affected. CBO estimates that nearly 5 million people currently covered by Medicare, Medicaid, and the Veterans Administration (VA) would then have an employer-sponsored plan as their primary payer. Another 8.2 million people would be expected to drop privately purchased individual health insurance plans (CBO 1991). These estimates of public coverage shifts are consistent, although somewhat lower than earlier estimates of 5–9 million publicly covered people who would be switched to a private plan (Morrisey 1991).

The CBO's private-switcher estimates include only those with individually purchased private policies. These people would switch to employer plans. The estimates exclude those with group coverage who would also switch. This is the case when, for example, a wife must be included under her own employer's plan. Earlier estimates put total individual and group switchers in the neighborhood of 14–29 million persons (Morrisey 1991, 29). Further, Jack Needleman et al. (1990) estimate that another 26 million people would be affected by an increase in benefits required of their existing health insurance plan by a more generous, mandated plan.

In short, lots of people are affected. If the CBO numbers are believed, the mandate would provide new coverage to 17.6 million people. Another 5 million would be shifted from public to private plans. Approximately 8 million would drop individual coverage. At least another 10 million group switchers would be affected, as would a large number of persons with currently inferior benefits.

The price of this expansion is high. Thorpe (1989) found that an employer mandate would have gross costs of about $42.5 billion; Needleman et al. (1990) estimated $39.4 billion in gross costs. Nevertheless, because of out-of-pocket expenditures and existing premiums currently paid by those covered under the new plan, the gross costs can be reduced. Further, there are savings in public program costs because of the shifting of workers to employer plans. A case can also be made for a saving from cost-shifting.[3] These savings lead to a net cost estimate of $10–$30 billion (Thorpe 1989; Needleman et al. 1990). CBO's (1990) analysis puts the net cost at $13 billion. The cost differences vary

---

3. Most of the estimates include such an estimate. I am skeptical of cost saving asserted to result from the reduction of "cost-shifting." See Morrisey (1991) for a discussion.

significantly because of the underlying assumptions of coverage, switchers, prices, and use of services.

It is important to note that few of the proposals involve employer mandates alone. Most also entail an expansion of a government program, usually Medicaid. A common Medicaid expansion is to provide eligibility for Medicaid coverage at zero premium to all those below 100 percent of the federal poverty line. Those between 100 and 200 percent of the poverty line are allowed to buy into the Medicaid program at a premium that reflects a percentage of their income. Here again the estimates vary significantly. If the recent CBO estimates are used, 84.9 percent of the currently uninsured get coverage—approximately 28 million people, for a net cost of $20 billion.[4] In these scenarios the cost of the mandate remains essentially unchanged, yet otherwise uninsured people are picked up by the Medicaid expansion and the buy-in.

Effects of an Employer Mandate

To examine the effects of a mandate on the labor market it is necessary first to sketch the economist's view of how labor markets work. The theory of labor compensation and adjustments for working conditions has a long history. The key insight is that compensation includes more than just the wage or salary. Adam Smith (1976, book I) discusses the trade-off, saying in part: "Honour makes a great part of the reward of all honourable professions. In point of pecuniary gain, all things considered, they are generally under-recompensed, as I shall endeavour to show by and by." The concept is also commonly understood today. Recall Bob Dole's quip on why he was running for vice president: "It's indoor work and no heavy lifting." Nonetheless, the principle tends to be lost in the debate over various approaches to health care reform.

The rigorous study of employer-sponsored health insurance, in this context, is relatively recent (Goldstein and Pauly 1976; Jensen 1986; Danzon 1989). Firms hire workers and, at the margin, pay them what they are worth. "Worth" is defined precisely as the amount of extra revenue that the firm receives from the efforts of the last worker in the job class. The firm would like to pay less, of course, but if it did so workers would work for other employers.

Why would an employer ever offer health insurance in this simple world? The answer is equally simple: it costs less to do so. More precisely, workers place some value on health insurance and are willing to accept a compensation bundle that includes health insurance *and* somewhat

---

4. See Holahan and Zedlewski (1989) for an excellent discussion of coverage and costs under alternative Medicaid expansion options.

lower wages rather than wages alone. If a firm finds it can get health insurance at a price lower than what the worker is willing to give up in wages, the worker is happy with the new insurance-wage bundle and the firm has lowered its labor costs.

Health insurance tends to be less expensive when purchased through an employer. There are three reasons for this. The first has to do with insurance underwriting. Employed people are healthier, on average, than those who are unemployed. Employment serves as a good signal of lower expected claims costs, and consequently an employer group can purchase coverage at lower cost than can an individual. The second reason has to do with the nature of the existing tax laws. Health insurance is not taxed as federal or state income, nor is it subject to FICA taxes. Thus if an employee were to value a dollar of health insurance as equivalent to a dollar of take-home pay, an employer need only spend a dollar on health insurance rather than a dollar plus tax on money compensation. Third, there are economies in the marketing and administration of group and employer-group plans relative to individually purchased insurance.

From the workers' perspective, wages adjust to reflect the change in the other form of compensation now provided. Other things being equal, more health insurance means lower money wages. Attempts to reduce health insurance—for instance, through the use of increased deductibles—require that workers be "made whole."

If health insurance lowers labor costs, why do not all firms offer this insurance? The answer is twofold. First, not all firms face the same costs of offering health insurance. Firms with high turnover face higher administrative costs, and smaller firms have higher administrative costs per worker. Further, as Chollet (1988) notes, small firms are particularly prone to adverse selection, including on occasion the employment of family members for the explicit purpose of insuring anticipated future medical expenses. Second, firms may be willing to offer health insurance, but minimum wage statutes prevent the compensating differential from taking place.

If some firms have lower labor compensation costs because they can offer health insurance more cheaply than others, why do not these lower-cost firms drive the others out of business? The answer is that different workers place different values on having health insurance. Several possible reasons can account for this. First, some workers prefer to spend their limited income on food and shelter rather than on health insurance. Even given the lower price of insurance available through an employer plan, they would prefer the cash. Second, some workers are less likely than others to become ill. If they do not expect to use the benefit, it is of little value to them, and they too would be more likely to prefer the cash. Third, some may be covered under a spouse's or a parent's plan, so the insurance is redundant. Finally, some have income and assets that may be near the Medicaid eligibility threshold in their state. A generous Medicaid program would then be a substitute for private coverage; they too would prefer the cash.[5]

This line of reasoning suggests that firms that incur relatively low costs of providing health insurance will attract persons with stronger preferences for coverage, and firms with higher costs of providing health insurance will attract workers who value insurance less intensely.

Implications and Misconceptions. This economic model has several implications. First, it suggests why we have not seen employers implement major restructuring of their health benefit plans. Suppose a firm could reduce its health care costs by contracting with only one hospital and one group of physicians. To be worth doing the innovation must not only cost less than the current insurance plan; it must save enough to allow the firm to compensate its workers in some other way for the restriction in choice, and still reduce total labor costs. These adjustments would ordinarily come in the form of increased wages. Because workers face an income tax on wages, however, the firm must be able to make the worker whole, after taxes. I suspect that little true innovation has gone on in employer health plans because it is difficult, in the current tax system, to find innovations that can meet this criterion.

This line of reasoning also highlights the misconception that firms offering health insurance subsidize firms that do not. Rather, the compensating differential model suggests that, adjusting for productivity, workers in both sets of firms are paid what they are worth. Those working in firms offering health insurance take their compensation in the form of lower wages and more (perhaps much more) health insurance. Workers in firms without health insurance take higher wages.

As Reinhardt (1989) notes, the model also challenges the view that U.S. international competitiveness would be enhanced by a tax-financed health insurance plan of some sort. If the government provided health insurance, then it would no longer be a vehicle for worker compensation; workers would get insurance whether they worked or not. But workers must still be paid the value of their marginal product. Profit seeking would lead employers to bid up the wages and other benefits they offer

---

5. A generous Medicaid program may be considered an oxymoron by some. Thorpe et al. (1989), however, show that setting the minimum benefit package at the level used by Minnesota, the most generous program, is expensive. Part of the cost arises from people's dropping private health insurance to take advantage of the public program.

in an attempt to keep their workers.[6] The net effect on U.S. competitiveness depends, among other things, on the actual cost of health insurance provided by the government relative to the cost of firm-purchased coverage and on the incidence of the taxes levied to pay for that coverage.

Effects of a Mandate. Now consider the effects of an insurance mandate on the labor market. The mandate has no effect on firms and workers with employer-sponsored benefits already in excess of those required. For the others, the mandate forces the firm to include health insurance in the compensation bundle. Workers are just as productive after the mandate as before. Therefore they will continue to be paid the value of what extra they produce. The theory implies that the wages or other benefits received by the worker must fall. Thus newly insured workers will pay for the mandate in the form of reductions in other forms of compensation, most notably wages.

There is an irony in this. One of the chief policy options for the expansion of Medicaid is the buy-in. Under it people between, say, 100 and 200 percent of the poverty line can purchase Medicaid coverage. The purchase price is linked to a maximum percentage of income, such as 3 or 5 percent.[7] This is done because it is feared that low-income individuals and families cannot afford high insurance payments and will not take advantage of the Medicaid buy-in option. These are the same people, however, who will pay for the employer mandate without benefit of any share of income limitation.

A second implication of the theory is that federal and state income tax payers will shoulder a significant share of the cost. The amount they pay depends upon the federal and state tax rates. Under current tax law, such payments are excluded from the personal income tax and from the FICA base. If the relevant federal income tax is 15 percent, the state income tax is 3 percent, and the combined FICA tax is 14.9 percent, then taxpayers would pay approximately one-third of the cost of the mandated health insurance benefits in the form of tax revenue forgone.

Third, the provisions of the mandating legislation that specify how the premium is to be split between employer and employee really designate the split between the currently uninsured worker and the taxpayer. Suppose the split is 80-20 for the employer. This implies that 80 percent of the cost of the premium will be paid by the worker with pre-tax dollars and 20 percent with after-tax dollars. In such a scenario

---

6. When the cost of the insurance program is identical whether mandated or imposed as a tax, the tax method is more distorting (Summers 1989).

7. For an excellent discussion of Medicaid expansions and the buy-in option, see Holahan and Zedlewski (1989).

with the tax rates noted above, taxpayers would pay for one-third of 80 percent of the premium; that is, 26 percent. Previously uninsured workers would pay 74 percent. Some mandate proposals contain provisions that require the employer to pay the entire premium. This does help the worker. But the help is in the form of a greater share of the cost being borne by taxpayers. In fact, 100 percent "employer-paid" health insurance is precisely the example in the previous paragraph.

Fourth, to the extent that wages are not able to fully adjust, unemployment results. Consider a stereotypic small firm not currently offering health insurance. I argued above that this firm did not offer coverage because it was more expensive. I also argued that the firm would attract workers for whom health insurance was less valuable. After the mandate, it would attempt to reduce wages to offset the insurance cost. Nevertheless, the small firm's insurance costs are higher; it must cut wages more than other firms to offset the coverage fully. Unfortunately, its workers value the benefits less intensely than others do. Some of these workers will migrate to other, stereotypically larger firms where, because of lower insurance costs, the insurance tax—that is, the compensating differential—is lower. Small firms will hire fewer workers at the higher level of compensation. Some workers will drop out of the labor force.

This provides a rationale for the often proposed subsidy for small employers. The issue, however, is not small employers but all employers who do not offer health insurance. The problem is that some workers will not accept the insurance tax; they drop out of the labor force and total compensation costs are bid up for those who remain. They are differentially bid up for those firms that rationally had not been providing health insurance. More fundamentally, however, the issue should be framed around the currently uninsured worker, not the firm. If society wants the individual to have coverage, the most efficient way to do this is to subsidize directly the individual's purchase of health insurance, not to subsidize particular types of firms.[8]

The unemployment effects are interesting. Evidence from minimum wage studies suggest that the effects will be relatively small and concentrated among part-time and teenage workers (Brown 1988). There are reasons to doubt even these effects. First, when the minimum wage is increased, the affected workers generally have no fringe benefits, and thus no compensating benefit differential can be applied. The whole effect must come through working conditions or unemployment. With mandated health insurance, wages can adjust. This significantly reduces

---

8. For a readable discussion of worker versus employer subsidies, see Pauly et al. (1991).

the unemployment effect. But the insurance mandate is more like a lump-sum tax applied to each worker than it is a minimum wage. The incentive is to reduce the number of workers. Hour reductions cut costs only if they result in employment below the minimum number of hours per week covered by the legislation. The model does suggest, however, that we should expect to see more workers with several "very" part-time jobs, an increase in the use of consultants, and the contracting out of certain tasks currently performed within the firm.[9]

A fifth implication deals with the interaction of mandated health insurance benefits with minimum wage laws. A worker employed at the minimum wage can legally face no compensating wage differential. Clearly for these individuals, reduced employment is the only mechanism for adjustment.

Finally, a case can be made that currently uninsured workers are generally made worse off as a result of an employer mandate. Following Wessels (1988), workers can be viewed as buying health insurance and other fringe benefits through their employers and paying in the form of lower wages. Workers continue to buy benefits until the last benefits purchased are just equal to the wages given up. If a health insurance mandate is imposed and if it requires the firm to offer or expand coverage, it must mean that the worker did not value the benefit enough to pay the wage price to obtain it.[10] Forcing coverage through the mandate, then, means that the worker must be giving up something of higher value—the wages—for something of lower value—the health insurance. The worker is made worse off. The taxpayer subsidy implicit in the mandate will not affect this result, because current workers have already made their decisions in the face of the existing tax subsidies. Additional subsidies to small firms may reverse this result. Whether they do depends upon the size of the new subsidy and the willingness of these workers to trade wages for health benefits. Those workers in firms unaffected by the special small-firm subsidy, of course, are not helped.

To summarize, employer mandates will generally be paid for by the worker in the form of lower wages. Under common features of mandates, the worker will pay approximately 75 percent of the cost of the mandated health insurance. Taxpayers will pay the other quarter. To the extent that wages cannot adjust, unemployment will result.

---

9. This argument of labor market segmentation is more general. For a fascinating discussion of firms specializing in a more homogeneous stock of labor to optimize fringe benefit offerings see Scott et al. (1989).

10. The worker may be misinformed, of course. That, however, raises a host of broader and deeper issues that will not be explored here.

Evidence of Compensating Differentials

Having argued that the principal effect of an employer mandate is to reduce the wages of currently uninsured workers, what evidence is there to support the view that compensating differentials exist? There is no evidence supporting compensating differentials with respect to employer-sponsored health insurance. But recent work in the areas of workers' compensation insurance and pensions suggests that compensating wage differentials not only exist but fully offset the costs of these fringe benefits.

Health Insurance. First, the bad news. The basic empirical argument in this and other examinations of wage-benefit trade-offs is that if one can properly control for differences in worker productivity, for the effects of taxes that make benefits cheaper as incomes rise, and for other relevant fringes and working conditions, then one should find the compensating differential. I have found two published empirical studies that examine wage reductions in the face of health insurance coverage in the workplace. Arleen Leibowitz (1983) used data from the Rand Health Insurance Experiment to estimate wage equations for participants in the experiment. She had data on available worker characteristics and had information on a variety of fringe benefits, including vacation, sick leave, accident insurance, and life insurance. Health insurance was measured as the total premium nominally paid by the employer. She found that wages were generally lower as a result of most of the benefits offered. The health insurance result, although not statistically significant, was positive. This implies that wages rise with health insurance.

The second study is by Alan Monheit and his colleagues (1985) at the National Center for Health Services Research. They used 1977 National Medical Care Expenditure Survey data to estimate employee-wage equations for each of five occupational categories. They included measures of education, work experience, sex, race, region of the country, and industry in which the worker is employed. Health insurance was measured as a dummy variable, taking the value one if *not* provided. In four of the five occupations, the health insurance variable was statistically significant and indicative of wages increasing with the presence of health insurance.

What Happened? There are good reasons to discount these studies, careful though they were. First, consider the problem. In simple comparisons one generally finds that higher wage workers have more benefits as well. One explanation is that the compensating differential theory is wrong. An alternative explanation is that more productive workers get both more money and more benefits. The studies may not adequately control for productivity differences.[11] Consider a firm that pays wages and benefits that are higher than its competitors'. It will have the "pick of the litter" of workers. That is, it will be able to select those workers who are better motivated, more dependable, more competitive, and more aggressive. These attributes are hard enough for a manager to measure, much less for a researcher limited to a few characteristics from a survey. The two available measures of productivity used by researchers are the number of years of schooling and the number of years in the occupation.

Suppose the researcher proceeds nonetheless and includes fringe benefits and badly measured productivity attributes in his regression. He will find a positive correlation between fringe benefits and wages. The reason is that the higher benefits are picking up the pick-of-the-litter attributes of the more productive and better paid work force. The study has not fairly tested the compensating differential story, because it has been unable to control sufficiently for differences in productivity across firms.

A second, analogous problem relates to income tax rates that increase with wages and salaries. At higher tax rates many benefits, health insurance included, become less expensive. Thus when people are more productive their total compensation rises, and the proportion they choose to take as tax-exempt fringe benefits increases as well.[12] Suppose one is unable to control for the marginal tax rate, but nonetheless runs a wage regression that includes health insurance. Health insurance will be correlated with higher tax rates, and the insurance variable will reflect the tax-wage relation as well as a compensating differential effect.

A third problem is also data-driven. To estimate the wage-benefit trade-off one needs firm-level data on benefits and job characteristics, but also individual characteristics on worker productivity and tax rates. Finding data that satisfy these conditions has been difficult in labor economics, particularly as it relates to health insurance.

In short, one explanation for the failure of Leibowitz and the Monheit team to find compensating differentials for health insurance is that they lacked sufficiently detailed data on taxes, benefits, job characteristics, and worker productivity. Based upon the pension literature and studies of workers' compensation, there is reason to believe this data tale might be true.

Workers' Compensation and Compensating Differentials. Research on workers' compensation insurance has come to support the compensating

---

11. This discussion borrows heavily on Smith and Ehrenberg (1983).
12. For empirical estimates, see Sloan and Adamache (1986).

differential story as the empirical attempts to examine the issues have had better data and become more sophisticated, better reflecting the complexities of real life. Like mandated health insurance, mandated workers' compensation insurance pays a worker in the event of illness or injury. It too should be paid for by reductions in workers' wages. The early literature, which consists of work conducted in the early and mid-1980s, found that attempts to find compensating differentials resulted in statistically insignificant findings, often pointing in the wrong direction.[13]

The best of the current work is that of Viscusi and Moore (1987). They carefully combined information on wages and job risks with detailed information on the workers' compensation formulas in use in the various states. They were the first and are still the only ones to calculate the amount a worker would receive if injured at the workplace, and to adjust this income for its tax-exempt nature. This is in contrast to the earlier studies, which were unable to use individual data and which had to rely on state or industry averages. This study thus offered major improvements in data quality.

Further, the authors were the first to link the workers' compensation benefit directly with the risk of injury. This was a key improvement. It said there should be only small compensating wage differentials, even under very generous workers' compensation programs, if the risk of injury or death was very small. Earlier studies estimated the average wage adjustment, regardless of the probability of receiving benefits.

Using 1977 data from the Internal Revenue Service together with pension survey data, Viscusi and Moore (1990) found that a one-dollar increase in the workers' compensation benefit resulted in a 12-cent-per-hour reduction in wages. The finding was statistically significant. Since the actuarially fair cost of the workers' compensation coverage is 5 cents an hour, the wage more than fully compensates the cost of the insurance. Since workers are risk-averse, the apparent overadjustment is also not unexpected. In later work they have buttressed this finding with a different data set for the years 1977 and 1983. They again found wage offsets that more than fully compensated the workers' compensation insurance.

Gruber and Krueger (1990) have also recently found wage adjustments that compensate workers' compensation insurance. They used 1979, 1980, 1981, 1987, and 1988 Current Population Survey data from privately employed carpenters, truck drivers, nonprofessional hospital employees, gasoline station employees, and plumbers. These are occupations with high workplace injury risks. While the results vary by

---

13. For an excellent review of this literature, see Moore and Viscusi (1990).

occupation, when combined they indicated that over 86 percent of the cost of workers' compensation insurance was borne by workers in the form of reduced wages.[14] The authors go on to suggest that mandated workers' compensation insurance is analogous to mandated employer-sponsored health insurance.

Pensions and Compensating Differentials. The chronology of empirical work in pension economics serves as a second excellent example of the returns to better data and more sophisticated analysis when searching for compensating wage differentials. Four studies serve to tell the story, although there were numerous others along the way.

Using 1966 data from 133 firms, Schiller and Weiss (1980) sought to observe compensating wage differentials for pension plans. They examined trade-offs of workers in four age cohorts. The results were discouraging. Young workers appeared to have wage effects that were much too large, while older workers had wage adjustments that were too small or even pointing in the wrong direction. Ehrenberg (1980) examined wages of police and firefighters in cities with populations of 50,000 or more. Using 1973 data he found support for compensating differentials among police but not firefighters, and he found no support for the theory using either group in 1974 or 1975. Smith and Ehrenberg (1983) analyzed data on a group of firms using the Hay Associates employee compensation program. This program carefully attempts to determine job characteristics of each position in the firm and actuarially to determine the value of each fringe benefit. Using creative statistical methods (in the best sense of that term) they attempted to determine the pension-wage trade-off. They found no support for the compensating wage differential story.

The problem with the pension literature turns out to be its narrow view of how the compensating wage differential is manifested (Brown 1983; Ippolito 1987). Suppose the value of a pension is proportional to one's age and tenure with the firm and wage at retirement. This is the usual case of a defined benefit plan in which a worker can retire at age sixty with twenty years of experience with the firm, and can receive an annual pension that is some percentage of the average salary in his last three years of work. If a worker has zero chance of dying, if the firm has zero chance of failing or otherwise terminating the pension, and if the worker has zero chance of being terminated, then the present value of the pension should be equal to the present value of the reductions in

---

14. If the Viscusi and Moore analysis is correct, this paper appears to suffer from a misspecification of the estimating equation, which appears to understate the compensating wage differential.

wages over the entire working life. This implies a lifetime trade-off. The early pension literature viewed the pension as being sold to the worker in the "spot market," where pension benefits earned in a given year had to be offset by a reduction in the year's wages. The proper view, according to the broader theory, is that there exists a "lifetime implicit contract" between the worker and the employer. That contract says if you stay with the firm for your working life you will receive an inflation-adjusted pension upon retirement.

This approach generates a number of testable implications. Most important for our purposes is that the value of the pension need not be equal to the forgone wages in any single time period. Second, it implies that workers will overpay for their accrued pensions in the early years of employment and underpay as they near retirement. Thus the pension ties the workers to the firm; if they leave too early they will receive a reduced pension.[15] Note that this prediction is consistent with the Schiller and Weiss paper discussed above, in which young workers paid "too much."

To my knowledge Montgomery and colleagues (1990) offered the first test of compensating differentials for pension in this lifetime model. They match 1983 Survey of Consumer Finances data (from the IRS) with detailed information on pension plans and demographic characteristics of individual workers. Using the standard spot market model, they find only a negligible trade-off between wages and pensions. But when lifetime wages were imputed and used in the models they found a coefficient of –.8, suggesting that 80 percent of the pension was offset by lifetime wages. Since workers do die before retirement, pension plans do fail on occasion, and workers are terminated before retirement, the 80 percent adjustment is plausible. Indeed, it is dramatic evidence of compensating wage differentials.

---

15. In practice this is exactly what a defined benefit pension plan does. Once vested, a worker will receive a pension that is some percentage of the average wage of the last few years of employment. Someone who leaves after vesting but before the intended retirement window will still receive the average of his last few years with the firm. If you would retire in the year 2010, quitting in the year 1990 means that your pension stops being inflation-adjusted. It will be based upon your income over the late 1980s.

The element of lifetime employment may seem atypical of the U.S. labor market. This is not the case. Over the 1963–1979 period more than 25 percent of workers were holding jobs that would last twenty years or more. The jobs held by middle-aged workers with ten years of tenure are pretty stable. Over the span of a decade only 20 to 30 percent of the jobs came to an end. Among workers aged thirty or above in 1980, about 40 percent were working in jobs that eventually would last twenty years or more (Hall 1982).

Summary and Conclusions

This chapter has examined the reform proposals that require employers to provide health insurance to their workers. First, it reviewed the estimates of the number of uninsured and insured people who would be affected by the mandates. The extent of coverage and the estimated costs were presented. Second, it put the reform proposals in the context of the labor market and argued that the proposals would result in a tax on uninsured workers—that is, that the cost of the expanded benefits would be borne largely by the workers themselves. Finally, the chapter examined the empirical literature on the extent to which wages really do adjust to the presence of fringe benefits.

The estimates suggest that approximately 34 million Americans are uninsured. Of this group, 80 to 85 percent are affiliated with the work force directly or through an employed family member. The most recent estimates suggest that just over half, or 17.4 million, of the uninsured would obtain coverage under a proposal that mandates coverage for those working more than ten hours a week in firms with twenty-five or more workers. Another 20 million would be affected by moving from a public plan to an employer plan, switching from an individually purchased plan to an employer-sponsored plan, or shifting from one employer plan to another. An additional large group of perhaps 26 million would find that their existing coverage would expand to reflect the minimum coverage in some plans.

The theory of compensating differentials implies that currently uninsured workers will pay for the mandated benefits in the form of lower money wages. Taxpayers generally will share in the cost of these benefits in the form of tax revenues forgone. Under existing tax laws the maximum taxpayer share is about one-third. Unemployment effects are likely to be small. They exist only to the extent that the cost of the benefits cannot be offset by reduced wages. This occurs if the affected workers do not value health insurance benefits very highly or if the minimum wage laws prevent the compensating differential from taking place.

No empirical literature shows the presence of compensating wage differentials for employer-sponsored health insurance. Nevertheless, there are conceptually straightforward but operationally complex reasons to be skeptical of these findings. Improved data and more sophisticated methodology in the areas of workers' compensation and pensions have found strong evidence of wage levels that compensate for more generous benefit plans.

At the very least, the review of the theory and related empirical work suggests that one cannot dismiss out of hand the compensating differential story. There is strong theory and a growing body of empirical literature that suggests workers will pay for the health benefits they receive. If workers do pay for health benefits they receive, then much of the policy proposals appear to be off the mark. The questions are not whether employers should pay their fair share, or whether small businesses or part-time workers should be subsidized or exempted. The questions should be:

- Does this society wish to compel individuals to purchase health insurance?
- If so, how much insurance and how much compulsion?
- Should general tax revenues be used to subsidize the purchase of health insurance?
- If so, how much of a subsidy, to whom should it be provided, and in what form?

The uninsured are certainly not as well organized as the elderly. Yet if the experience of the Medicare Catastrophic Coverage Act teaches anything, it is that when people are compelled to pay for expanded insurance coverage, they do not necessarily see themselves as better off. Before we risk again proceeding down the wrong path, perhaps we should try to answer the right questions.

References

Blendon, Robert J., and Jennifer N. Edwards. "Caring for the Uninsured: Choices for Reform." *Journal of the American Medical Association* 265 (1991): 2563–65.

Brown, Charles. "Comment." In *The Measurement of Labor Cost*. Edited by Jack E. Triplett. Chicago: University of Chicago Press, 1983.

———. "Minimum Wage Laws: Are They Overrated?" *Journal of Economic Perspectives* 2 (1988): 133–46.

Chollet, Deborah J. "A Profile of the Nonelderly Population without Health Insurance." In *Government Mandating of Employee Benefits*. Washington, D.C.: Employee Benefits Research Institute, 1987.

———. "Uninsured Workers: Sources and Dimensions of the Problem." Paper presented at the annual meeting of the Allied Social Sciences Associations, New York, 1988.

Congressional Budget Office. *Selected Options for Expanding Health Insurance Coverage*. Washington, D.C.: U.S. Government Printing Office, 1991.

Danzon, Patricia M. "Mandated Employer-Based Health Insurance: Incidence and Efficiency Effects." Discussion paper no. 66. Philadelphia: Leonard Davis Institute for Health Economics, University of Pennsylvania, 1989.

Ehrenberg, Ronald G. "Retirement System Characteristics and Compensating Wage Differentials in the Public Sector." *Industrial and Labor Relations Review* 33 (1980): 470–83.

Foley, Jill D. *Uninsured in the United States: The Nonelderly Population without Health Insurance.* EBRI Special Report SR–10. Washington, D.C.: Employee Benefit Research Institute, 1991.

Goldstein, Gerald S., and Mark V. Pauly. "Group Health Insurance as a Local Public Good." In *The Role of Health Insurance in the Health Services Sector.* Edited by Richard Rosett. Chicago: University of Chicago Press, 1976.

Gruber, Jonathan, and Alan B. Krueger. "The Incidence of Mandated Employer-Provided Insurance: Lessons from Workers' Compensation Insurance." Working paper 3557. New York: National Bureau of Economic Research, 1990.

Hall, Robert E. "The Importance of Lifetime Jobs in the U. S. Economy." *American Economics Review* 72 (1982): 716–24.

Holahan, John, and Sheila Zedlewski. *Insuring Low-Income Americans Through Medicaid Expansion.* Report 3836–02. Washington, D.C.: The Urban Institute, 1989.

Ippolito, Richard A. "The Implicit Pension Contract: Developments and New Directions." *Journal of Human Resources* 22 (1987): 441–67.

Jensen, Gail A. "Employer Choice of Wage Supplements." Working paper. Chicago: University of Illinois at Chicago, 1986.

Leibowitz, Arleen. "Fringe Benefits and Employee Compensation." In *The Measurement of Labor Cost.* Edited by J. E. Triplett. Chicago: University of Chicago Press, 1983.

Monheit, Alan C., Michael M. Hagan, B. L. Berk, and Pamela J. Farley. "The Employed Uninsured and the Role of Public Policy." *Inquiry* 22 (1985): 348–64.

Montgomery, Edward, Kathryn Shaw, and Mary Ellen Benedict. "Pensions and Wages: An Hedonic Price Theory Approach." Working paper 3458. New York: National Bureau of Economic Research, 1990.

Moore, Michael J., and W. Kip Viscusi. *Compensation Mechanisms for Job Risks.* Princeton, N.J.: Princeton University Press, 1990.

Morrisey, Michael A. "Health Care Reform: A Review of Five Generic Proposals." In *Winners and Losers in Reforming the U.S. Health Care System,* EBRI Special Report SR–11. Washington, D.C.: Employee Benefit Research Institute, 1991.

Moyer, M. Eugene. "A Revised Look at the Number of Uninsured Americans." *Health Affairs* 8 (1989): 102–10.

Needleman, Jack, Judith Arnold, John Sheils, and Lawrence S. Lewin. *The Health Care Financing System and the Uninsured.* Washington, D.C.: Lewin-ICF, 1990.

Pauly, Mark V., Patricia Danzon, Paul Feldstein, and John Hoff. "A Plan for 'Responsible National Health Insurance.'" *Health Affairs* 10 (1991): 5–25.

Reinhardt, Uwe E. "Health Care Spending and American Competitiveness." *Health Affairs* 8 (1989): 5–21.

Schiller, Bradley R., and Randall D. Weiss. "Pensions and Wages: A Test for Equalizing Differences." *Review of Economics and Statistics* 62 (1980): 529–38.

Scott, Frank A., Mark C. Berger, and Dan A. Black. "Effects of the Tax Treatment of Fringe Benefits on Labor Market Segmentation." *Industrial and Labor Relations Review* 42 (1989): 216–29.

Sloan, Frank A., and Killard Adamache. "Taxation and the Growth of Nonwage Compensation." *Public Finance Quarterly* 14(1986):115–37.

Smith, Adam. *The Wealth of Nations.* Reprint edition. Chicago: University of Chicago Press, 1976.

Smith, Robert S., and Ronald G. Ehrenberg. "Estimating Wage-Fringe Benefit Trade-offs: Some Data Problems." In *The Measurement of Labor Cost.* Edited by Jack E. Triplett. Chicago: University of Chicago Press, 1983.

Summers, Lawrence H. "Some Economics of Mandated Benefits." *American Economic Review* 79(1989):177–83.

Swartz, Katherine. "The Uninsured and Workers without Employer-Group Health Insurance." Working paper, The Urban Institute, Washington, D.C., 1988.

Thorpe, Kenneth E. "Costs and Distributional Impacts of Employer Health Insurance Mandates and Medicaid Expansion." *Inquiry* 26 (1989):335–44.

Thorpe, Kenneth E., Joanna E. Siegel, and Theresa Dailey. "Including the Poor: The Fiscal Impacts of Medicaid Expansion." *Journal of the American Medical Association* 261(1989):1003–07.

Viscusi, W. Kip, and Michael J. Moore. "Workers' Compensation: Wage Effects, Benefit Inadequacies, and the Value of Health Losses." *Review of Economics and Statistics* 69(1987):249–61.

Wessels, Walter J. "The Effect of Minimum Wages in the Presence of Fringe Benefits: An Expanded Model." *Economic Inquiry* 18(1980):293–313.

151

7

The Dilemma of Affordability—Health Insurance for Small Businesses

Catherine G. McLaughlin

The medically uninsured population continues to be a subject of policy and research interest. This interest stems in part from the fact that this population is large—between 13 and 18 percent of the nonaged population—and growing in size (Moyer 1989; Butler 1988). In addition, more than one-third are children, and three-quarters are working adults and their dependents, historically considered the "deserving poor" (Short, Monheit, and Beauregard 1989). Therefore much of the research and several of the proposed solutions aimed at reducing the number of medically uninsured individuals have focused on the so called working uninsured.

More than one-half of these uninsured working individuals are employed by firms with twenty-five or fewer employees (Short, Monheit, and Beauregard 1989, 13). Little is known about these individuals or, more important, about their employers. Although many of the small-business owners we interviewed pronounced themselves "the backbone of American industry," they have been neglected by most researchers. Until recently, the few surveys of small businesses that had been conducted were of limited use—often relying on restrictive membership lists for their sample and experiencing very low response rates. The studies were consistent, however, in their estimates of lower rates of health insurance coverage among small businesses (ICF, Inc. 1987; Hall and Kuder 1990; Health Insurance Association of America 1991).

Questions remain about which small businesses do not offer health insurance, why they do not offer health insurance, and whether there is a private-sector solution. That is, is there some way to increase employment-based private health insurance in the small-business market? Or are the supply or demand barriers such that some form of governmental intervention is needed if policy makers want to reduce the

152

number of uninsured individuals? Clearly the ability of any proposed policy to cause a notable reduction in the number of working uninsured depends on whether the correct incentive is being sent to a population likely to respond. Without a sound understanding of whether and what private market failures may exist, any policy enacted is likely to be ineffective.

The Myths about Why Small Businesses
Do Not Offer Health Insurance

Although many reasons for the lack of insurance in the small-business market have been put forward, most fall into the four following categories:

1. *Lack of products*. It has been suggested that there are too few insurers with a book of business in this market (Committee on Small Business 1987). Many of the large national insurers have stopped marketing to these businesses, usually citing nonprofitability, and those that do offer a product usually limit their small-group business.

2. *Lack of information*. Even if products are out there, there may be a problem getting information about these products to small-business owners and their employees. Small businesses have no benefit managers; the typical owner-manager is usually not well-versed in the details of health insurance, is not aware of what is out there, and does not have the time to look.

3. *Lack of demand*. The small-business employee is younger than the typical large-business employee, with a lower level of educational attainment and a higher turnover probability (Monheit and Short 1989). Small businesses may not need to offer health insurance to attract their desired employees. The "young invincibles" may not perceive a need for health insurance and therefore are not willing to give up *any* wages to get health insurance.

4. *Lack of affordable products*. In addition to being younger, the typical small-business employee is also lower paid. Workers in large companies earn approximately 35 percent more than those in small businesses (Brown, Hamilton, and Medoff 1990). At the same time, small group premiums are 10–40 percent higher for small employers, because of higher loading factors and perceived higher risks (ICF, Inc., 1987; GAO 1991). With approximately one-half of the employees earning less than $5.00 per hour, the opportunity cost of trading wages for available health insurance packages may be too high (Monheit and Short 1989). Not only is the premium higher; since only 25 percent of the health insurance premium paid by employers is tax deductible for unincorporated

153

businesses (sole proprietors and partnerships), which compose approx-imately 40 percent of the small businesses in our sample, the tax advantage for employers is smaller for many as well.

Clearly the reason for the large number of working uninsured in the small-business market would influence what intervention is appropriate and whether a private-market solution is viable. If lack of information is the primary cause, for example, establishing some sort of clearinghouse and distributing concisely written descriptions of packages available is a rather straightforward solution. But if insurance companies are not willing to market a product to the small-business community at a price that employees are willing to pay, then little hope exists for a private-market solution without some kind of subsidy.

The Evidence about Why Small Businesses
Do Not Offer Health Insurance

In 1985 the Robert Wood Johnson Foundation (RWJF) committed $6.5 million to the Program for the Medically Uninsured, to investigate who the uninsured are for fifteen projects and to design and test variations on a market approach (see appendix 7–A). Lawrence D. Brown of Columbia University and I are evaluating that program. In addition to putting together information gathered by the project staff about the fifteen projects, we surveyed more than 1,300 small businesses—those with twenty-five or fewer employees, working seventeen or more hours per week—in four project sites—Denver, Flint, Tampa, and Tucson. We also surveyed forty-three insurers in those same four sites, as well as eleven national companies with a large book of business in the small-group market. Even though several of the RWJF projects are still too new to evaluate fairly, several lessons have been learned from the projects and surveys that give insight into the causes for the lower rates of insurance in the small-business market.

Lack of Products. A number of the projects found that there is a substantial supply of insurance products available to small businesses. In 1986 the project staff in San Francisco found more than 150 products in the Bay Area alone (Bay Area Health Task Force 1988). Contrary to claims that HMOs will not offer a small-group package, the staff found that many HMOs in the area marketed directly to small business. Insurance experts on the advisory panel estimated that there are at least 2,000 different options available from the various sources selling health insurance. The results of a 1986 survey of eighty-four insurance companies conducted by the Wisconsin project staff portrayed the

TABLE 7–1
ESTIMATED PERCENTAGE OF FIRMS OFFERING HEALTH INSURANCE,
BY SIZE OF FIRM, 1990

	2–5	6–9	10–25
Tucson	40	52	77
Tampa	51	62	71
Flint	51	53	85
Denver	49	82	95

NOTE: Size of firm is measured as number of persons working more than thirty-four hours per week.
SOURCE: Small Business Benefits Survey, 1990.

small-group market as "extremely competitive, with a wide range of available products which were aggressively marketed to employers" (Wisconsin Department of Health and Social Services 1988). A broad array of small-group products was also found in a 1990 survey by the Colorado Division of Insurance. In part in response to these and similar findings, most of the RWJF projects decided not to develop their own products.

As we found in our employer surveys, however, there exist several gaps in the markets supposedly flush with small-group policies. First, many of the small-group policies are available only for firms with ten or more employees. Repeatedly our respondents said they had trouble obtaining insurance because they had fewer than ten full-time employees. In three of the four sites, we found a notable difference in the percentage of firms with fewer than ten employees that offer health insurance (table 7–1).

Second, specific businesses and their employees may have difficulty in finding products. Because of certain insurance industry underwriting practices, some individual employees are excluded because of preexisting conditions. In some cases the excluded individual causes the entire firm to be considered ineligible; in other cases the premium for the entire group is increased. In addition, approximately 15 percent of small firms fall into industries that are routinely redlined, the practice that excludes firms that the insurers consider uninsurable. The Colorado Division of Insurance found that preexisting-condition exclusions and redlining constituted a major problem for many small firms attempting to purchase insurance (Colorado Department of Regulatory Agencies 1990).

Our survey of insurers found systematic exclusions of certain businesses. We received copies of underwriting guidelines from thirteen of the insurers. In eleven of these cases, the guidelines included lists of industries considered ineligible. As explained by one insurer, these industries are considered "not acceptable because of the hazardous nature of the industry, the general high turnover of the employees within the industry, or the presence of certain underwriting problems." Another added, "Some industries are known to present high employer [sic] turnover, frequent claims submissions, older age content, and/or hazardous working conditions. These types of firms are not desirable risks for the plan." Other insurers will insure these industries, but they will add a substantial surcharge to the usual premium—as high as 60 percent. Certain companies with hazardous working conditions already pay high workers' compensation premiums—as high as $50 for every $100 of payroll for Denver construction firms—adding to the financial burden.

Many of the industries listed are typically made up of small businesses. So although the list may be relatively short, workers employed by small businesses may be disproportionately affected by these underwriting principles. The restricted businesses mentioned in at least nine of the cases were as follows:

- bars, taverns, liquor stores
- buses, limousines, taxi services
- construction
- entertainment—theaters, music studios, radio stations
- government agencies and municipalities
- hairdressing salons, beauty and barber shops
- hospitals and other allied medical services, nursing homes, and physician offices
- junkyards and salvage operations
- logging and sawmills
- mining operations
- security, detective, and collection agencies
- trucking firms

Although fewer than 3 percent of the respondents to our small-business survey said they were turned down because of their type of business, several mentioned difficulties in finding an insurer. For example, one employer in Denver reported: "For the longest time I couldn't find one. Who would insure us? It's hard to get insurance in the trucking business." Several of the agents we interviewed stressed the difference between "offering" a package to particular small groups—that is, being willing to price an insurance product to a small business that comes to the agent requesting coverage—and "marketing" a package, or actively seeking purchasers.

The third gap in coverage exists for part-time workers. With only one exception, the fifty-four health insurance companies we interviewed

TABLE 7–2

ESTIMATED PERCENTAGE OF EMPLOYEES WITH EMPLOYMENT-BASED HEALTH
INSURANCE, BY HOURS WORKED, 1990

	Part-Time (17–29 hrs.)	Full-Time (30 or more hrs.)
Tucson	19.5	45.0
Tampa	27.2	54.6
Flint	14.0	48.6
Denver	16.5	61.2

SOURCE: Small Business Benefits Survey, 1990.

restricted benefit availability to full-time employees, usually defined as working at least thirty hours per week. Small businesses typically have a larger proportion of part-time workers (Short, Monheit, and Beauregard 1989). In our sample of small-business employees, the percentage of full-time workers with employment-based health insurance was two to three times greater than the percentage of those working fewer than thirty hours with insurance (table 7–2).

Because of the types of businesses and workers excluded, there may be a lack of products for some small businesses and some of their employees, but availability is not the problem for all. Few of our respondents mentioned this as an important reason for not offering health insurance to their employees.

Lack of Information. In their study of small businesses, the Denver project staff found that only 17 percent of the employers without insurance complained that a lack of information was a problem (Denver Department of Health and Hospitals 1988). In fact some of our survey respondents complained about getting too many calls about health insurance, estimating that they received two to three calls per week from insurance agents.

Information dissemination may need improvement, however. The difficulty is not necessarily the volume of information available, but rather that the market is characterized by misinformation and inadequate methods of getting the needed information to purchasers. Several surveys also revealed that small-business owners do not always trust insurance agents. In our survey, a common complaint was summarized by one employer as, "Most health insurance companies for the small business are all crooks." Another frequently expressed concern was about the instability of insurers and the churning of the market. As expressed by one employer in Tampa, "You are with a company for six months and then something happens to them. They have affordable rates

157

and all the agents sell it out, and when the claims start coming in they can't pay them and go out of business, or it takes three–four months to pay the claim, and you are left high and dry, or they want to get out of the state, and so they double the premium to get rid of you."

The San Francisco project staff discovered that a key problem for small businesses centered on the lack of usable information upon which to base a purchasing decision. Employers complained about the paucity of "good" information enabling them to evaluate different plans; insurers also stated that there is insufficient usable information. In response to this the staff developed a guidebook of available health insurance products, and they maintain an employer hotline, which employers can call for referrals or information. As of May 1991 more than 3,000 calls had been placed to the hotline, resulting in approximately 255 businesses purchasing insurance for about 875 individuals (Alpha Center 1991).

Although lack of information or misinformation can serve as a barrier, fewer than 25 percent of the employers we surveyed who do not offer health insurance indicated that an unbiased source of information about available health insurance packages would play an important role in influencing their decision to offer insurance.

Lack of Demand. Several of the projects found that there is a fairly hard-core group of small-business owners who do not want to provide health insurance benefits to their employees. Usually these employers state that this lack of coverage reflects a lack of demand on the part of their employees, that they can recruit employees without it, and that most of their employees are covered elsewhere. In a West Virginia survey of small businesses, 53 percent of the firms not offering insurance said they were not interested in doing so (Pollard et al. 1988). In a San Francisco survey, 45 percent of the employers not currently offering insurance indicated they would not be interested in doing so (Bay Area Health Task Force 1988). In Tennessee, 39 percent of the interviewees said they were not interested in offering health insurance, with several offering the opinion that the *job* was the benefit and that the employee was lucky to be working (Tennessee Primary Care Association 1987).

More than half the employers in our survey who do not offer insurance indicated they were not interested in doing so. Almost 20 percent of these firms used to offer health insurance. Consistent with this claim of no interest, when asked to indicate if any of six possible programs would influence them to offer health insurance—including access to an unbiased source of information, administrative help, and financial aid to the firm or employee—employers who had indicated they were not interested in offering insurance were consistently less enthusiastic about any of the programs than were the other employers who do not currently offer health insurance. For each of the six programs, 10–20 percent of those not interested in offering insurance indicated that it would influence them to offer a plan, whereas 50–75 percent of the other employers indicated that the program would influence their decision.

The majority of employers who do not offer health insurance said an important reason was that their employees were not interested, either because they had coverage through another source, such as a spouse's policy, or because they would rather have higher wages. Lack of demand on the part of a subset of employees can result in the entire firm being without coverage, since most insurers require 75 percent or even 100 percent participation by eligible employees in small firms. Although we did not get information from the employees about their preferences, we did gather information about whether they were covered through another source and about their wages.

Not surprisingly, a significantly higher proportion of workers in firms that do not offer health insurance have insurance through another source—approximately 75 percent versus 30 percent in firms that offer insurance to their employees. Most employers not offering insurance claim that their employees do not want insurance because of other coverage. Interestingly, though, when asked about individual employee coverage, approximately 25 percent of these employers noted that fewer than 50 percent of their employees had insurance coverage through another source, and on average employers did not know whether an employee had other coverage for close to 20 percent of their employees.

Unfortunately we do not know whether these employers are in fact responding to the demands of their workers, or their employees sought coverage from another source because the employer would not offer health insurance, or they were willing to take this uncovered job only because they knew they could get insurance through another source.

It is also possible that individuals who do not want to trade wages for health insurance seek jobs in firms that do not offer health insurance. Consistent with the young-invincible theory, we found that young (under twenty-five years of age) unmarried workers are more likely to work for firms that do not offer insurance and are less likely to have either employment-based insurance or to be covered through another source.

More than 80 percent of the firms that offer health insurance to their employees indicated that an important reason for offering health insurance was the need to keep their employees. According to our survey results, 60–75 percent of workers who are offered a health insurance plan by their employers elect to participate. Of the 25–40 percent who choose not to participate, 70–80 percent have coverage through another source.

In all four survey sites, those workers who have employment-

TABLE 7–3
AVERAGE WAGE BY INSURANCE STATUS, 1990
(dollars per hour)

| | With Health Insurance | | |
	Employment-based	Other source[a]	Without Health Insurance
Tucson	11.26	9.28	6.97
Tampa	11.20	9.22	7.73
Flint	9.89	9.02	7.49
Denver	12.64	9.86	9.19

a. Do not participate in employment-based benefit plan, but noted as having insurance through another source, such as a spouse's policy.
SOURCE: Small Business Benefits Survey, 1990.

based health insurance earn more than those who have insurance through another source, who in turn earn more than those who have no insurance (table 7–3). Of course, without better controls for other factors that determine total compensation, it is impossible to say what the trade-off is between wages and health insurance and other fringe benefits. Those firms offering health insurance not only pay higher average wages but are also more likely to offer other fringe benefits to their workers, such as paid vacation, sick leave, long-term disability insurance, life insurance, and a retirement plan (table 7–4).

Lack of Affordable Products. While the evidence on lack of demand is inconclusive, without exception all of the studies reviewed cite cost as the primary reason why employers do not offer health insurance. In our survey, 80 percent of the employers offering insurance indicated that an important factor in influencing their decision to offer was that they found an affordable plan; 85 percent of the employers not offering insurance said that high premium cost was an important reason they did not offer. Half of the 300 employers who added comments to the end of the questionnaire complained about the high and rising cost of health insurance. Many were as concerned about the rapid increase in premiums as the actual level, often citing doubling of premiums after one or two years of initial enrollment.

Most employers claimed that they could not pass on these higher operating costs to their customers. Although most could not define price elasticity of demand, they clearly understand the concept. One employer in Tampa put it this way: "As a pub serving alcoholic beverages, we pay very high fire, liability and workmen's comp insurance. We also have a

TABLE 7–4

AVERAGE WAGE AND PERCENTAGE OF COMPANIES OFFERING SELECT BENEFITS,
FOR FIRMS WITH AND WITHOUT HEALTH INSURANCE, 1990

	Tucson		Tampa		Flint		Denver	
	With	With-out	With	With-out	With	With-out	With	With-out
Wage	$11.30	$7.75	$10.89	$9.14	$10.87	$9.31	$12.18	$9.67

Percentage of Companies Offering Benefits

Paid vacation	68	45	80	55	66	50	69	45
Sick leave	51	23	68	34	47	24	56	32
Long-term disability	21	3	29	5	31	8	28	6
Life insurance	33	3	63	3	45	4	47	7
Retirement	26	3	26	6	27	7	24	6

SOURCE: Small Business Benefits Survey, 1990.

very extensive licensing and operating fee. Beer drinkers are notoriously cheap—they will go where the prices are best." Many small businesses face competition not only among themselves, but also with large companies offering the same product. In addition to benefiting from certain economies of scale that lower their operating costs, those large companies also enjoy lower premiums for the same health insurance package and higher tax advantages.

Many small businesses are operating on low profit margins. The failure rate among small businesses is relatively high—in any given year, approximately 20 percent go out of business. The average age of firms offering insurance was only slightly higher than that of those not offering insurance, but those offering insurance were significantly larger and richer, as measured by revenue per full-time equivalents (table 7–5). Approximately 25 percent of the firms that do not offer health insurance report grossing less than $30,000 per employee.

Employers who do not offer health insurance claim their workers are not willing to take a pay cut to get health insurance. Those that do offer insurance claim that rather than cut wages if faced with another premium increase, they will have to cut down on the number of employees. With average monthly premiums ranging from a low of $112 to a high of $496 per enrolled employee, which translates into a cost of 70 cents to $3.10 per hour for health insurance, many low-wage employees have little room within which they can pursue wage-fringe

TABLE 7–5

AVERAGE NUMBER OF FULL-TIME EQUIVALENTS, REVENUE PER FTE, AND AGE OF
BUSINESS, FOR FIRMS WITH AND WITHOUT HEALTH INSURANCE, 1990

	Tucson		Tampa		Flint		Denver	
	With	With-out	With	With-out	With	With-out	With	With-out
FTE	7.1	4.6	6.4	4.8	6.9	5.9	7.2	3.8
Rev/FTE	$90	$66	$106	$74	$86	$66	$84	$84
Age	16.6	15.5	15.5	12.3	21.0	19.9	16.4	15.0

NOTE: FTE is full-time equivalent; Rev/FTE is revenue per FTE, in thousands; and Age refers to age of business, in years.
SOURCE: Small Business Benefits Survey, 1990.

benefit trade-offs. Not surprisingly, proportionately more employees earning $5 or less per hour are without employment-based health insurance (table 7–6). For these individuals, the opportunity cost of health insurance may be too high.

What to Do?

The results of the RWJF projects and of our surveys indicate that if policy makers want to make substantial reductions in the number of working, uninsured individuals, a variety of public and private interventions may be needed. For some subset of this population, various private-sector solutions are possible. For example, because of current underwriting practices, certain individuals and certain businesses face a lack of products. The Tampa program is underwriting only 3 percent of its enrollees, and a few RWJF projects are "taking all comers." If the early utilization data are any indication, the experiences of these groups indicate that certain underwriting practices may be based on inaccurate data. In this case, changing insurers' views or reforming the small-business insurance market may result in increased coverage. For other firms, increased dissemination of unbiased and useful information about insurance products already available to them may lead to improved working of the market.

It is doubtful, however, that these rather simple, low-cost interventions will make a substantial dent in the number of medically uninsured individuals. For some workers and their families, the cost of health insurance is "too high"—that is, they are not willing or able to ratchet down their wages to obtain health insurance. Most of the RWJF projects offer subsidized health insurance premiums. In several cases these

TABLE 7–6
DISTRIBUTION OF EMPLOYEES, BY HOURLY WAGE AND PARTICIPATION IN
EMPLOYMENT-BASED HEALTH INSURANCE, 1990
(percent)

	Tucson		Tampa		Flint		Denver	
	Yes	No	Yes	No	Yes	No	Yes	No
<$3.80	1.0	5.2	3.1	3.3	2.2	6.7	2.0	4.0
$3.80–5.00	6.8	24.8	5.3	18.7	14.9	27.5	2.5	13.7
$5.01–10.00	50.9	50.8	47.8	55.6	40.8	45.7	40.2	55.6
$10.00–15.00	21.3	13.5	23.5	13.4	26.8	12.8	26.5	17.2
>$15.00	20.0	5.7	20.3	9.0	15.3	7.3	28.8	9.5

SOURCE: Small Business Benefits Survey, 1990.

subsidies come from the state, in other cases the subsidies stem from reduced rates offered by providers. In Florida, for example, the state is providing reinsurance, which lowered the premium by approximately 25 percent. In Michigan the state paid for 33 percent of the premium for qualified employees. In Salt Lake City the hospitals agreed to a lower rate for project participants, lowering the premium by 40 percent.

The program in Tampa has been very popular to date, with approximately 17 percent of the small firms without health insurance enrolling. In other cases, however, even the subsidized premiums were not considered low enough by the small businesses in the area. The project staff of the RWJF program in Utah has found that even with the 40 percent discount, they are having problems convincing small-business employers to purchase insurance for their employees. The program in Flint, Michigan, was able to enroll fewer than 100 firms. The programs in Denver and Tucson, with indirect subsidies from the public sector, have enrolled fewer than 5 percent of the small businesses that were not offering health insurance.

A variety of other low-cost policies with limited benefits have been offered to small businesses, with few takers (Hinds 1991). These low enrollments could be the result of several factors: the subsidy is not large enough to make the premiums affordable (several employers in both Flint and Tampa discussed the state-subsidized program and indicated that even at those lower premiums, they would go out of business offering the insurance); employers are skeptical about how long the subsidy will last (in Flint, several employers expressed doubt about the state's willingness and ability to continue the subsidy); some individuals may not be willing or able to sacrifice any wages for health insurance.

It is not clear what size of subsidy would be needed to make substantial reductions in the number of uninsured individuals, but it is not likely that these subsidies would come from the private sector alone. Some public intervention, either through subsidies or some form of play-or-pay tax program, seems inevitable *if* policy makers want to reach low-income workers. Many of the employers we surveyed expressed very strong negative views toward government intervention in general; for example, "Please let's keep all those control-and-power greedy politicians out of running our businesses and lives," and, "I don't want government getting involved with the health insurance issue. Any time they get involved they mess things up." Nevertheless, the only two proposed programs that met with favorable response from more than two-thirds of the firms not currently offering insurance made either the company or the employees eligible for government assistance with premium costs. The firms said these programs would influence them to offer insurance.

Although the young are more likely to be in small firms that do not offer insurance, the not-so-young, not-so-invincible still account for the overwhelming majority of these employees, and 40 percent of them do not have coverage through another source. Although lack of insurance may lead to underutilization of certain health care services, many working, uninsured individuals and their families do receive some health care services, often in hospital emergency rooms and often resulting in uncompensated care. A new study also suggests that, despite the availability of an uncompensated care pool for paying hospitals, uninsured persons admitted to the hospital for heart attacks face a higher risk of dying (Young and Cohen 1991). Reducing the number of working uninsured would not only improve the efficiency of the market, but also reduce such untoward health effects. Our results indicate that merely reforming the small-business insurance market and encouraging small-business owners to provide health insurance will not make a significant dent in the number of working uninsured.

Appendix 7–A
List of Robert Wood Johnson Foundation Project Locations

The fifteen Robert Wood Johnson Foundation Health Care for the Uninsured Program projects are located in fourteen states. Several projects established demonstrations in multiple sites within the state. They are as follows:

- Alabama (Birmingham)
- Arizona (Tucson and Phoenix)
- California (San Diego)

- California (San Francisco)
- Colorado (Denver-Boulder CMSA, Fort Collins, and Colorado Springs)
- Florida (Tampa-St. Petersburg-Clearwater MSA, and Tallahassee rural areas)
- Maine (Bath-Brunswick and Skowhegan-Somerset)
- Massachusetts (Boston)
- Michigan (Flint and Marquette)
- New Jersey (statewide)
- Tennessee (Memphis)
- Utah (Salt Lake City)
- Washington (statewide)
- West Virginia (statewide)
- Wisconsin (Appleton)

References

Alpha Center. *Health Care for the Uninsured Program Update.* Washington, D.C.: Alpha Center, July 1991.

Bay Area Health Task Force. *Final Report.* San Francisco: United Way of the Bay Area, May 1988.

Brown, Charles, James Hamilton, and James Medoff. *Employers Large and Small.* Cambridge: Harvard University Press, 1990.

Butler, Patricia A. *Too Poor to Be Sick: Access to Medical Care for the Uninsured.* Washington, D.C.: American Public Health Association, 1988.

Colorado Department of Regulatory Agencies, Division of Insurance. *Health Insurance Availability and Affordability in Colorado: A Report on Underwriting and Pricing Practices.* Denver: Division of Insurance, 1990.

Committee on Small Business, House of Representatives. *The Health Insurance Problem: Alternative Strategies to Expand Coverage among Small Businesses.* Washington, D.C.: U.S. Government Printing Office, December 1987.

Denver Department of Health and Hospitals. *Survey of Small Employers in the Denver Metropolitan Area.* Denver: Denver Department of Health and Hospitals, Health Care for the Uninsured Program, Shared Cost Option for Private Employers (SCOPE), September 1988.

General Accounting Office. See United States General Accounting Office.

Hall, Charles P., Jr., and John M. Kuder. *Small Business and Health Care: Results of a Survey.* Washington, D.C.: National Federation of Independent Businesses, 1990.

Health Insurance Association of America. *Health Care Financing for All Americans.* Washington, D.C.: Health Insurance Association of America, 1991.

Hinds, Michael deCourcy. "Movement to Sell Basic Health Plan is Found

Faltering." *New York Times* (November 10, 1991).

ICF, Inc. *Health Care Coverage and Costs in Small and Large Businesses, Final Report.* Washington, D.C.: ICF, Inc. Prepared for the U.S. Small Business Administration, April 1987.

Monheit, Alan C., and Pamela Farley Short. "The Economics of Health Insurance Offerings by Small Firms." Chicago: Paper presented at the Annual Meeting of the American Public Health Association, October 23, 1989.

Moyer, M. Eugene. "Data Watch: A Revised Look at the Number of Uninsured Americans." *Health Affairs* 8(Summer 1989):102–10.

Pollard, Cecil, Valerie Frey-McClung, Stephanie Pratt, and Paul M. Furbee. *Health Insurance Coverage: A Study of Small Business in West Virginia.* Morgantown: West Virginia University, Department of Community Medicine, September 1988.

Short, Pamela Farley, Alan C. Monheit, and Karen Beauregard. *A Profile of Uninsured Americans.* Washington, D.C.: Department of Health and Human Services. DHHS Publication no. 89–3443, September 1989.

Tennessee Primary Care Association. *Marketing Assessment: Developing a Managed Care Plan for the Uninsured in Tennessee.* Nashville: Tennessee Primary Care Association, May 1987.

United States General Accounting Office. *Private Health Insurance: Problems Caused by a Segmented Market.* Washington, D.C.: United States General Accounting Office, Report to the Chairman, Subcommittee on Health, Committee on Ways and Means, House of Representatives. USGAO Publication no. GAO/HRD–91–114, July 1991.

Wisconsin Department of Health and Social Services. *Annual Progress Report, Small Employer Health Insurance Maximization Project: Making the Market Work.* Madison: Wisconsin DHSS, Division of Health, 1988.

Young, Gary J., and Bruce B. Cohen. "Inequities in Hospital Care: The Massachusetts Experience." *Inquiry* 28 (Fall 1991): 255–62.

8
Regulating the Content of Health Plans

Gail A. Jensen

Among the fastest-growing areas of regulation affecting the market for health insurance are state-mandated benefits. These state laws prescribe the terms of coverage for group health insurance purchased from Blue Cross–Blue Shield (BCBS) and commercial insurers. Mandates often apply to the coverage of particular providers, such as chiropractors, psychologists, and optometrists; to particular services, such as mammography screening, alcohol treatment, and drug abuse treatment; and to persons who must be insured by the plan, such as children with disabilities and terminated workers. This chapter describes the scope of these regulations, considers the question of why they exist, summarizes what is known about their effects in insurance and medical care markets, and raises a current policy issue concerning these regulations.

State-mandated benefits are important for three reasons. First, they have recently evolved into a major category of insurance regulation. At last count, there were approximately 850 mandates across the states (*Health Benefits Letter* 1991b), a number up from almost none in 1970 and roughly double the number in 1980. The rate of enactment of *new* mandates has dropped off somewhat since 1988; however, if modifications to existing mandates are included in the tally, then the rate of mandate enactment is still running strong.

Second, mandates can have some undesirable effects on employers' provision of insurance. Mandates may increase a firm's cost of offering group health insurance and, consequently, its cost of hiring labor. When cost increases, an employer may act in ways that attempt to deflect that cost. The firm, for example, may reduce workers' insurance benefits in nonmandated areas, require workers to pay a larger share of the premium, lower workers' wages, or reduce their other fringe benefits. If mandates are sufficiently burdensome, the firm may decide that insurance is simply not worth it, in which case it would decline to offer it at all. If the firm is large enough, it might self-insure. Section 514 of the 1974

167

Employee Retirement Income and Security Act (ERISA) gives self-insured plans an exemption from all state laws pertaining to insurance. Thus, by self-insuring, a firm is able to avoid all costs associated with mandates.

Third, by expanding insurance coverage, mandates may increase demand for various types of medical care. The prices for those services and total expenditures for those services may rise as a consequence. When an expansion of insurance coverage is involuntary, as it is for some groups under mandated benefits, then the value that consumers place on the additional medical services they purchase will be less than the incremental cost of bringing those services to market. From a consumer's standpoint, the marginal benefits of the expansion in coverage will be less than marginal costs. The increased expenditures for those services will be economically inefficient as a result, and society will incur a dead-weight loss.

The next section discusses the evolution of state-mandated benefits and some recent legislative developments in this area. The third section considers why the states mandate insurance coverage and the extent of empirical support for the different theories. The fourth section examines the known consequences of mandates: Who is affected? What do mandates cost? Do small firms forgo insurance as a result? Do large firms self-insure to avoid them? How do mandates affect medical service markets? The final section summarizes my findings and considers a federal-level policy question regarding these state regulations.

The Scope of State Insurance Regulations

Growth in Mandated Benefits. State governments have been regulating the terms of coverage for group plans for over two decades. Although the very first mandate, a requirement that dependent coverage include insurance for mentally and physically handicapped children, was enacted by Massachusetts in 1956, mandates in other content areas and other states did not appear until the mid-1960s (Blue Cross–Blue Shield 1989).

Some states then began requiring that coverage be extended to certain groups of persons who might otherwise find it difficult to obtain insurance. Handicapped children and newborns from the date of their birth were two such groups. Legislative activity was minimal and until the early 1970s restricted largely to mandates that broadened beneficiary groups. At that time several states began requiring policies to cover various nonphysician practitioners, such as psychologists, podiatrists, and dentists. Mandates for the coverage of particular services and conditions were not common until the late 1970s and early 1980s.

FIGURE 8–1
TRENDS IN MANDATED HEALTH CARE BENEFITS, 1970–1990

Number of Mandates

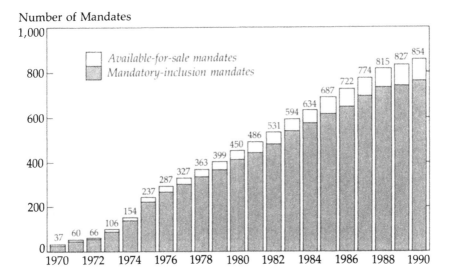

SOURCE: Data for 1970 through 1989 are from Blue Cross–Blue Shield 1989; and for 1990 from *Health Benefits Letter* 1991a.

Figure 8–1 shows the number of mandates enacted across all states for each year from 1970 to 1990. The collective total has risen from 37 in 1970 to 854 in 1990.[1] The mid-1970s and early 1980s were two peak periods of legislative activity, with an average of about 60 new mandates enacted per year between 1974 and 1976 and about 50 enacted per year between 1982 and 1984 (see figure 8–2). The rate of growth has dropped off slightly since then, with about 35 to 40 new mandates per year. In 1990, 27 mandates were newly enacted. As both figures show, nearly all mandates are mandatory-inclusion laws, a characteristic true in 1970 as well as today.

The typical state has about fifteen to seventeen mandates; however, there is considerable variation across states, as shown in figure 8–3. Delaware, South Carolina, Idaho, and Vermont have fewer than eight, while Connecticut, Maryland, and California have thirty or more. States with the most got an early start enacting them. Recent legislative activity

1. Data for 1970 through 1989 are from Blue Cross–Blue Shield (1989) and the 1990 count updates this source using *Health Benefits Letter* (1991a).

169

FIGURE 8–2
Number of New State-Mandated Benefits by Year, 1970–1990

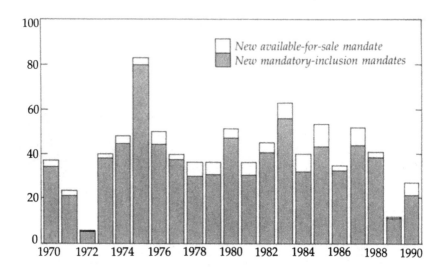

New available-for-sale mandate
New mandatory-inclusion mandates

Source: Data for 1970 through 1989 are from Blue Cross–Blue Shield 1989; and for 1990 from *Health Benefits Letter* 1991a.

has been concentrated in states that up until a few years ago had almost no mandates.

There are two types of mandated benefits. The more common category consists of minimum coverage standards for all group policies in a state. These laws, called "mandatory-inclusion" mandates, require that every policy sold contain certain provisions specified by the state, for example, twenty-eight days of inpatient alcohol rehabilitation coverage. The second category consists of laws that require insurers to offer certain coverages for sale; the decision of whether to purchase them is left to the buyer. These laws are called "available-for-sale" mandates. Distinguishing between the two is important, because only the first type has possible negative consequences for insurance and medical care markets.

As noted earlier, mandates can apply to providers, services, or beneficiary groups. Table 8–1 reports the most common mandates of each type, suggesting that available-for-sale mandates tend to be more common when particular services, rather than providers or beneficiary groups, are considered. This is indeed the case.

Usually all purchased group contracts in a state, regardless of

170

FIGURE 8–3

MANDATED HEALTH CARE BENEFITS BY STATE, 1990

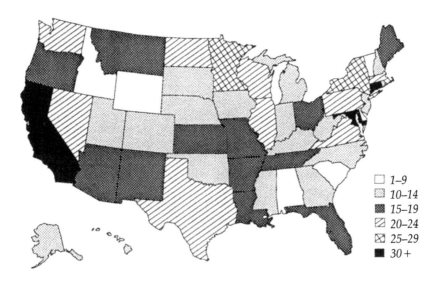

☐ 1–9
▨ 10–14
■ 15–19
▨ 20–24
⊠ 25–29
■ 30+

SOURCE: *Health Benefits Letter* 1991a.

vendor, must comply with mandates, with certain exceptions. In five states, however, some mandates apply to commercial insurers but not to Blue Cross–Blue Shield plans.[2] In other states health maintenance organizations (HMOs) are exempt from some mandates. In Minnesota, for example, while HMOs are not required to cover various nonphysician providers, other insurers must do so (State of Minnesota 1988).

Other Laws Affecting Group Coverage. All states tax commercial premiums, twenty-six tax BCBS premiums, and a few tax HMO premiums. The typical tax is 2 to 3 percent. Technically it is levied on insurers, not employers. Like other business expenses, however, the cost tends to be passed on to purchasers in the form of higher prices. Most states that operate risk pools for "uninsurable" individuals levy an additional tax on group plans, the revenues from which help subsidize pool premiums.

---

2. These are Delaware, Pennsylvania, Rhode Island, Virginia, and West Virginia (Blue Cross and Blue Shield 1989).

TABLE 8–1

MOST COMMON PROVIDER, BENEFIT, AND EXTENSION MANDATES, 1990

Required Coverage	Number of States with a Mandate	Number of States Requiring Mandatory-Inclusion	Number of States Requiring Available-for-Sale
Provider mandates			
Chiropractors	39	38	1
Psychologists	38	38	0
Optometrists	32	31	1
Dentists	28	28	0
Podiatrists	27	27	0
Benefit mandates			
Alcoholism treatment	39	29	10
Mammography screening	33	29	4
Mental health care	28	18	10
Drug abuse treatment	24	20	4
Maternity	20	19	1
Extension mandates			
Newborns	48	48	0
Handicapped dependents	34	34	0
Conversions to nongroup coverage	33	33	0
Continuation coverage for dependents	28	28	0
Continuation coverage for employees	25	24	1

Source: Author's tabulations based on data from *Health Benefits Letter* (1991a).

Other state laws also affect the terms of coverage in group plans. All states set minimum reserve requirements for insurers, to ensure their financial solvency. Usually it is set at 20 to 30 percent of premiums, and like premium taxes, it may vary according to the type of insurer. To protect consumers, states often require contract disclosures, bonding, auditing, and standardized printing of the terms of contracts. Finally, states have established coordination-of-benefit regulations for determining who shall pay and how much when someone is covered by more than one plan.

Recent Legislative Developments. Some state legislatures have begun to reconsider whether mandates are really in the best interests of their constituents. In 1989 and 1990 seventeen states passed twenty-two new

TABLE 8–2
EXPERIENCE OF THE FIRST FOUR MANDATE EVALUATION LAWS, 1984–1986

State	Year of Passage	Number of Mandated Health Care Benefits[a] Enacted		
		During four years before passage	In the year of passage	During four years after passage
Washington	1984	5	2	4
Arizona	1985	2	5	4
Oregon	1985	4	1	8
Pennsylvania	1986	0	4	5

a. These counts refer only to the number of "mandatory inclusion" mandates, that is, mandates that stipulate that every policy sold must include the coverage in question.
b. For Pennsylvania, which passed its evaluation law in 1986, the prior and post periods each cover three years instead of four.
SOURCE: Author's tabulations based on data from *Health Benefits Letter* (1991a).

laws that recognize, in one way or another, that mandates may impose too heavy a burden on insurance purchasers. These mandate awareness laws fall into three categories: mandatory financial and social impact evaluations, ERISA equalization requirements, and small-firm waivers of mandated benefits.

Mandate evaluations. A number of states have started requiring an assessment of the potential effects of any proposed legislation. Washington was the first to do so in 1984, and since then fifteen more states have followed suit (*Health Benefits Letter* 1991a). The states have widely different provisions for how these evaluations are to be carried out. Reportedly, Pennsylvania, Hawaii, and Maine have the most thorough reviews (Scandlen 1989).

Whether these laws have slowed the passage of mandates at all is questionable. Indeed, data on the experience of states that have evaluated their legislation for at least four years suggest that the opposite has happened (see table 8–2): in three of the first four states to pass such a law, the rate of mandate passage actually increased following the call for evaluations.

ERISA equalization laws. Three states have passed legislation restricting their ability to mandate benefits unless the coverage can also be required of self-insured plans. Nebraska enacted its ERISA equalization law in 1986, with Illinois and Indiana each passing one in 1990. Indiana has since overridden its law, however, by mandating mammography screening for purchased plans (Blue Cross and Blue Shield Association 1991).

Mandate waivers for small businesses. Several states have become concerned with the potential burden of mandates for small employers. In 1990 five states began allowing small employers who previously did not offer insurance to offer bare-bones coverage exempt from most, if not all, mandates,[3] and in 1991 at least nine more states began granting similar exemptions. The size cutoff is set at twenty-five workers in most of these states and in a few at fifty workers. Although most mandates are waived, the legislation nonetheless usually specifies that a plan contain at least a few minimum coverages. Prenatal services, well-child care, a week or two of hospital in-patient care, and a few physician visits are among the services that must be covered.

Many of the bare-bones laws passed in 1991 are attempting to do more than simply waive most mandates for small firms. Some exempt these firms from state premium taxes, others provide a tax credit for providing health insurance (usually $25 per employee per month), and a few provide a stand-alone premium subsidy. In several states the legislation also contains provisions that address underwriting and rating practices in the small-group market. Underwriting refers to an insurer's process of rejecting or accepting prospective customers, and if accepted, a determination of the terms under which the group will be insured. An important underwriting provision that appears in nearly half the bills passed is a requirement for the guaranteed renewability of policies. Many of the bills also set minimum standards for an insurer's loss ratio in this market.

Why States Choose to Mandate

Why Mandate? There are two schools of thought on why the states have passed these laws, and they are not mutually exclusive. After briefly describing these two theories, this section then examines the empirical support for them.

Public interest explanations. One explanation is that the states have intervened to correct certain shortcomings in the market for group insurance. McGuire (1981) discusses two such possible shortcomings. First, insurance purchasers may have unknowingly undervalued the

---

3. In Washington the availability of this coverage is not restricted solely to previous non-offerors; rather, the insurance plan of any firm with under twenty-five workers is exempt from all state mandates (*Health Benefits Letter* 1991b).

benefits of some types of care or the risk of needing particular services, such as mental health care. In this case, a mandate may, *if chosen appropriately,* pull up a population's demand for coverage to a level more in line with what it would have been if buyers had only been well informed to begin with.

Another is the possibility of "adverse selection" in the market for special coverages. Adverse selection occurs when buyers, in this case employment groups, vary in their riskiness, but insurers are unable to price coverage according to risk. When adverse selection is present, the price for a special coverage—alcoholism treatment, for example—tends to reflect the cost for high-risk buyers, such as groups with higher rates of alcoholism, because these buyers have the strongest demand for coverage. Lower-risk groups either choose less extensive coverage or forgo it entirely. Although they would prefer more, they are unable to purchase it except at actuarially unfair rates. In this sense, adverse selection creates a market shortcoming: low-risk groups cannot buy as much coverage as they want at a fair price.

With adverse selection, a mandate may, again *if chosen appropriately,* improve on the competitive market outcome. It is possible to show theoretically that there may be a range of coverage levels, which, if mandated, would improve the well-being of both low-risk and high-risk purchasers.

With either type of shortcoming, however, how would government ever know if the optimal level had been mandated? It would not, most likely, nor have any means to find out. This is an important point, for, if chosen incorrectly, a mandate could make consumers worse off. Without a good knowledge of the problem, setting a mandate may be like Russian roulette: it might pay off (in improving consumer welfare), but then again it might not. And even if market shortcomings are significant, we should consider whether interventions *other than* a mandate can achieve an improved outcome. Given purchaser ignorance, for example, might education be more efficient?

Political interest theory of mandates. An alternative view is that states mandate coverage because doing so serves the political interests of legislators.[4] State legislators balance the competing interests of constituencies in deciding whether to enact a particular mandate. Because their ultimate goal is reelection, they act in the way that best trades their vote on passage for support at election time. Very small interest groups may wield considerable influence with legislators if they are either politically

---

4. This notion of regulation stems from the work of Peltzman (1976) and Stigler (1971).

energized or well financed. In contrast, large, politically diffuse groups may go unheard.

Proponents of a mandate include: (1) the health care providers who stand to reap enormous financial benefits after its passage; (2) patients who currently lack such coverage but whose demand for the service is continually high; (3) large self-insured firms; (4) the state, if expanded private coverage would reduce its own strained expenditures, as in the case of mental health care and certain other services; and (5) some legislators themselves, who may view the state's expenditure offset as new funds to spend in more politically attractive ways or who simply view mandates as an off-budget means of providing more services without raising taxes. Large self-insured firms, which actually offer most mandated coverages, are likely to be among proponents for two reasons. First, the law may give them an advantage *vis-à-vis* small competitors that do not self-insure, because it increases competitors' labor costs but not their own. Second, a mandate might indirectly lower their premiums because there are fewer opportunities for biased selection (that is, higher risks migrating to generous large-firm plans) and some enrollees for whom large-firm coverage is secondary (for example, spouses with primary coverage elsewhere) now draw down benefits first in their primary plan.

Opponents of a mandate include insurers, who lose flexibility in designing benefits, and small businesses that may not want or may be unable to afford the extra coverage. Most small businesses tend not to be well organized or well represented at the state level.

Empirical Tests of Regulatory Theories. The public interest explanations do not lend themselves to a direct empirical test. One can and should ask, however, what evidence there is that the shortcomings, which mandates supposedly correct, really exist in the first place. Are employment groups and insurers, for example, really ignorant of the benefits of certain coverages or unwilling to recognize them? In most firms a benefits manager selects the particular features of the plan. Normally his duties include staying informed about coverage matters and workers' needs. Are these specialists really ill-informed? No studies indicate that they are.

The case for adverse selection with respect to special coverages is extremely weak. The one piece of evidence for it is anecdotal from the late 1960s. At that time, Aetna and BCBS apparently were offered simultaneously to federal employees. Aetna experienced rapidly increasing claims when it offered more generous coverage for mental health care than did BCBS. To avoid attracting a disproportionate share of risks, Aetna then reduced its mental health coverage (McGuire 1981).

Much more research tests the political interest theory. Lambert and

McGuire (1990) examined the determinants of mandates for mental health care and psychologists' services. Using state-level data spanning 1968 through 1983, they estimated two models for the determinants of mandate enactment; one explained whether a state passed a mandate for mental health care during the period, and the other explained whether a state passed a mandate for psychologists' services during the period. For each of the models passage was hypothesized to depend on the strength of proponents, the strength of opponents, the political environment in the state, and the demographics of constituents. The variables used to operationalize these constructs varied depending on the mandate. The authors found some evidence that groups that would have had a stake in enactment indeed influenced a mandate's passage in the way expected. The probability of passage was positively responsive to the provider lobby and to the size of the state's own mental health budget. The strength of their evidence for these two findings, however, was not great. Their finding that states appeared to have acted in their own interests, for example, was found only for the passage of mental health mandates, not mandates for psychologists' services. (The political interest theory would have predicted both.) The statistical significance of their provider interest variables was also sensitive to the parametric specification used. Significance apparently dropped appreciably when population size was omitted from the model.

Morrisey and Jensen (1991a) examined the enactment of mandates for alcohol and drug abuse treatments and, like Lambert and McGuire, mandates for mental health and psychologists' services. Conceptually their models were similar to those developed by Lambert and McGuire; they included variables reflecting the influence of various interest groups, the state's political system, and its socioeconomic characteristics. They found some support for a provider-interest explanation, but this finding was limited to mental health mandates and even there lacked statistical significance. Their strongest finding was evidence of a legislative "snowball" effect; that is, the more insurance mandates a state had already passed, the more likely it was to pass yet another. These authors too found that their results were sensitive to specification.

Both studies suggest that the politics of mandates are difficult to explain. For mental health care and psychologists' services, there is modest support for the political interest theory, but when applied to alcohol and drug abuse mandates, the same theory does not fit very well.

Evidence on the Effects of Mandates

What are the consequences of mandates? The literature has addressed several aspects of this question, including their cost, their effect on a firm's ability to afford health insurance, and their potential role in the recent trend to self-insure. Before reviewing these studies, we consider the question of who is affected by a mandated benefit.

Those Affected by Mandates. Group policies sold by BCBS, commercial insurers, and HMOs typically must comply with mandated-benefit requirements. In most states, however, the persons covered by these plans are only a small portion of the population. Not covered are persons in self-insured plans, persons in publicly funded plans such as Medicaid and Medicare, those with individually purchased coverage, and the uninsured. The distribution of the population nationally by type of insurance suggests the situation in the typical state. Sixty-three percent of the civilian population has employment-based group health insurance (Nelson and Short 1990), but less than half these people (44 percent) have BCBS or commercial coverage (Sullivan and Rice 1991). Thus, only about 28 percent of the population is covered by "purchased" group insurance.

Not all of these persons, however, are affected by a mandated benefit; only those who would *otherwise lack* the benefit are affected. Persons in plans offered by small and mid-size firms are probably more affected, because benefits in these plans normally tend to be lean (DiCarlo and Lippert 1990). Larger firms often already offer the coverage in question and indeed may exceed a state's required minimum. Employer surveys have shown this to be the case for mandated mental health benefits in Washington and Pennsylvania (Frank 1989). Thus, while one's initial perception might be that mandates cover the vast majority of a state's population, in fact, the opposite is the case. Only about a quarter of the population or less gains access to a special coverage with a mandate, and most of those that do are likely tied to small or mid-size firms.

Cost of Mandates. The cost studies have employed a variety of both cost measures and estimation methods. The majority have focused on the cost of mandates to employers. The effect of mandates on an employer's group premium is important because, in principle, it measures the extent to which other forms of compensation must be reduced as a result. In competitive markets where each firm behaves so as to maximize profit, total compensation per worker (the value of wages and fringe benefits combined) tends to be equal to workers' marginal revenue product. If a firm pays any less than this amount, it cannot attract the work force it needs, and if it pays any more, it will be unable to recoup that cost in its output market (for example, through a higher product price). Thus, if one form of compensation is increased, another must be reduced to offset the increase. In this way workers themselves indirectly pay for state-mandated benefits; they do so in the form of lower wages and other fringe benefits. The empirical evidence on compensating differentials, all things considered, tends to support this logic (Morrisey 1992). Thus, by examining how much mandates add to employer premiums, we can gauge the burden they impose on workers.

Share-of-claims estimates of employer cost. Several studies have tried to estimate how much mandates add to the cost of group coverage. Two approaches have been used. The first has been to calculate directly the share of insurance claims in those coverage areas mandated by a state. Using this method, researchers found that Maryland's mandates accounted for 11 percent of claims in 1984 (Dyckman and Anderson-Johnson 1989), Virginia's accounted for 21 percent of claims in 1988 (Mathews 1991), Iowa's mandates in two areas (mental health and chemical dependency) accounted for 5 percent of claims in 1987 (Power and Ralston 1989), and Wisconsin's mandates in three areas (mental health, chemical dependency, and chiropractic services) accounted for 7 percent of claims in 1989 (Krohm and Grossman 1990). The second approach has been to rely on the opinion of actuaries. Based on actuarial estimates, Maryland's mandates accounted for 12 to 17 percent of costs in 1984 (Health Insurance Association of America 1985), and Massachusetts' accounted for 13 percent of costs in 1991 (Blue Cross and Blue Shield of Massachusetts 1991).

A few studies, although not directly concerned with mandates, also provide some additional estimates of the share of claim costs in various areas. Mental health and substance abuse, in particular, have received some attention. Frank, Salkever, and Sharfstein (1991) reported that, within large self-insured plans, mental health care accounted for 8 percent of all claims in 1986 and 9 percent of all claims in 1988. Substance abuse accounted for 3 percent of claims in both years. In another sample of firms observed in 1988, mental health care accounted for 10 percent of employers' total claims (A. Foster Higgins & Company, Inc. 1988).

It is inappropriate to interpret any of these "share-of-cost" statistics as indicating the cost of mandates to employers. Clearly, the estimated share (in those areas mandated) cannot *all* be due to regulation, because some of those coverages would have been provided anyway. The following section suggests an alternative and more relevant notion of cost, the "marginal cost" of mandates. Before a discussion of this, however, one other problem with these estimates should be noted. Share-of-cost estimates fail to account for possible spillover effects between different areas of an insurance plan. In particular, a mandated coverage will tend to reduce patients' demand for substitute services and increase their demand for complementary services. The changes in claims associated with these utilization shifts need to be accounted for in any estimate of cost-per-group contract. There is some evidence that mental health care, for example, reduces expenditures for other types of health care (Goodman 1989), in which case a share-of-cost estimate would likely overstate the cost of mental health coverage.

Hedonic price estimates of employer cost. The appropriate measure of added cost is an employer's "marginal cost," that is, the difference between his actual plan cost and the cost that he would have incurred in a mandate-free setting. None of the mandate studies cited above have used this concept. A few studies, however, give us a partial glimpse of the marginal cost of mandates. Although not concerned with mandates, per se, they provide estimates of the price employers pay for frequently mandated coverages.

Consider a particular mandate. Its marginal cost to an employer is either zero, if the benefit is already offered, or the price of adding it to the plan. Marketwide, marginal cost is the product of the number of firms adding the coverage and the price per plan of adding it. Thus, knowledge of prices of a coverage provides half the information needed to assess the marginal cost of mandating it.

Jensen and Morrisey (1990) estimated the marginal prices for various features based on the actual cost experience of plans. They estimated so-called hedonic pricing models for group health insurance. A hedonic price model is one that describes how the price of a product—in this case, the premium for group health insurance—varies with the specific characteristics of that product. In their models premiums varied with the actual benefit provisions in the plan, with the size and demographic characteristics of the group covered, and with the plan's funding medium. Data on large private sector firms surveyed between 1981 and 1984 were used for the analysis.

Several benefits were found to be quite expensive. The coverage for treating chemical dependency, for example, increased family premiums by 8.8 percent on average. Coverage for a psychiatric hospital stay increased premiums by 12.8 percent. Adding benefits for psychologists' visits increased them by 11.8 percent, and adding benefits for routine dental services, by 15 percent. These estimates may slightly overstate an employer's cost of complying with a mandate in one of these areas because the sample firms offered very generous benefits all around and may have offered richer coverage than what a state would typically prescribe. Nonetheless, this study too suggests that mandates may be expensive for firms that would otherwise offer no-frills coverage.

Employer cost-of-continuation-of-coverage requirements. Although no studies have examined how much state continuation-of-coverage mandates have cost employers, the recent experience under the 1986 Consolidated Omnibus Budget Reconciliation Act (COBRA), the federal requirement that is similar in some respects to these state laws, provides some clues to the effects of continuation-of-coverage requirements.[5] The state laws are similar to COBRA, except that the eligibility periods tend to be shorter and the state laws usually apply to all firms offering coverage, not just firms with twenty or more workers, which is the group to which COBRA applies. According to three surveys of employers, persons who elect COBRA coverage cost much more to insure than active workers. Claims for COBRA enrollees range from one-third to twice as high as those for normal enrollees (Charles D. Spencer and Associates 1990; Towers Perrin, Inc., 1991). Like the federal law, state laws typically limit an employer's permissible charge to the group rate or an amount close to it (for example, 102 percent). Thus, employers pay a large subsidy for each continuation enrollee.

Such adverse selection undoubtedly raises the total group premium. Although no studies have estimated the incremental premium, it would likely depend on the size of a group's subsidy per enrollee, the frequency with which workers are eligible for continuation coverage, and the frequency with which they elect it when eligible. The three surveys mentioned above provide some information about the last of these: they found that approximately one in five eligible persons actually chose it.

A continuation-of-coverage mandate also imposes a transaction cost on a firm, that is, the cost of communicating continuation rights to eligible persons, collecting premiums from these enrollees, and in some cases monitoring their right to continued eligibility. Although probably small in relation to incremental premiums, the transaction cost is not insignificant. Estimates for 1990, for example, are in the range of $150 to $240 annually per COBRA enrollee (Charles D. Spencer and Associates 1990; Towers Perrin, Inc., 1991).

The systemwide cost of mandates. Although relevant, the marginal cost to employers is only one aspect of cost. As McGuire and Montgomery (1982) have noted, the broader cost of a mandate is important for a

---

5. COBRA requires that firms with twenty or more workers continue eligibility for coverage among workers and their dependents who would otherwise lose eligibility because of either reduced employment, the death of a covered spouse, or divorce or separation from a covered employee. Workers and their dependents who would lose eligibility because of reduced employment are allowed to continue participation for eighteen months. Survivors or dependents who lose coverage because of divorce or separation are allowed participation for thirty-six months. Continuation enrollees are charged a premium no greater than 102 percent of the group rate.

number of reasons. First, some part of the cost to employers may be a savings to other payers. Existing users of mental health services, for example, who previously paid some or all of their expenses out of pocket, may have to pay less under a mental health mandate. Similarly, patients whose expenses were previously paid by the state may gain private coverage under a mandate. In each instance, there is no new cost systemwide; rather, the cost is simply shifted among payers.

Second, part of the cost of mandates is paid by parties other than those employers who expand coverage because of the law. The most visible additional cost is incurred by persons whose insurance is expanded. This group's demand for the service will increase, causing out-of-pocket expenses to rise. These extra out-of-pocket expenses occur provided the new insurance is less than full coverage, as is normally the case. There are other indirect but potentially important effects of additional coverage as well. By broadening some patients' insurance, the mandate increases aggregate market demand for the service in question, which should cause the price of the service to rise.[6] If individual demands are inelastic, as they are for most health care services, then each person's total expenditures will rise because of the price increase. Thus, total prices as well as the expenditures of parties not initially affected by the law should increase because of a mandate.

Third, offset effects may be associated with a new coverage, which occur "outside" the markets for insurance and health care services altogether or which occur in these markets but at some future date, and these effects too influence a mandate's systemwide cost. Generous alcohol benefits, for example, could conceivably improve productivity and reduce the reliance on nonalcohol-related health services in the long run. If such offsets indeed occur and are large enough, then a mandate may perhaps pay for itself in the broader scope of things.

McGuire and Montgomery (1982) were the first to take a systemwide view of the cost of mandates. After examining how mental health mandates affect the quantity and price of mental health services, they estimated how much mental health expenditures rise with a mandate. Using state-level data for 1978, they found that a mandate increased per capita expenditures for psychotherapy by 10 to 20 percent. A more recent study by Sternlieb and Beaton (1986), also based on state data, reached a similar conclusion concerning mandates for mental health care and alcohol treatments. Sternlieb and Beaton then determined whether mandates affected the proportionate sharing of expenditures among

---

6. The price increase occurs unless supply is completely elastic, which is unlikely given the high entry costs for most health professions and licensing restrictions in most states.

payers or the rates of mental illness and alcoholism within a state. Both types of mandates had the effect of shifting treatment cost to the insured private sector. With an alcohol mandate, for example, the private sector absorbed about 15 percent more of total expenditures than without a mandate. Neither the prevalence of mental illness, as proxied by a state's suicide rate, or the incidence of alcoholism appeared to be affected by the presence of a mandate, however.

Only one study has conducted a prospective evaluation of the cost impact of particular legislation. Frisman, McGuire, and Rosenbach (1985) estimated the total costs to Massachusetts of expanding the benefits stipulated in its existing mental health mandate. Their study illustrates all too well the practical difficulties involved in actually implementing the concept of total cost for a mandated benefit. One noteworthy finding was that more than half the increase in insurers' cost under the new mandate would have been shifted costs from other payers (primarily patients and the state) rather than new costs to society.

Mandates and the Affordability of Insurance. Close to two-thirds of the uninsured live in families headed by a worker employed in a small firm.[7] This was true in 1977 and again the case in 1987 (Short, Monheit and Beauregard 1989). When the employers of uninsured workers are asked why they do not provide health insurance, the overriding reason given is that they cannot afford it (Malholtra et al. 1980; Dennis 1985; Sullivan 1990). By making insurance more expensive, state-mandated benefits may have priced some of these firms out of the group-coverage market. Small businesses are especially vulnerable to this possibility because they face much higher premiums to begin with and because self-insurance is not viable for them.

Two studies have explored whether mandates are responsible for some portion of the uninsured, and both conclude that they are. The first, a study by Goodman and Musgrave (1988), used state-level data to estimate the effects of mandates on the percentage of a state's population without coverage. They found that in 1986 each mandated benefit increased the percentage of uninsured by about 0.17 percent, holding other factors constant. Goodman and Musgrave used their model to predict that 14 percent of the uninsured in 1986 lacked coverage because of mandates.

In another study, Jensen and Gabel (in press) modeled the extent to which mandates and other state insurance regulations discouraged small firms from providing health benefits in 1985 and in 1988. Since individual

---

7. A small firm is defined as a firm employing twenty-five or fewer workers.

firms, rather than whole states, were the units of observation, this analysis provides more direct estimates of the effects of mandates. The authors found that most individual mandates did not significantly lower a firm's probability of offering insurance but that taken collectively, they did. In their totality state mandates caused a significant drop in a small firm's propensity to offer coverage. Altogether, state mandates accounted for about one-fifth of noncoverage. The most troublesome mandate appeared to be a state continuation-of-coverage rule, that is, a COBRA-type requirement that terminated workers be allowed to participate in the firm's plan. (Such mandates were common before COBRA, and they still exist.) As shown earlier, continuation mandates appear to result in acute adverse selection and hence raise premiums. In small firms, which typically have high worker turnover, these effects could be especially severe.

Mandates and Self-Insurance. As noted earlier, ERISA exempts self-insured plans from all aspects of state insurance regulation. Whether the growth of state-mandated benefits spurred firms to self-insure during the 1980s has been the subject of several studies.

Reported reasons for self-insuring. When asked whether mandates contributed to their decision to self-insure, most benefit managers answer "yes, but mandates were not the major factor" (Health Insurance Association of America 1986; State of Minnesota 1988; Krohm and Grossman 1990). Earning interest generated from the plan's claims reserve, instead, was often the primary motive. Indeed, the most rapid growth in self-insurance occurred when real interest rates were high in the early 1980s. Small firms, however, gave avoiding mandates as a fairly important reason for having self-insured (State of Minnesota 1988), quite likely because small firms often provide less generous coverage than large firms and thus mandates will more often represent new costs to a small firm.

Mandated coverages within self-insured plans. If mandate avoidance were a factor, then we should find that self-insured plans less often contain mandated coverages. Several studies have looked at this possibility, but the findings are mixed. Three state-specific studies suggest that most larger firms that self-insure do not avoid mandated coverages but that smaller firms do. In Minnesota nearly all small firms that self-insured in 1987 tended to exclude from their policies five of the state's mandates that the survey specifically asked about (State of Minnesota 1988). Medium to large self-insured firms, however, tended to include them. In both Iowa (Power and Ralston 1989) and Wisconsin (Krohm and Grossman 1990), self-insured firms also tended to offer benefits in mandated areas equal to or greater than those found in purchased plans.[8]

National data, though, are less conclusive. Data from the mid-1980s on larger private sector firms, for example, show that self-insured plans were less likely to contain coverages in those areas frequently mandated (Jensen 1988; Jensen and Gabel 1988). In 1985, subscribers in self-insured plans less often had coverage for alcohol treatment, drug abuse treatment, home health care services, clinical psychologists' services, and coverage of a stay in a psychiatric hospital, when compared with subscribers in either commercial or BCBS plans. Since then, self-insured plans have apparently caught up in their provision of alcohol and drug abuse treatments (Jensen and Morrisey 1991). Whether they have done so in other areas is unclear.

Effects of mandates on the decision to self-insure. One study has examined whether a firm's decision to self-insure actually correlates with the level and scope of mandates in its state. Jensen et al. (1992) estimated the impact of state mandates on firms' decisions to convert to self-insurance during the 1980s. They found that most mandates had a positive but statistically insignificant effect on the likelihood of conversion and that even when considered collectively, mandates were statistically insignificant.

Another category of state insurance regulation, however, played an important role. Greater taxation of purchased plans strongly encouraged self-insurance. Both premium taxes and state risk-pool taxes had positive and significant effects on the likelihood of conversion. In the early 1980s the presence of a state continuation-of-coverage requirement also greatly encouraged self-insurance, but this was not so later in the decade. One interpretation is that when COBRA took effect in early 1986, self-insurance was no longer an escape route to avoid offering continuation rights; hence the incentive effect of the state laws dissipated.

Effects of Mandates in the Market for Services. By expanding insurance for some people, mandates influence the demand for medical services. A shift in demand, in turn, may cause the price of services and expenditure levels to change. Nearly all studies of the effects of mandates in the markets for services have focused on mental health–related mandates. Frank (1989) provides a careful review of these studies. In this section I highlight the major findings of his review and discuss some recent research not covered there.

---

8. Power and Ralson examined coverage in three areas (mental health, alcoholism, and drug abuse), which were under consideration for being mandated in Iowa at the time.

Several studies have assessed the effects of a mandate for mental health coverage in the markets for both psychologists' and psychiatrists' services. They suggest that a mandate indeed stimulates the demand for both services and increases total expenditures on mental health care. McGuire and Montgomery (1982), for example, found that the presence of a mental health mandate increased statewide demand for psychologists' visits by 18 to 25 percent in 1978 and for psychiatrists' visits by 9 to 12 percent in that year. Its effect on prices in both markets, however, was negligible. Based on data over a much longer period (1970–1978), Frank (1985) found that the presence of this mandate increased statewide demand for psychiatric services by 12 to 22 percent and increased psychiatrists' fees by 9 percent. A study by Sternlieb and Beaton (1986), based on more recent data but less sophisticated methods, found that the presence of a mental health mandate increased the price per mental health treatment but had no effect on the number of treatments statewide (either inpatient or outpatient). All three studies apparently imply a rise in mental health expenditures, even though they disagree about its source.

There is additional evidence of a demand shift for individuals. Using data on individuals from the National Medical Care Expenditure Survey (NMCES), Horgan (1986) found that the presence of a mental health mandate significantly increased the demand for mental health care, even after accounting for its expansion effect on insurance coverage. Her study suggests that part of a mandate's effect may work indirectly through a change in attitudes: people may come to view their consumption of mental health services as more socially acceptable once the state has "sanctioned" that consumption through a mandate.

One other study, by Mitchell et al. (1986), used physician survey data to examine whether a mandate for health coverage affects the demand facing an individual psychiatrist. They found no effect on the psychiatrist's visits, income, or fee. These findings are not necessarily inconsistent with the other studies, however. In the long run, any excess provider profits in the first few years after a mandate's enactment might be bid away by new psychiatrists entering the market. It is quite possible that their effects on both aggregate demand and individuals are significant but insignificant on individual providers.

The market effects of alcohol treatment mandates have been examined by Sternlieb and Beaton (1986) and Morrisey and Jensen (1991b). The first authors found that an alcohol mandate tended to raise the price per alcohol treatment but not the number of treatments per capita, results similar to those found in their analysis of mental health mandates. The second authors found some evidence suggesting an increased social acceptance of treatment under a mandate. Specifically,

Morrisey and Jensen found that self-insured firms in 1989 were significantly more likely to offer alcohol coverage in states that mandated it than in states that did not, controlling for other factors that would have influenced the coverage decision.

Some studies have investigated whether a mandate in one area affects the demand for services in another. It is expected that for categories of care with substitutes, an insurance mandate in one area decreases demand in the other substitute areas, whereas for complementary categories of care, the opposite occurs. A mandate for psychologists' coverage, for example, has been found to have significant indirect effects on psychiatrists. Frank (1985) found that it reduced the demand for psychiatrists' services by 15 percent and the fees they charge by 9 percent, suggesting that psychologists and psychiatrists are substitutes. Mitchell et al. (1986) also found a significant decrease in the demand for psychiatrists' visits in the presence of a psychologists' mandate. Both studies imply reduced expenditures on psychiatrists' care. Such indirect cost savings are apparently one offset effect of a mandate for psychologists' services. Other mental health professionals have been found to be substitutes for psychiatrists as well. Fairbank (1989) found that a Massachusetts mandate for the coverage of clinical social workers reduced psychiatrists' market share of outpatient mental health business in the first year following enactment.

The issue of whether much broader substitutions in health care occur, and the nature of intertemporal interdependences among alternative categories of care, also bears on the question of the offset effects of a mandate. Some research has shown that mental health care reduces expenditures for nonmental health–related care (Goodman 1989), suggesting that mandates in the mental health area may produce some expenditure offsets outside mental health. Alcohol treatment, in contrast, has been found to increase expenditures for nonalcohol-related care and to lead to higher total costs years later (Goodman 1991). Thus, it appears that one cannot generalize regarding possible offsets under a mandate but rather that the situation depends on the specific coverage in question.

Summary and Policy Considerations

This chapter has considered what we know about the extent and scope of state-mandated benefits, why the states have enacted these laws, and their consequences for insurance and medical care markets. Ten observations emerge from the review:

- In recent years state-mandated benefits have evolved into a major category of insurance regulation.

- Patterns of mandate enactment across the fifty states conform only modestly to a political interest theory of regulation. When applied to the passage of mandates for mental health care or psychologists' services, the theory fits moderately, but when applied to alcohol and drug abuse mandates, it does not fit at all.

- Although some workers and their families gain access to a special service with a mandate, most of a state's population is often unaffected. Mandates have no effect on the uninsured, persons in self-insured plans, and persons who already have such coverage. Most of those affected are tied to smaller firms offering modest health benefits.

- Mandates often raise the price employers pay for insurance. It is likely that these additional costs are ultimately paid by workers in the form of lower wages, lower levels for other fringe benefits, or lower employment.

- Some small firms forgo coverage altogether because of mandates. An estimated one-fifth of small firms that now do not offer insurance would do so in a mandate-free environment.

- Some existing health care costs are shifted onto private insurance plans when a mandate is enacted. Looking solely at employers' additional premiums tends to overstate the cost of mandates because it ignores these savings to other payers.

- Mandates fueled only a small portion of self-insurance during the 1980s. Most self-insured plans contain mandated coverages, and firms' decisions to switch to self-insurance are only weakly correlated with the level and scope of state mandates.

- Continuation-of-coverage requirements are very burdensome. Of all the state mandates, these are the most influential in a small firm's decision to offer insurance and in a larger firm's decision to self-insure. There is a serious adverse selection problem with continuation enrollees; very high risk individuals stay on in a plan, while low risks drop out.

- State premium taxes too have a strong effect on insurance choices. The higher the tax, the more likely it is that a small firm forgoes coverage and that a larger firm chooses self-insurance, thereby escaping all state oversight.

- Mandates shift demand for newly covered services and increase expenditures for those services. In a few areas, such as mental health care, there may be a modest offset of expenditures in other areas after a mandate is enacted.

Recent legislation in several states suggests that some lawmakers have become sensitive to the possible consequences of mandates. Twenty-two states have now passed "mandate awareness" bills, most in 1989 and 1990. Nearly all either call for an impact statement on proposed mandates before their enactment or lift mandated benefits for small firms newly entering the insurance market. Although it is far too early to tell whether the various mandate-waiver programs will be successful, the studies reviewed in this chapter suggest that they will be. A comparative evaluation of these new programs is clearly in order.

From a health policy standpoint, mandates raise an important issue concerning the differential treatment of different types of insurance plans. By interpreting ERISA as preempting state laws for self-insured but not purchased plans, the courts have created a two-tier regulatory system for employer-sponsored health insurance. On one tier are purchased plans under state scrutiny. They pay state taxes, must comply with, what is now, a large number of rules on the content of coverage, and maintain state-specified reserves to prevent insolvency. On another tier are self-insured plans over which the states have no oversight. They pay no taxes, are exempt from all state mandates, and need not follow sound actuarial practices. By avoiding the costs of regulation, self-insured firms can, in principle, attract workers with compensation packages that cost less than those offered by firms that do not self-insure. Thus, non–self-insured firms are at a competitive disadvantage in labor markets *vis-à-vis* self-insured firms. Because non–self-insured firms tend to be smaller, ERISA's exemption has arguably weakened the ability of small firms to compete effectively against large ones.

Most observers agree that when ERISA was enacted, this dual regulatory treatment of insurance plans was a fully unforeseen and unintended consequence (Fox and Schaffer 1989). With a majority of persons now in self-insured plans, federal policy makers must consider whether to maintain the current regulatory vacuum for self-insured plans that ERISA created or to change federal law so that health insurance plans are treated equally, regardless of self-insurance status. With regard to the equal treatment question, federal policy could take two directions. One would be to eliminate ERISA's exemption for self-insured plans; the other would be to expand it to all employer-sponsored insurance plans. The first would leave health insurance regulation with the states, where it largely was until the self-insurance boom of just a few years ago. The second strategy would essentially turn regulation over to the federal government.

The question of what to do with ERISA's exemption is one that must now be addressed, regardless of whether we maintain our current system of voluntary employer coverage or move on to something new. State mandates have evolved into such a major category of regulation that if we ignore the issue, then we have essentially permitted a major component of U.S. health policy, one that now affects a majority of Americans, to be formed by accident.

References

A. Foster Higgins & Company, Inc. *Health Care Benefits Survey, 1988.* Princeton, N.J.: 1988.

Blue Cross and Blue Shield Association. "State Mandated Health Insurance Benefit Laws Enacted through April 1989." Washington, D.C.: Office of Government Relations, State Services Department, May 1989.

————. "State Health Benefit and Provider Mandates." *Issue Review.* Washington, D.C., July 1991.

Blue Cross and Blue Shield of Massachusetts. "Mandated Benefits: Impact on Group Master Medical Rates (based on second quarter 1991)." Boston, Mass., 1991.

Charles D. Spencer and Associates. *Spencer Research Reports on Employee Benefits.* Washington, D.C., July 1990.

Dennis, William J., Jr. *Small Business Employee Benefits.* Washington, D.C.: National Federation of Independent Businesses, 1985.

DiCarlo, Steven, and Clare Lippert. "Types and Characteristics of Health Plans." *Providing Employee Health Benefits: How Firms Differ.* Washington, D.C.: Health Insurance Association of America, 1990.

Dyckman, Zachary, and Judy Anderson-Johnson. "The Cost of Mandated Health Insurance Benefits: The Maryland Experience." Paper presented at the 1989 American Public Health Association Annual Meeting, Center for Health Policy Studies, Columbia, Md., October 1989.

Fairbank, Alan. "Expanding Insurance Coverage to Alternative Types of Psychotherapists: Demand and Substitution Effects of Direct Reimbursements to Social Workers." *Inquiry* 26 (1989): 170–81.

Fox, Daniel M., and Daniel C. Schaffer. "Health Policy and ERISA: Interest Groups and Semipreemption." *Journal of Health Politics, Policy, and Law* 14 (1989): 239–60.

Frank, Richard G. "Pricing and Location of Physicians Services in Mental Health." *Economic Inquiry* 23 (1985): 115–33.

————. "Regulatory Policy and Information Deficiencies in the Market for Mental Health Services." *Journal of Health Politics, Policy, and Law.* 14 (1989): 477–502.

Frank, Richard G., David S. Salkever, and Stephen S. Sharfstein. "A Look at Rising Mental Health Insurance Costs." *Health Affairs* 10 (1991): 116–23.

Frisman, Linda K., Thomas G. McGuire, and Margo L. Rosenbach. "Costs of Mandates for Outpatient Mental Health Care in Private Insurance." *Archives of General Psychiatry* (June 1985): 558–61.

Goodman, Allen C. "Estimation of Offset and Income Effects on the Demand for Mental Health Treatment." *Inquiry* 26 (1989): 235–48.

Goodman, Allen C., Harold D. Holder, and Eleanor Nishiura. "Alcoholism Treatment Offset Effects: A Cost Model." *Inquiry* 28 (1991): 168–78.

Goodman, John C., and Gerald L. Musgrave. "Freedom of Choice in Health Insurance." Dallas, Texas: National Center for Policy Analysis, November 1988.

Health Benefits Letter. "Mandated Benefits: Mixed Signals From the States." Alexandria, Va.: Scandlen Publishing Inc., March 13, 1991a.

———. "Bare Bones Health Insurance: An Emerging Consensus in the States." Alexandria, Va.: Scandlen Publishing Inc., May 23, 1991b.

Health Insurance Association of America. "Maryland Mandates Report." Washington, D.C., 1985.

———. "The Competitive Marketplace: Commercial Insurers and Blue Cross Blue Shield." Washington, D.C., 1986.

Horgan, Constance M. "The Demand for Ambulatory Mental Health Services from Specialty Providers." *Health Services Research* 21 (1986): 291–319.

Jensen, Gail A. "Effects of State Mandated Benefits on Employers: Preliminary Findings From Research in Progress." Testimony before the Governor's Task Force on Health Plan Regulatory Reform, State of Minnesota, St. Paul, Minn., June 1988.

Jensen, Gail A., and Jon R. Gabel. "The Erosion of Purchased Health Insurance." *Inquiry* 25 (1988): 328–43.

———. "State Mandated Benefits and the Small Firms' Decision to Offer Health Insurance." *Journal of Regulatory Economics,* in press.

Jensen, Gail A., and Michael A. Morrisey. "Employer-Sponsored Insurance for Alcohol and Drug Abuse Treatment, 1988." *Inquiry.* 28(1991): 393–402.

———. "Group Health Insurance: A Hedonic Price Approach." *The Review of Economics and Statistics* 72 (1990): 38–44.

Jensen, Gail A., Michael A. Morrisey, and Kevin D. Cotter. "State Insurance Regulation and the Decision to Self-Fund." Working paper, Department of Economics, Wayne State University, August 1992.

Krohm, Gregory, and Mary H. Grossman. "Mandated Benefits in Insurance Policies." *Benefits Quarterly* (fourth quarter 1990): 51–60.

Lambert, David A., and Thomas G. McGuire. "Political and Economic Determinants of Insurance Regulation in Mental Health" *Journal of Health Politics, Policy, and Law* 15(1990): 169–90.

Lichtenstein, Jules H., and Hazel A. Witte. "Government and the Special Circumstances of Small Employers." *Rescuing American Health Care: Market Rx's.* Washington, D.C.: NFIB Foundation, 1991.

Malholtra, Suresh, Kenneth M. McCaffree, John M. Wills, and Jean Baker. *Employment Related Health Benefits in Private Nonfarm Business Establishments in the United States,* vol. I. Final report for the U.S. Department of Labor under contract No. J-9-P-7-0150, Seattle, Wash.: Battelle Human Affairs Research Centers, 1980.

Mathews, Roderick B., Senior vice president, Blue Cross–Blue Shield of Virginia, personal communication to author, July 1991.

McGuire, Thomas G. *Financing Psychotherapy: Costs, Effects, and Public*

Policy. Cambridge: Ballinger Publishing, 1981.

McGuire, Thomas G., and John T. Montgomery. "Mandated Mental Health Benefits in Private Health Insurance Policies." *Journal of Health Politics, Policy, and Law* 7 (1982): 380–89.

Mitchell, Janet B., et al. *Psychiatric Office Practice Study.* Washington, D.C.: National Institute of Mental Health, 1986.

Morrisey, Michael A. "Mandated Benefits and Compensating Differentials: Taxing the Uninsured." In this volume, 1992.

Morrisey, Michael A., and Gail A. Jensen. "Determinants of Mandates for Alcohol, Drug, and Mental Health Coverage." *Employer Sponsored Insurance for Alcohol Abuse.* Final report under grant #1-RO1-AA08391-01 for the National Institute for Alcohol and Alcohol Abuse, Rockville, Md., 1991a.

———. "Employer Demand for Alcohol Abuse Treatment and Related Health Insurance Coverages, 1989." *Employer Sponsored Insurance for Alcohol Abuse.* Final report under grant #1-RO1-AA08391-01 for the National Institute for Alcohol and Alcohol Abuse. Rockville, Md., 1991b.

Nelson, Charles, and Kathleen Short. *Health Insurance Coverage 1986–88.* Current Population Reports, Household economic studies Series P-70, no. 17. Washington, D.C.: Bureau of the Census, March 1990.

Peltzman, Samuel. "Toward a More General Theory of Regulation." *Journal of Law and Economics* 19 (1976): 211–40.

Power, Mark, and August Ralston. "State-Mandated Group Health Insurance Coverages." *Benefits Quarterly* 5 (1989): 1–10.

Rothschild, Michael, and Joseph Stiglitz. "Equilibrium in Competitive Insurance Markets: An Essay in the Economics of Imperfect Information." *Quarterly Journal of Economics* 90 (1976): 629–49.

Scandlen, Greg. "Overview of the Evaluation Process: Bringing Order to the Mandate Debate." Paper presented at the Conference on Mandated Benefits, Charleston, S.C., May 1989.

Short, Pamela, Alan Monheit, and Karen Beauregard. "A Profile of Uninsured Americans." National Medical Care Expenditure Survey Research Findings 1, DHHS Publ. #PHS-89-343. Rockville, Md.: National Center for Health Services Research and Health Care Technology Assessment, September 1989.

State of Minnesota. *Health Plan Regulation.* Office of the Legislative Auditor, St. Paul, Minn., February 1988.

Sternlieb, George, and W. Patrick Beaton. *Mandated Health Care Benefits: The Cost of Insurance Coverage of Alcohol, Drug Abuse and Mental Health Treatment.* Center for Urban Policy Research, Rutgers University, April 1986.

Stigler, George J. "The Theory of Economic Regulation." *Bell Journal of Economics and Management Science* 2 (1971): 1–21.

Sullivan, Cynthia B. "Why Employers Do Not Offer Coverage." *Providing Employee Health Benefits: How Firms Differ.* Washington, D.C.: Health Insurance Association of America, 1990.

Sullivan, Cynthia B., and Thomas Rice. "The Health Insurance Picture in 1990." *Health Affairs* 10 (1991): 104–15.

Towers Perrin, Inc. "COBRA Survey Results." *Medical Benefits.* July 30, 1991, p. 3.

Commentary on Part Two

William J. Dennis

I am associated with the National Federation of Independent Business (NFIB) Foundation. The foundation, in turn, is affiliated with the National Federation of Independent Business, the nation's largest small- and independent-business trade group. My remarks, therefore, focus on smaller firms.

There are a number of ways to enhance access to health care through the private system and small employers. I agree with Catherine McLaughlin's findings in chapter 7: that focused information and the exclusion of industries are problems for small employers. A plethora of health care information is available to them. Unfortunately, much of it is not very useful. Small employers are usually not sophisticated buyers of health insurance. The terminology is alien to them. The rate-setting process is often incomprehensible. And a comparison of products, particularly with out-year-premium volatility, is very difficult.

McLaughlin is also correct with respect to the exclusion of industries. Some insurers exclude one type of firm. Other insurers will include that type of firm but exclude others. Differences in exclusions often confuse small employers, who assume that if they are excluded by one or two companies then they are excluded by all. There is also an under-appreciated problem regarding exclusion of new firms and their employees.

The access problem, however, is really a cost problem. Countless surveys of small employers conclude that cost is the primary reason they do not offer employee health insurance. According to the Small Business Administration, 1.7 million self-employed people themselves lack health insurance.

Who doesn't provide health insurance? NFIB data established a direct relationship between the amount an employer earns from the business and his or her provision of employee health insurance. Those who take out less than $10,000—and, unfortunately, there are too many of those—offer employee health insurance less than 30 percent of the time. Yet, among those who take out over $70,000, the figure is well over

90 percent. I do not believe that surprises anyone, but its relevance for the policy debate is obvious.

Analyzing NFIB survey data, we also found that the number of nonproviders who say they would not offer health insurance under almost any circumstance is about 15 percent. McLaughlin reported that in some of her surveys and the surveys she has reviewed, that percentage is closer to half. This is an important discrepancy that we cannot resolve here.

It is necessary, however, to examine not only how many owners respond this way, but the size of their firms. The very smallest are most likely to say they would not provide insurance under almost any circumstance. That means the number of employees working for these employers is very small.

If cost is the critical factor, are there ways to reduce costs for small employers? Obviously there are. First, government could stop cost-shifting in the Medicare and Medicaid programs. That would be helpful.

Second, the industry could move to a universal claims form, better coordination of benefits, and other measures of that nature. I do not know how much that would eventually cut premiums, but it would clearly cut the hassle, which is always important when dealing with small firms.

I question proposals for small-group reform, however. As Blue Cross notes, these reforms would actually increase the cost of coverage for some small firms. This would be particularly true if the ERISA preemption were still in effect and no other cost reduction steps were taken.

If we eliminated state mandates, costs could be reduced. Gail Jensen in chapter 8 estimates that one in six small, nonproviding employers would probably have insurance if we were in a mandate-free environment. That is 18 percent of somewhat less than 2 million businesses. If one wants to improve access, this would be a good place to start. Unfortunately, the number of mandates seems to be growing rather than shrinking.

Reform of medical malpractice is another reasonable step. We can also cap the tax exclusion, not because it would directly cut premium costs, but because it would begin to make the consumer-patient more aware of prices charged. In the long term this is the most important thing to be done.

We can also grease the system with useful consumer information on prices and outcomes. The Department of Health and Human Services has begun to publish some outcomes information. Why should private insurers not provide consumers information about individual doctors and other providers, particularly with regard to prices for common procedures?

I do not consider employer-mandated insurance as improving access to the private system. But even if one accepted that employer mandates constitute a private approach, it would not take long for them to become a government program.

I have done some rough calculations on the so-called Mitchell bill, a play-or-pay approach. Under the proposal, between 1 million and 2 million small employers would find it financially advantageous to pay the penalty and opt for public coverage. There would also be those who initially would not find it financially advantageous to opt for public coverage, but who later would, as health care costs and insurance premiums rose faster than employee wages.

Look at the Massachusetts experiment. It originally planned a flat $1,500 per employee penalty for those not provided health insurance. By the time the program was scheduled to be operational, prices had risen so that every employer would have found it financially advantageous to go into the public program. So mandates do not represent a private approach at all. They represent a public approach, or a halfway house, to a one-payer or, more likely, socialized system.

Michael Morrisey asks a critical question in chapter 6: "Does this society wish to compel individuals to purchase health insurance?" That question is critical because it is at the heart of a play-or-pay mandate.

Small employers, who had not previously provided insurance, will pick up the tab in the short term under an employer mandate. But in the long term, it will be absorbed by employees, many of whom have relatively low incomes. Do we want to force low-income individuals to purchase their insurance through forgone wages and lost job opportunities?

As is pointed out above, a direct relationship exists between employer income and the provision of employee health insurance. The effect is that relatively poor employers are matched with relatively poor employees, and relatively wealthy employers are matched with relatively wealthy employees. Under a play-or-pay approach, therefore, neither relatively wealthy employers nor relatively wealthy employees subsidize the health insurance of low-income employees. Yet relatively poor employers, those most affected by a mandate, often cannot absorb the short-term costs. That leaves these employers no alternative but to eliminate employees or terminate business operations.

If we adopt a play-or-pay system, we ought to be honest with the people who are going to receive the benefits and pay the costs. In sum, there is no lack of things to do in order to increase access through the private sector. The issue is whether we have the political will to do so.

Donald W. Moran

Like many in the active adult population, I am a musical technophile. As a young man I banged around with electric guitars and amplifiers to produce sounds that differed from what one could achieve in a purely acoustic environment.

Twenty-five years later the technical frontier in music has become digital, typified by electronic controllers and computer-based sequencers linking synthesizers, drum machines, and the like. As a consequence the home recording studio of today reverberates to sounds never before heard in nature. In order to illustrate some important points about the current health care reform debate, I will use the organizing metaphor of electronic music to suggest similarities between the way electronic music is produced and the way the current health care reform debate is conducted.

The biggest effect of the evolution to digital music is that musicians have become far more conscious of the underlying acoustic mechanics of sound, a phenomenon based on complex analog wave forms. These electronic instruments permit users to monkey around with the wave forms that naturally occur, to produce totally new sound waves. One can use the new digital technology to place a natural wave form on the screen and then use synthesis software and technology to change subtly—or dramatically—such features as the attack of each note, the shape and period of the wave, and the rate and character of the decay in the note after the onset of the attack.

The imperative for health care reform comes and goes in our politics in a cyclical manner that exhibits many of the characteristics of acoustic waves. About every fifteen years, events conspire to cause many elements of our society—consumers, businesses, and public-policy makers—rapidly to coalesce around the proposition that the U.S. health care system is in imminent danger of collapse, and that only extensive changes in the structure of our private health care financing system will remedy this otherwise intractable problem. The "attack" phase of each cycle is unusual for its initial amplitude, as well as for the staying power of the issue in the public press, the business news, and public-policy debate. Usually within twelve months of the onset of each cycle health care reform moves from the back burner to the front of the stove, where it persists as a major public issue for several years.

The "decay" period of the wave ranges from four to five years after each acute attack. It is typified by a transformation of the debate from one about the need for greater access to one about cost containment as a prerequisite to any expansion of insurance coverage for Americans. Eventually health care policy gives way to another issue in the seemingly endless arguments between payers and providers of health care about control of resource allocation in the existing system—arguments in which the access issue is sidelined.

The reasons for these endless cycles, as in acoustics, is the inherent circularity of many of the underlying, dynamic forces that generate the wave behavior. In health policy these circular generating functions are both real and rhetorical.

On the real side, although underlying health care costs seem to rise inexorably, the apparent rise in cost for businesses and consumers is influenced by what insurance analysts call a "property casualty cycle" on top of trends in insurance premiums. The period from 1988 to 1990 saw a faster-than-normal rise in the apparent cost of health care in the form of increases in health care premiums at rates four to five times the underlying rate of inflation in the general economy. This phenomenon naturally stimulated substantial concern among those paying the bills. In such circumstances, since not all Americans or businesses are equally influenced by these trends, policy analysis naturally turns to a distributional analysis that identifies the problems of those who are least able to cope with the inexorable rise in cost.

At this point the rhetorical generators take over. The persisting lack of health insurance for many Americans, in both good times and bad, leads many to conclude that there is an inherent market failure in the private health care financing system that must be remedied by a powerful dose of nonmarket forces. In terms of the acoustic analogy this view of the world is the "synthesizer hypothesis," the premise that active intervention from outside nature can create a new generating function that will produce a more pleasing outcome than would obtain were the normal cycle of events permitted to run its course. The existence of this book, analyzing a wide range of proposed nonmarket interventions into the private health care financing system, is testimony to the substantial number of adherents to the synthesizer hypothesis who are in public policy circles.

Nevertheless, my purpose is to suggest that the synthesizer hypothesis is really the synthesizer illusion, and that the impetus for radical transformation of the U.S. private health care financing system may be reaching its cyclical peak.

In this conclusion, I am not suggesting that all is well in the world of the private health insurance system, which is under considerable stress. Rather my conclusion is based on the premise that the commonly perceived problems in our present health care financing system are so intrinsic to the structure of the system as to doom to failure any halfhearted attempt at reform.

As Michael Morrisey clearly indicates in chapter 6, labor markets based on voluntary exchange will not significantly generate insurance in the near future for those who do not now have it. The reason is that a significant number of Americans, rightly or wrongly, value other forms of compensation more highly, and they will not willingly surrender those other forms.

Another perspective on this conclusion comes from chapter 7, Catherine McLaughlin's work. The Robert Wood Johnson experiments show that offering high levels of support to small businesses for health insurance produces mixed results at best. Such a strategy is thus unlikely to be universally efficacious in changing employer behavior.

A further retardant to private financing reform is the unenviable track record of the nonmarket interventions that have been employed in the private insurance market. Gail Jensen's work in chapter 8 drives home the fact that most purely regulatory interventions at best yield mixed interpretations and results. Policy analysts are relieved that public-sector interventions have not done as much damage as they theoretically might have done.

Furthermore, the uninsured population is so heterogeneous, churning so frequently in and out of various employment, that employment-based strategies miss their target. Even within the population subgroups at greatest risk for uninsurance, the demand for insurance may vary more systematically by employee occupation than the supply of insurance varies by type of firm—or even firm size.

Many who share my gloomy view of the prospects for markedly enhancing access through reform of employer-based insurance cite the foregoing analysis as an argument against the continuation of private insurance, and in favor of a fully public system. Despite the appeal of such conclusions, however, it is possible to conclude that the prospects for successful nationalization of the health care financing system are even more bleak.

The infeasibility of substituting public financing mechanisms for those of our troubled private system is structurally intrinsic to the system. The nation's employers spent roughly $170 billion in 1991 dollars to support the existing system of employer-financed insurance. Were I the designer of a universal public program, I would view that $170 billion as an insoluble dilemma; given the likely state of the public purse in the forseeable future, I could not bear to give up that $170 billion. Attempting a dollar-for-dollar substitute for those resources would more than double the present governmental commitment to health care at all levels—a practical impossibility in budgetary terms.

Yet attempting to fashion public-sector solutions preserving that $170 billion by maintaining a regulated private insurance system would further distort behavior in a system whose distorted behavioral incentives create the perception of market failure today. As long as employers and employees have the freedom to make utility-maximizing choices, they may do so in ways that will raise the cost of the undertaking. The ability of private actors to maximize their own utility reduces the target efficiency of solutions designed to provide insurance to those who would otherwise not have it, since some resources must be expended to prevent those who *do* now have it from devolving their present spending commitments onto whatever public program is created.

At Lewin/ICF we estimated that it would cost roughly $13 billion in 1991 dollars to increase the level of health care consumption by the uninsured in the United States to a level equivalent to that enjoyed by the average insured American. This amount is relatively modest in comparison with total U.S. health spending, because the uninsured consume on average about two-thirds of the dollar value of health care consumed by the insured public.

To expand coverage to the uninsured while maintaining existing employer spending, however, most proposed mechanisms, ranging from purely regulatory mandates to the pay-or-play hybrids, require a reallocation far higher than $13 billion to achieve the putative $13 billion objective. The need to specify minimum-benefits packages, for example, to ascertain whether some minimum level of insurance is being offered, means that any existing plan falling short of those standards in any particular will have to be averaged up.

The magnitude of this effect is easy to underestimate, since many supposedly generous private-sector health plans have areas in which their coverage is limited. The traditional benefits offered to auto workers by Big Three auto makers, for example, is commonly perceived as being of "Cadillac quality"; despite this perception, that package offers only very limited coverage of routine office visits. Any minimum-benefit package that required significant benefits in this area, therefore, would require significant upgrades on the existing benefits in such plans.

A significant portion of these upgrades would redound to the benefit of those who are presently insured. Many ambitious reform proposals bearing price tags in excess of $60 billion in new federal program commitments would generate more than three-quarters of those costs in the provision of coverage to those who now have insurance elsewhere.

As policy makers come to grips with the significant fiscal implications of these strategies, the debate rapidly becomes transformed from the arena of access to that of cost containment, since most of the action in these proposals pertains to those who presently have insurance. This displacement of the locus of debate, to borrow again from the language of digital signal processing technology, "closes a filter" and removes all information content associated with anything other than mechanisms for cost control.

The political system is unable to achieve consensus on cost-containment mechanisms sufficient to finance tens of billions of dollars worth of new benefits to the newly or the previously insured. Unfortunately for proponents of reform, this means the duration of the cost-containment debate is long relative to the duration of maximum emphasis on the access issue. After the elevation of insurance access issues in the 1960 presidential campaign led to the enactment of Medicare and Medicaid in 1965, the remainder of the cycle, from 1966 to 1974, was preoccupied with controlling the health care cost explosion that immediately followed. The high energy portion of the great national health insurance debate of 1974–1976 was even shorter. After Jimmy Carter was elected, in part on a national health insurance platform, the Washington health policy community spent the majority of the 1977–1990 period preoccupied with cost-containment questions at the expense of access.

Although the volume of debate on access questions was higher in 1991 than it had been for the previous fifteen years, perhaps the debate will soon be transformed into one about cost containment as a prerequisite for action on any other front. Nonetheless, the rhetoric associated with the 1991 cyclical peak in interest regarding access will probably persist for some time. For it is a fundamental principle of acoustics that, as long as the frequency of the cycle remains constant, the pitch will remain the same.

Stephen Zuckerman

The chapters and the discussants have focused on the process of purchasing health insurance through the present employer-based system. I will, however, now shift gears and reflect on the title of part two—"What Should Be the Role for the Private Sector in Improving Access to Health Care?" The issues involved here extend beyond access to insurance.

The decision to use the health care system is often made independently of prior decisions regarding the purchase of insurance. Emergencies and unexpected illnesses arise requiring treatment that cannot be delayed. Moreover, society is unwilling to deny care to seriously ill patients, even when they are uninsured and cannot afford to pay. This is the special nature of health care. Analyses of the present system, its obvious shortcomings, and development of future policies must never lose sight of this.

My commentary focuses on four points. First, some new subsidies will be required to improve access for those currently receiving inadequate services. Second, building on the employer-based structure is a reasonable next step. Third, exploring alternatives to the standard, fairly rich package of health insurance benefits is appropriate. Finally, improving access without developing explicit policies aimed at controlling costs is not desirable.

The issue of subsidies to improve access is implicitly raised by Michael Morrisey in chapter 6, who suggests that it may be rational for low-wage workers and their employers to agree to a compensation package that does not include health insurance. For these workers, not having insurance is the best option, given their earnings constraint and current health care costs.

Although there is truth in this conclusion, the decision regarding the purchase of insurance should not be viewed only from a purely private perspective. Health care in the United States has a free-rider problem. Individuals without health insurance believe that services will be available when they need them, even if they do not pay. There is a public-good dimension to health care, since individuals behave as if the system can provide services in emergency situations without being overburdened or imposing extreme costs. One of the goals of mandates—on either employers or individuals—is to eliminate this free-rider problem.

Morrisey questions whether it would be desirable to compel workers to incur a tax on their wages to purchase health insurance. Obviously, it would be futile to try to improve the welfare of these workers by imposing a mandate and tax when they do not have sufficient earning capacity. If there were a mandate, compensation packages would likely include lower wages in exchange for health insurance. But Morrisey's consideration of the adverse effects of mandates for insurance fails to recognize that mandates *not* to consume health care services—that is, not to get sick—are clearly impractical.

Individuals lacking employer-based health insurance have three basic options for financing services they may need. They can purchase private insurance in the nongroup market. They can pay for these services out of pocket; for many minor, acute illnesses it may be possible even for low-wage workers to do this. Or they can seek the largess of health care providers—namely, receive services in the form of uncompensated care. Uncompensated care may be the most viable option for serious illnesses.

When uncompensated care is provided, the individual receives a patchwork of subsidies—from taxpayers who fund public hospitals, from other payers in the system who may pay unfairly high rates, and from philanthropies. If our society is not willing to deny emergency or critical care then these ad hoc subsidies will continue. A basic goal of health system reform is the development of a more efficient and equitable approach to providing subsidies for individuals who do not have adequate access.

All of the proposed ideas for reform—a Canadian-style system, a pay-or-play approach, a less flexible, straight employer mandate, or the provision of individual subsidies through the tax system—include some form of redistributive subsidies to provide better balance in access to care. These will always be necessary to provide mainstream insurance, as opposed to ad hoc subsidies, to individuals without the means to pay for it. Questioning whether to provide these subsidies is relevant only if we are willing also to question the feasibility of not providing services, and we do not appear willing to do this.

The present system subsidizes the purchase of health care for virtually everyone in the employer-based system. These subsidies are now being skewed toward individuals with high incomes. Some change in this approach is warranted on equity grounds. In seeking alternative approaches, however, some favor administratively simpler policies. But neither equity nor efficiency should be traded for simplicity. It is important to avoid providing subsidies to all small firms, if the objective is to assist low-wage workers who otherwise could not purchase coverage. Many employees of small firms are highly compensated.

The second theme of my commentary relates to the desirability of retaining employer-based coverage. If the nature and degree of the across-the-board subsidy for health insurance were to change, employer-based groups might no longer be the desired mechanism for purchasing coverage. Under the present system, however, they work for most of the privately insured. Since this is a sizable constituency, they may be able to block policies that seek to eliminate this system and to replace it with anything else. Initially policies should be developed that would leave this basic administrative structure intact for most people.

This is a transitional security blanket. If a different structure were to appear more efficient, it could evolve over time. If, for example, the public backup mechanism accompanying a pay-or-play system succeeds in providing coverage and controlling costs, it may reduce or eliminate the role of private insurers. The battle over these fundamental choices can be fought at a later stage of the reform process.

A willingness to retain the employer-based system does not imply it is without problems. Some problems seem small enough to tolerate. People change jobs, they change insurance. But since most care is provided on a fee-for-service basis, changing insurers does not mean changing physicians. Sometimes complex choices face multiple-job households, yet for the most part people seem willing to make these choices within the system.

Certain aspects of the employer-based system, however, should be addressed. Small firms and certain others face initial underwriting practices that increase insurance costs well above the actuarially fair price within the community. Also, there are often strict preexisting condition exclusions. And by basing rates on the experiences of small numbers of workers, insurers effectively undermine the nature of insurance—that is, the pooling of risks to spread costs of unpredictable events. We need insurance market reforms that would require community rating of premiums, especially for small employers. Despite the problems with community rating pointed out by Roger Feldman and Bryan Dowd in chapter 4, community rating would make employer-based insurance a more viable option for many firms.

Gail Jensen in chapter 8 highlights the potential problems of mandating benefits that must be included in every health insurance policy, and she raises the important issue of exploring alternatives to the present standard benefit package. Despite the arguments in favor of keeping mandates—social needs exceeding private demand, the potential for adverse selection with certain benefits, and the potential for political maneuvering—the standard package should not be viewed as etched in stone.

Insurance is often seen as protection against the costs of infrequent and unpredictable events, and therefore many people interested in purchasing coverage may believe most policies presently include much that is unnecessary. Fewer covered services, much higher deductibles, and variable copayments could all be features of policies that move us away from health care prepayment—the way many policies now operate—and closer to insurance for catastrophic and unforeseen events. Reducing some of the tax subsidies received by higher-income workers may create demand for alternative insurance products.

To the extent that mandates block this type of product variation, they limit options at a time when no single solution is apparent; in fact, finding solutions may involve experimentation that the present mandates inhibit. One argument against relaxing mandates is that individuals will end up with costly coverage that provides fewer benefits. But if the saving in cost is not sufficient to motivate purchase of a reduced array of benefits, there should be no buyers.

Despite the interest in expanding access to care for the uninsured, this should not be undertaken without serious attention to controlling costs. Unless the redistribution in tax subsidies for health insurance is massive—taking many benefits away from high-income, well-insured individuals—the provision of access to some form of insurance to the presently uninsured is likely to increase the aggregate demand for health care services. This would drive up costs, given the history of this market. And given the already increasing burden of health care costs on those currently able to afford insurance, cost control should be on an equal footing with improving access.

Is there a single approach to cost-containment that will work? Some believe it is managed competition. Others adhere strongly to regulation by a single payer, or at least to control by a single entity. If incentives and rate controls do not work, there are policy makers who would support explicit rationing. The bottom line is that there will not be agreement on an approach, and experimentation should be encouraged. But no policy should be expected to work unless there are some penalties for failure, such as if providers' incomes fall and legislators have to raise taxes or cut benefits. It is unlikely that policies that do not feature an explicit constraint on spending will force the hard choices required to limit the growth in health care costs.

The Role of the Private Sector

Discussion of Part Two

RICHARD KRONICK, University of California, San Diego: I have a question about internal cross-subsidies within firms for Michael Morrisey. Some firms contribute more for health insurance for married people than for single people. I know of no firms with compensating wage differentials to pay the single people more. Similarly, most firms pay more—certainly self-insured firms do—for older workers than younger. But I am not aware of compensating wage differentials on the basis of age. There are cross-subsidies between single and married and probably between older and younger within firms, although the age differential is a little less clear.

I also see cross-subsidies among income classes within firms. Most of the people making, say, $10,000 a year in large firms have health insurance. Seventy-five to 80 percent of $10,000-a-year workers in large firms have employer-sponsored insurance. Would a $10,000-a-year worker gladly give up some $2,000 of income for health insurance? Most people, I think, would consider it a very bad trade—having the cash would be preferable.

The question is, Are these $10,000-a-year workers with health insurance really giving up wages, or do better-paid workers at the firm subsidize the health benefits offered the lower-wage workers? And the corollary is, If that is true, will it change the way we think about subsidies to lower-income workers in small businesses who obviously do not have other workers around to compensate for their benefits?

MICHAEL A. MORRISEY, University of Alabama, Birmingham: The short answer is, I don't know. The longer answer is that I suspect it has something to do with the compensating differential for pensions. A young worker in the firm pays too much for health insurance—there is too much of a compensating differential. But as an older worker approaches retirement, the compensating differential is smaller. In the aggregate, though, it balances out. To the extent that workers are tied to the firm over their lifetime—and a surprisingly large number of people stay with one firm—some sort of lifetime compensation may occur at the firm.

Some new research looks at market segmentation as a result of fringe benefits, particularly health insurance. It suggests that some firms have been making their work force more homogeneous by contracting out services. To the extent that the janitorial crew, for example, has a different demand for health insurance than other workers in the firm, hiring them through a cleaning service rather than directly may allow the firm to tailor its benefit package to a relatively homogeneous group of employees.

Many other things are going on in labor markets, but I suspect that part of what we are trying to determine empirically has to do with those sorts of issues.

DONALD W. MORAN, Lewin/ICF: Another complexity in sorting out the evidence on compensating differentials is that compensation for full-time employees is different from that for part-time employees in many particularly large, retail establishments. In a large national account such as K mart, all the full-time employees may have relatively higher wages and be routinely covered for health insurance. Their average wage structure looks much more typical of white-collar America. By contrast, in the individual stores, the great majority of checkers and other employees may be part-time workers excluded from the benefits plan.

HAROLD S. LUFT, University of California, San Francisco: The benefits for both pensions and workers' compensation are roughly scaled to wages— a worker gets paid back about what he was earning. In contrast, health insurance, while it may be scaled to age, is not scaled to income. So it is not clear to me that the same kind of wage offsets, if there are any, would occur for the health insurance. Just because my earnings are twice someone else's, I will not then use twice as much health care, but I will get twice the pension. We cannot assume that what happens with pensions and workers' compensation will happen with health insurance.

ROGER FELDMAN, University of Minnesota: Small business insurance is said to cost 10 to 40 percent more than a comparable group policy. Before we involve the government in addressing this problem, we need to know whether it represents a real market failure or whether it is one of the unavoidable costs of selling insurance to this market.

Possibly the disparity could be explained by prosaic factors such as small businesses' contracting out services that the large businesses include somewhere else in their accounting system.

I want to skewer one straw man: I do not think the higher insurance costs for small groups are due to higher-risk premiums being charged. If this were true, we would see higher profit margins, and in fact the opposite is the case.

207

CATHERINE G. MCLAUGHLIN, University of Michigan: I have several comments on your point. First the Government Accounting Office report is the source of the 10 to 40 percent differential. That office found that much of the difference could be explained by differences in the administrative costs above the actuarially fair (risk-adjusted) premium.

In the Robert Wood Johnson Foundation projects, we found in several cases attempts to reduce the administrative costs. In Arizona, for example, the state Medicaid program supplied many administrative tasks so that the insurer did not have to do them. This shifting of duties reduced the premium by several percentage points.

In Florida, the state was planning to do all the marketing and all the sales, collect the premiums, process the claims, and take care of virtually all the administration—all of which reduced the premium by only a few percentage points. What really reduced the premium in Florida, however, was that the state offered the reinsurance. The result was a 24 percent reduction in premiums. So I think that the difference in the premiums charged is only to a small degree attributable to administrative costs.

In response to Roger Feldman's comment about the actuarially fair premium, we did find that most insurers believe that the small-group business is a much higher-risk population because of adverse selection. They believe that employers offer health insurance either when they have to hire the workers they want or when they want to cover an ailing family member or business associate. Insurers respond by offering higher premiums in part because of higher perceived risk.

Just recently, Lincoln National announced that it would try to sell off most of its group health insurance policies because they were unprofitable. The *Wall Street Journal* article about this subject said that many large insurers were selling off their health insurance. The last sentence of that article noted that Lincoln National did not plan to sell off its small group business: the company intended to keep small firms of fifty and fewer employees. The data, then, may not support the claim of lower profit margins in the small business insurance market.

STEPHEN ZUCKERMAN, Urban Institute: I think that insurers are concerned about getting hit by one or two illnesses within a small firm. Their concern about this risk is consistent with the fact that reinsurance had the biggest impact in Florida. So the risks may not necessarily be rated across firm sizes.

DAVID DRANOVE, Kellogg Graduate School of Management, Northwestern University: For any number of reasons, we can make the argument that it is more costly for small firms to obtain insurance under current markets.

That begs the question of why we would want to subsidize the purchase of insurance by small firms. After all, small steel manufacturers pay more for iron than large steel manufacturers do, but we do not subsidize the purchase of iron by small manufacturers. Unless we were making a policy statement that we like small firms better than big firms, or we are favoring them to offset costly state mandates, I do not see any reason to subsidize small insurance purchasers simply because it is less efficient for small firms to purchase insurance.

Ms. MCLAUGHLIN: Somebody said earlier that one reason is the externalities—that is, the external costs borne by society because of the uninsured. For example, as a society we are not willing to turn away the car accident victim who shows up in the emergency room and does not have health insurance. As long as we are not willing to make that kind of denial, then we do have an issue of externality. It is then not a matter of whether to subsidize but a matter of whom we are subsidizing.

MR. DRANOVE: If we think the externality argument is a reasonable argument for why everybody should have insurance, we can mandate that every employer provide insurance. But if being small makes a company less efficient at fulfilling that mandate, I do not see why being small should be subsidized.

MR. KRONICK: I think if we were to mandate that every employer provide insurance, then we get back to the problem that Mr. Morrisey has laid out for us: it is a very large tax on low-wage workers. If we should subsidize low-wage workers, why subsidize only low-wage workers in small firms and not in large firms? That gets back to the question that I started with: are low-wage workers in large firms already being subsidized by higher-wage workers in the form of different compensating wage differentials? While probably not any of us knows for sure, we could argue that we need to subsidize low-wage workers in small firms because there is no one else to subsidize them.

HEATHER J. GRADISON, American Enterprise Institute: Why should employers subsidize workers' insurance at all? We might ask Mark Pauly to comment on that.

MARK V. PAULY, Wharton School, University of Pennsylvania: If we want everyone to have insurance, we should require everyone to have insurance, pay a subsidy that we deem fair to each level of the income distribution directly to the individuals, and then be done with it. Let them get their insurance however they can.

MS. GRADISON: Take the employer out?

MR. PAULY: No, the employer could be used as a vehicle through which individuals obtain insurance if they wish, but our proposal would remove the obligation from the employer, especially the low-income employer who does not have much money anyway, of arranging to finance that insurance.

MS. GRADISON: What about the point made earlier with regard to the income of a low-wage worker faced with the option of increasing his or her income from $10,000 to $12,000 a year without health insurance or just adding the health insurance? Do we have any idea what the insurance would be worth to such a worker?

MR. PAULY: I estimate an average individual policy this year to be about $1,400 a year and an average family policy to be about $3,000 or more. For a low-wage worker the marginal tax rates are fairly low, in the 15 to 20 percent range. For someone at $10,000 a year after taxes, then, an individual policy at $1,000 or a family policy at $2,500 would be real money. They might reasonably be expected to prefer the extra $2,000 in wages even if they have to pay $150 to $200 in additional taxes.

MR. MORAN: This debate could go in an endless circle, so let me try to close the circle with the following comment. Part of the confusion we face in this debate is caused by what is now covered in the typical health insurance policy. In either the public or the private market, the cost of health insurance contains some adjustment for the risk of serious adverse health events. But that is not all. Contained in the cost of health insurance as well is the cost of what might be called "installment financing for predictable consumption." This part of the cost is not really insurance at all but is for things such as preventive care that we as a matter of policy or equity have decided people should have.

The biggest single difference in health care consumption between the uninsured and the insured is not emergency hospitalization, but rather the kind of consumption expenditures that we as a society seem to have collectively decided that we want people to have. Part of this debate is not so much a health insurance debate as it is a debate about income security. Do we believe that some people have adequate income to purchase particular kinds of items or services that we expect they ought to? The debate really does not have much to do with risk pooling at all.

PART THREE

What Can Reform Achieve in Health Care Cost-Containment?

9

Innovations and Impediments in Private Sector Initiatives

Jack A. Meyer

We face three problems in health care today. First, the real cost of care is rising sharply and continuously. Second, access problems are widespread and are becoming more serious as the "free care" system and hidden subsidies dry up. Third, we have for too long delayed the effort to define and measure the quality of the health care services we are buying, to gauge the relative ability of different providers to deliver those services, and to use that information to purchase care selectively, in consumers' best interests.

Powerful forces are pushing health care costs upward. New medical technology is being developed at a rapid pace. Federal tax subsidies underwrite the overconsumption of health care services even as they leave large segments of low- and moderate-income families out in the cold. Demographic trends—most notably the aging of our population—will increasingly add to health care costs in the future. Threats to our public health, including AIDS and drug and alcohol abuse, drive costs higher. Our medical malpractice system raises costs through the practice of "defensive medicine"—ordering extra tests and procedures, for example, to protect the physician should there be litigation. And regulation is driving up the price of health insurance by loading the benefit package and by placing unreasonable limits on efforts by purchasers and insurers to foster managed care.

Business, labor, and government need to change the way they purchase health care. To underpin this effort we need greater investments in outcomes-research and evaluation, to help providers determine standards of appropriate care. Without such standards, bill payers are underwriting an unknown mix of appropriate, useless, and even deleterious care.

A corresponding investment must be made in obtaining information about the performance of specific providers in delivering effective care. Who does it best? Who does it worst? This information also should be made public, to help educate consumers and purchasers. Thus we should equip purchasers to buy prudently through a three-stage strategy: (1) basic research on health care outcomes and appropriateness of various procedures under different circumstances; (2) the development of case-mix-adjusted information on the relative effectiveness of providers; and (3) public dissemination of this information.

Unless we fundamentally restructure our health care system, we will see a continuation of administered prices under government programs, cost-shifting, risk selection, and consumer vulnerability. This will lead us inexorably to a system of national controls on spending and technology. Such controls are not the best way to solve the problems of cost, access, and quality. This chapter describes a different approach that will better meet the following goals for our health care system:

• All Americans should have regular access to good quality health care for basic needs.

• The productivity of the health care system should be improved to provide better health outcomes more efficiently, so that we get more health care for each dollar spent.

• The quality of health care should be improved by measuring providers' performance and strengthening the incentives to eliminate unnecessary or harmful procedures without discouraging innovation.

Reforming the Health Care System

A market-oriented reform strategy that makes use of incentives for providers and consumers to change their behavior is the best approach for meeting all the goals listed above. Proposals for more centralized control of the health care system could certainly provide universal access to health care and put a lid on total spending. But that approach will not meet the goals of improving the productivity of the system and the quality of care it delivers, as well as would a market reform strategy. Such a market-based strategy must include changes in public policies in addition to actions by private purchasers and providers to implement managed care.

The general principles that should guide such an approach are as follows:

• No one should go without needed health care because it is unaffordable—everyone should have ready access to at least some basic level of services.

• To achieve this, everyone should have some basic level of health insurance coverage. Government subsidies of coverage or care should be based on financial need, and should be carefully designed not to distort employer or employee incentives to purchase prudently.

- Cost discipline should be built into all efforts to improve access to care and should be achieved through incentives rather than controls.
- These incentives should steer patients and providers toward the use of managed care and away from open-ended financing arrangements. They should also steer patients toward providers who produce the best outcomes at a competitive cost level.
- Providers of health care should be paid in a way that rewards those delivering good quality and value and penalizes those delivering poor quality and value.
- Measures of medical necessity, appropriateness, effectiveness, and efficiency must be agreed to and implemented in order to define quality and ascertain who is doing the best job of providing it.
- The United States should maintain a pluralistic, decentralized delivery system to stimulate innovation in basic medical research and in the delivery and financing of health care. We should not freeze the system or block new competitors from entering the market.

Restructuring the Delivery System through Managed Care

A new wave of managed-care initiatives is emerging around the country, as some leading private purchasers work with providers to restructure the delivery of health care. These initiatives incorporate some of the best features of previous cost-control efforts, such as rigorous utilization review, selective contracting with providers, and case management. New Directions for Policy (1991) recently completed a major study of such initiatives and published the results in a report entitled "Private Sector Initiatives: Controlling Health Care Costs."

While the term "managed care" has been widely used to describe a variety of unsuccessful past efforts to control costs, these new wave initiatives show real promise of being successful. After studying these efforts we have determined that each exemplifies one or more of the following principles:

- measuring and comparing provider quality—medical necessity, appropriateness, effectiveness, and efficiency
- purchasing on the basis of value—contracting with providers who deliver the best quality at a reasonable cost
- using strong financial incentives—for employees to use preferred providers and for providers to deliver quality care cost-effectively
- managing health care—guiding patients to appropriate services provided in cost-effective settings
- emphasizing prevention and wellness—health promotion, preven-

215

tive care, and employee assistance programs

In the following sections, each of these principles is discussed at greater length.

Measuring Provider Quality

Until recently, quality has been the missing element in purchasers' efforts to control costs. But now employers increasingly see quality as the key to costs and are designing ways both to measure it and to find out who is providing it. The potential gains here are suggested by Honeywell's controlled experiment with the Mayo Clinic. The company discovered that Mayo-style medicine, widely recognized as top quality, would have saved Honeywell more than 30 percent of its health care costs if its Minneapolis employees had been treated there.

Honeywell will pursue this discovery by trying to induce more employees to use exclusive provider organizations (EPOs), organized on the group or staff model that the company believes is most effective at delivering Mayo Clinic-style medicine. It has already chosen providers in Minneapolis, its corporate headquarters city, and it believes that group and staff-model HMOs may prove highly competitive as the company seeks to establish EPOs at its other locations.

The most sweeping effort to measure and compare the quality of care delivered by different providers is the Greater Cleveland Health Quality Choice Project, where the providers themselves have joined with corporate purchasers to agree on a system for doing this. Usable measures of providers' relative performances are not yet fully developed. But as the system is refined and adopted collectively by purchasers and providers in enough communities, quality-based purchasing could eventually have a significant impact on costs.

Perhaps the most intriguing quality initiatives have less to do with the niceties of measuring quality and more to do with the process of delivering it. Honeywell and the Cleveland employers are seeking providers who will dedicate themselves to continual efforts to improve the quality of care they deliver.

Purchasing Value

Purchasers seeking to measure quality are also laying a foundation for buying health care on the basis of its value; the higher the quality and lower the cost, the better the value. Value-based purchasing is now starting to spread through the corporate sector, as purchasers look for providers that deliver good quality rather than simply discount their fees. And they find that good quality is often provided at a lower cost, not a lower price.

Cleveland Health Quality Choice is certainly a value-based purchasing model, and employer coalitions around the United States are now starting value-based purchasing programs for their members. These include groups in Denver, Milwaukee, Seattle, and St. Louis.

Other employers are contracting with third parties—usually insurers—to pursue such initiatives for them. Allied Signal's national contract with CIGNA, Southwestern Bell's regional one with Prudential, and Chevron's national contract with American PsychManagement for mental health and substance abuse services are all attempts to find cost-effective providers of good quality care and then to channel employees to them.

Employee Financial Incentives

Allied-Signal provides the strongest financial incentives for getting its employees to use CIGNA's network providers. These include cost-sharing for nonusers, with income-related deductibles up to $1,500 and copayments of 20 percent for all covered services—versus virtually first-dollar coverage for those who stay within the network.

Southwestern Bell and Chevron also have strong incentives for employees to use their contract networks, and Xerox uses differential cost-sharing to induce employees to enroll in HMOs that are part of its new HealthLink managed-care programs.

Managing Health Care

Although many employers and insurers are ostensibly pursuing a managed-care approach, health care could actually be managed much better than it now is and could benefit purchasers through both lower costs and improved quality. Honeywell's health-services advisers are an in-house corps of first-level case managers, while the company also contracts with outside experts for more involved cases, such as organ transplant recipients and mental health patients.

Chevron has contracted with a third-party organization to build and manage a network of mental health and substance abuse providers for its employees around the United States. The company is now pursuing a similar arrangement with Metropolitan Life for all other kinds of care, following in the path already blazed by Allied-Signal with CIGNA and by Southwestern Bell with Prudential. Similar arrangements are springing up elsewhere in both the private and public sectors.

Prevention and Wellness

Wellness programs have been heralded as another wave of the future for some time now, yet only a small proportion of companies have adopted them. The future may be about to arrive, however, thanks to the recent publication of results from a study by Johnson & Johnson of its Live for Life program. Johnson & Johnson has provided a bottom-line justification for such programs in the corporate world by showing that savings from reduced medical care expenses and absenteeism in the workplace have been nearly double the amount of program costs. The company is now marketing the program to other employers, and the market should grow as business comes to realize more fully the value of a healthier work force.

Honeywell has a strong employee assistance program (EAP) that seeks to deal with such personal problems as drug abuse before they become expensive medical cases. EAP staff counsel employees and, if appropriate, refer them to treatment programs. Honeywell has shown its EAP to be cost-effective in reducing the use of inpatient psychiatric care, and the company encourages heavy utilization of its services as a good investment in the health and productivity of its work force.

Policy Barriers

The promising models presented in this chapter are still bucking public policies that push health care costs upward. These include open-ended federal tax subsidies, state-mandated benefits, the medical malpractice system, and anticompetitive laws and regulations. Lowering these policy barriers must be part of any cost-control strategy.

Federal Tax Policy. Employees are allowed to exclude from their taxable incomes the full amount of employer contributions to their health insurance. Since most employers do not cap their contributions at fixed dollar amounts, this tax policy encourages the choice of costlier, more comprehensive insurance plans, which then increase the use of medical services.

The tax subsidy emerging from this provision of the law is also very poorly targeted to financial need. It goes mainly to middle- and upper-income households, even while about half the poor receive no government help with the purchase of health insurance. A ceiling should be placed on this tax subsidy, and the additional revenue should be contributed to a stronger effort to help lower-income households purchase health insurance.

Mandated Benefits. More than 800 state benefit mandates exist today, compared with only forty-eight in 1974. These requirements to cover specified services and providers drive up the cost of all health insurance plans and make coverage less affordable for many small employers. Some states now require a cost-benefit analysis of all new proposed mandates. More promising, though, are actions by several states to waive all such requirements for small employers offering coverage for the first time.

Anticompetitive Regulations. All the states have responded to the emergence of managed-care plans by allowing preferred provider organizations and selective contracting. But some have put constraints on the consumer cost-sharing and utilization-review features needed to make these arrangements work—and save money. More than 200 bills imposing restrictions and requirements on managed care have been introduced in states in the early 1990s.

Many states have passed laws limiting the differential in fees that insurers can negotiate with providers, preventing larger discounts from customary charges. And some states have hampered the formation of preferred or exclusive provider organizations by limiting the extent of cost-sharing that can be imposed on consumers for using out-of-plan providers. This strikes at the heart of these arrangements, which were designed to create powerful financial incentives for consumers to use the selected providers who were chosen because they were judged more efficient. By keeping plans from financially penalizing the use of nonpreferred providers, these regulations perpetuate the relatively unrestricted choice of any provider, no matter how costly or inefficient.

The latest, more subtle devices used by a few states to limit alternatives to the traditional free-choice system are laws requiring purchasers to contract with any provider willing to meet the terms and conditions of the contract. This effectively abolishes purchasers' rights to contract selectively with providers of their own choice. All such barriers to a more competitive and efficient medical system raise costs and drive up total expenditures.

Some states also restrict the ability of employers and insurers to review utilization of health care services. In some instances certain medical procedures have been exempt from review altogether. This kind of legislation is the product of lobbying by provider groups seeking to protect their traditional practices. Some rules may be justified to ensure that the people performing reviews are qualified. If the rules are so strict as to make it difficult and costly to perform any review at all, however, providers' actions will be unchecked. More health care services will be used, resulting in higher spending. Often these "credentialing" requirements protect the status of a particular group because they leave the group as the only check on itself.

219

The anticompetitive laws described here should be repealed. This would breathe new life into and reinforce the promising actions of purchasers to control the costs described earlier.

Medical Malpractice System. Malpractice laws raise health care costs directly, through insurance premiums paid by health care providers and then passed on to consumers, and indirectly, through the practice of defensive medicine—tests and procedures that presumably would not be performed if there were less fear of litigation.

The American Medical Association has estimated that malpractice premiums constitute 4.5 percent of total spending for physician services. Total malpractice premiums for doctors and hospitals make up about 1 percent of all health care spending. Even greater than the price tag of insurance premiums are the indirect costs of defensive medicine practiced to avert or defend against potential litigation. The portion of health care dollars that can be attributed to defensive medicine is estimated between 5 percent and 20 percent. Another estimate puts the amount at 15 percent of all expenditures for physician services.

Trends in malpractice premiums and practice patterns for obstetrical care highlight the effect of defensive medicine. Between 1982 and 1987, average premiums for obstetricians more than tripled—from $11,000 to $37,000 per year. During the same period the rate of Caesarean sections, which cost two-thirds more than normal deliveries, jumped by a third. And an increasing proportion of physicians no longer practice obstetrics as a result of professional liability costs.

Even if the threat of litigation were reduced, curbing defensive medical practices would be difficult. Some such medicine is undoubtedly helpful, and much is now standard practice. Moreover, patients have come to expect that every potentially helpful test or procedure be performed. To control the practice of defensive medicine, more research on medical outcomes will be needed, and medical practice guidelines will have to be formulated.

In addition, tort reform will be needed to put a check on defensive medicine. Proposals include: setting guidelines for jury awards based on the age of the victim and severity of the injury, along with limits on pain-and-suffering components to jury awards; greater use of pretrial arbitration; the use of collateral source offsets; and a rethinking of the use of contingency-fee arrangements for attorneys.

A Caveat on Managed Care

The initiatives cited in our report represent the best of what private purchasers are doing about health care costs, but their potential should not be overstated. They still represent the efforts of a relatively small number of companies, with most employers remaining far behind these leaders in changing the way health care is purchased and delivered. If "smart" purchasers are merely shifting costs, then we have to get all purchasers to buy smart so there will be no place for costs to be shifted.

The employers described in our report have reduced the rate of their cost increases well below the curve for most employers. But this means their costs are still rising 10 percent to 15 percent annually, instead of 20 percent or more.

Some of the forces driving up health care costs lie beyond the control of purchasers and will have to be addressed by changes in public policies. Nevertheless, purchasers can do much to improve the performance of the health care system, especially if they work with providers.

Other Parts of a Reform Strategy

While aggressive pursuit of managed care will improve the productivity of the health care system and the quality and cost-effectiveness of services delivered, it is not a complete prescription for system reform. It must be accompanied by strategies for expanding access through universal insurance coverage. There are two basic strategies for expanding access under a market reform approach: Medicaid expansion or tax credits; and reforms in Medicaid and the private insurance market.

Medicaid Expansion and Tax Credits. A critical part of an incentive-based package must be a major effort to arm all consumers with adequate purchasing power to afford basic health insurance and ensure that a mechanism is in place for them to buy that coverage.

The funding can be provided in at least two ways. A refundable federal income tax credit could provide all low-income Americans with enough money to purchase at least basic coverage. A broad version of this approach would substitute this credit for the current exclusion from income tax of employer contributions to employees' health insurance. Under this approach all Americans would receive the credit, which would be earmarked for health insurance—that is, it could be used only to purchase a qualified health insurance plan. This idea was first proposed by Alain Enthoven (1980). A narrow version of the tax credit approach involves providing a refundable credit equal to the full cost of a basic insurance package for the poor, with a gradually diminishing subsidy for the near-poor.

An alternative approach would be to expand Medicaid. This would provide joint federal and state funding for states to provide Medicaid coverage for a greater share of the poor, and it would allow near-poor

221

people to buy in to Medicaid with reasonable financial contributions related to their incomes.

One important caveat should be noted. The newly earmarked public assistance must be scaled down sharply and phased out at some point, such as 150 percent of the federal poverty line. This type of phasing down may have to be combined with a maintenance-of-effort requirement for employers, to keep them from dumping workers onto the Medicaid rolls. Widespread dumping of private insurance is a significant risk under various play-or-pay employer-mandate proposals. These proposals are billed as private-sector oriented, but in reality they may lead to a form of national health insurance through the back door.

Whether assistance to low-income households takes the form of Medicaid expansion, tax credits, or some combination of the two, it must be financed. One financing option for paying a part of the cost is to place a ceiling on the amount of employer contributions to health insurance that may be excluded from federal income tax liability by employees. According to 1991 Congressional Budget Office projections, a cap of $325 a month for family coverage and $150 a month for individual coverage (in 1992 dollars) would raise an estimated $71.9 billion in new federal revenues over the 1992–1996 period.

In addition to the obvious improvement in equity that would result from putting a ceiling on this tax benefit and using the proceeds to help the poor get coverage, there are potential efficiency gains as well. Consumers will have a financial incentive to select the health plan that best controls costs. Above some limit, selecting the high-cost plan will expose the consumer to a small tax liability. Other financing options include higher taxes on alcohol and tobacco products, a consumption tax, and reductions in government outlays elsewhere in the budget.

Medicaid Reform. Medicaid must be reformed as it is expanded. In the past, Medicaid cost-control has exemplified our fixation with suppressing providers' prices while paying insufficient attention to their practice patterns. Medicaid payments per unit of service are pathetically low, while inappropriate care in emergency room settings and unnecessary referrals to specialists abound. For example, the median Medicaid payment for obstetrical services over the course of a pregnancy, including a vaginal delivery, was $738 in 1989, compared with private-sector payments that have been estimated to average $4,334, or about six times as much as Medicaid pays.

Incentives for primary care doctors to participate in the program must be improved by paying more reasonable fees. Greater use of managed-care approaches is necessary, to steer recipients toward care in the most cost-effective setting while avoiding unnecessary or inappro-

priate care. Finally, more risk-sharing arrangements should be established between providers and the government.

Private Insurance Market Reforms. An important aspect of regulatory
reform involves setting some new ground rules for the private insurance
industry. The social contract in which the healthy subsidize the sick
through an insurance pool is breaking down in the United States, and
high-risk patients are in danger of being screened out of insurance or
offered coverage at unaffordable rates.

The problem can be addressed through such measures as requiring
open enrollment and minimum-benefit provisions for qualified health
plans; the latter would have to be kept minimal, to avoid the problem of
state mandates. Limits would be set on the premiums that high-risk
patients could be charged. Insurers would be prohibited from using
medical underwriting to set premiums for each individual and would
be required to ensure renewability of policies to employee groups. The
use of preexisting-condition requirements to limit insurance coverage
would apply only once for each person, as opposed to being renewed
each time the individual takes a new job.

Reducing risk selection may also require a program of reinsurance
under which private health insurers are themselves reinsured against
extremely large outlays per patient. It will be important to spread the
cost of reinsurance premiums over all payers in the community.

Tax Incentives

Under current tax law, self-employed people and unincorporated
businesses cannot avail themselves of the tax preferences afforded to
employees, who are permitted to exclude from taxable income the full
value of their employers' contributions to their health insurance.
Although the social value and fairness of this tax preference are
debatable, we ought to apply it to proprietors on a like basis if we are
going to keep it.

We should also consider some temporary tax incentives to induce
small firms not currently providing health insurance to offer it, and to
make significant financial contributions. This could be accomplished
through a temporary, fixed-dollar tax credit that would phase out after
two years. These approaches concentrate on creating incentives for
employers to provide and fund health insurance. This approach can be
sharply contrasted with one that requires firms simply to pay for health
coverage without paying any attention to affordability. Flat employer
mandates simply move the problem from the government's budget to
employers' budgets and represent another form of cost-shifting. Most

injured by this process would be relatively low-wage workers, who would be seen as dispensable. For these workers, the cost of the insurance represents a high percentage added on to their earnings—creating an incentive for employers to find ways to do without them.

Conclusion

This chapter has presented a case for adopting an incentive-based, market-oriented strategy for reforming the U.S. health care system. This strategy has two major parts: restructuring the health care delivery system through the aggressive pursuit of managed-care principles described here, including removal of public policy barriers to the spread of managed care; and expanding access to care, to achieve universal coverage by combining Medicaid expansion or universal tax credits for the purchase of health insurance with private insurance market reform. A market-oriented strategy of this kind is the best way to achieve the three goals listed in the introduction for our health care system: (1) universal access to good quality health care for basic needs; (2) a more productive health care system that provides better outcomes more efficiently; and (3) improved quality of care, through identifying and rewarding effective providers.

References

Enthoven, Alain. *Health Plan*. Addison-Wesley Press, 1980.
New Directions for Policy. "Private Sector Initiatives: Controlling Health Care Costs." Washington, D.C., March 1991.

10

Medicare as the Basis for All-Payer Provider Payment Reform

Karen Davis

Rapid increases in health care costs have been the dominant problem in the health care system for the past two decades. Over this period considerable experimentation has occurred in approaches to curb the growth in health outlays, either by moderating the rise in prices or by utilizing health care services. Despite some isolated successes of these efforts, health care expenditures have risen far faster than the gross national product and far faster than most payers of health care services are willing to pay in the long term (Davis et al. 1990).

The U.S. experience is increasingly viewed as unsatisfactory in the light of the international experience. The United States is the only major industrialized nation without universal health coverage for its population. More than 33 million Americans lack public or private health insurance coverage. Access to health care is uneven and inequitable. The uninsured are much less likely to receive appropriate health care, contributing to the poorer health status of the U.S. population compared with other nations. Despite the failure to ensure universal health insurance coverage, the United States devotes a far greater share of its gross national product to health care than do other nations (Schieber and Poullier 1991).

Interest is growing in comprehensive reform of the U.S. health system, to ensure universal health insurance coverage and to limit total health expenditures. Universal health insurance legislative proposals also provide for the establishment of global budgets for health care, or the establishment of prospective expenditure targets or ceilings on health outlays (Congressional Research Service 1991). Typically these proposals retain a central role for fee-for-service private practice of medicine but establish a mechanism for setting the rates for services provided by hospitals, physicians, and other providers within the context of a total expenditure limit.

This chapter reviews recent trends in health expenditures, with

225

special attention to the effectiveness of public sector efforts to curb rising outlays. It describes some of the major legislative proposals to establish all-payer provider payment systems and limits on health expenditures, and it concludes with a discussion of the merits of building on Medicare's provider payment system to control costs under a universal health insurance system.

Trends in National Health Expenditures

The Congressional Budget Office has calculated annual rates of real growth in health expenditures for hospital and physician services over the period from 1970 to 1989.

Trends in National and Medicare Hospital Expenditures. After deflating for inflation in the economy as a whole (using the GNP fixed-weighted price deflator), we find that hospital expenditures increased at an annual rate of 7.2 percent in the period from 1970 to 1980 (see figure 10–1). This rate of increase slowed in the 1980s but still increased substantially faster than prices in the economy. In the period from 1980 to 1985 real hospital expenditures increased at an annual rate of 4.8 percent, and in the period from 1985 to 1989 at an annual rate of 4.6 percent.

The slowdown in hospital expenditure growth is one of the few bright signs in the fight against rising health care costs—although many would find the trends even in the 1980s unacceptably high, since hospital expenditures continued to grow faster than the gross national product.

The trend in Medicare hospital expenditures has been particularly striking. In the 1970s real Medicare hospital expenditures increased at an annual rate of 10.6 percent. In the first half of the 1980s this slowed to 7.3 percent, and in the period from 1985 to 1989 real Medicare hospital expenditures increased at an annual rate of 2.5 percent. Clearly, the decelerating trend in Medicare expenditure growth is a major factor in the general slowdown in national hospital expenditure growth.

Growth rates on a per capita basis are even lower. As shown in figure 10–1, real national hospital expenditures per capita increased at an annual rate of 6.3 percent in the period from 1970 to 1980, while real Medicare hospital expenditures per beneficiary increased at an annual rate of 7.0 percent. During the period from 1980 to 1985, real national hospital expenditures per capita increased 3.7 percent annually, while Medicare continued to exceed the national rate of increase with a 5.4 percent real annual increase per beneficiary. But in the second half of the 1980s, while real national hospital expenditures per capita continued to increase at 3.6 percent, real Medicare hospital expenditures per benefi-

FIGURE 10–1

AVERAGE ANNUAL GROWTH RATES OF REAL NATIONAL AND MEDICARE EXPENDITURES FOR HOSPITAL AND PHYSICIAN SERVICES, TOTAL AND PER CAPITA, 1970–1989

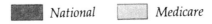

■ National ▢ Medicare

Total Expenditures

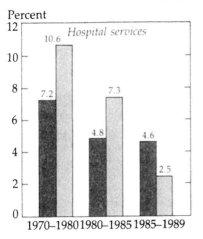

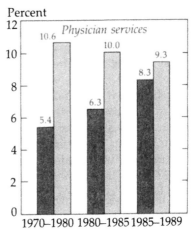

Per Capita/Per Enrollee Expenditures

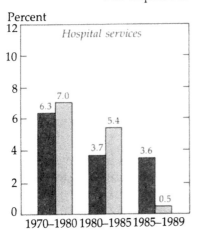

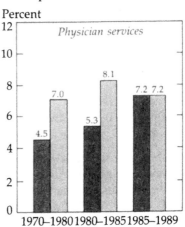

NOTE: Real expenditures are calculated using the GNP fixed-weighted deflator.
SOURCE: Congressional Budget Office calculations, based on data from the Health Care Financing Administration, Office of the Actuary, 1991.

227

ciary slowed to a 0.5 percent annual rate of increase.

These trends reflect the success of the Medicare prospective payment system for hospitals, introduced in the fall of 1983, in slowing the rate of increase in Medicare hospital outlays. The Medicare prospective payment system for hospitals was important for several reasons. It based payments to hospitals on a fixed rate, depending on the diagnosis-related group of the patient, rather than on the actual cost of caring for the patient. This created a major incentive for hospitals to increase efficiency, to eliminate unnecessary services, and to discharge patients as soon as possible. By establishing a limit on the rate of increase in Medicare payments per patient over time, the Medicare prospective payment system has also had a major impact on controlling the growth in hospital outlays for the care of beneficiaries.

Trends in Real Hospital Expenses and Interventions to Control Costs. It is also interesting to examine trends in growth in real hospital expenditures according to time periods, based on national policies to control health care costs. With several colleagues at Johns Hopkins University, I analyzed trends in real community hospital expenses during seven time periods:

- 1950–1965, characterized by rapid growth in private health insurance
- 1965–1971, the early years of Medicare and Medicaid
- 1972–1974, during the Nixon Economic Stabilization Program of wage and price freezes on the economy
- 1975–1977, following the lifting of ESP controls
- 1978–1980, when the Carter administration hospital cost-containment legislation was under consideration, and the hospital industry mounted a voluntary effort to control costs
- 1981–1983, when a market approach to controlling health care costs was emphasized
- 1984–1986, under the Medicare prospective payment system (Davis et al. 1990)

As shown in figure 10–2, we found that increases in real community hospital expenses rose at an annual rate of 8.3 percent during the private health insurance expansion period; accelerated to 11.6 percent in the Medicare and Medicaid expansion period; slowed to 6.1 percent under the Nixon Economic Stabilization Program; accelerated to 8.7 percent following the lifting of ESP controls; fell to 3.1 percent during the Carter hospital cost-containment debate; jumped to 7.8 percent in the early 1980s in the absence of any national policy to control costs; and fell to

FIGURE 10–2
AVERAGE ANNUAL RATE OF INCREASE IN
REAL COMMUNITY HOSPITAL EXPENSES, 1950–1986
(percent)

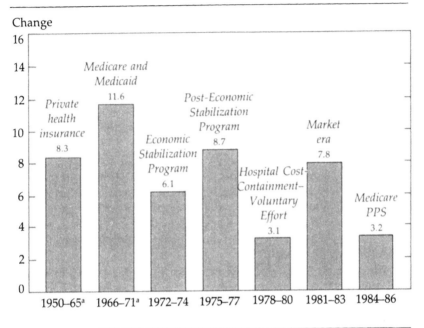

a. Annualized.

SOURCE: Karen Davis, Gerard Anderson, Diane Rowland, and Earl Steinberg, *Health Care Cost Containment* (Baltimore, Md.: The Johns Hopkins University Press, 1990).

3.2 percent after Medicare prospective payment limits were introduced.

Clearly, while rising hospital costs have continued to be a major problem over the past several decades, increases have been affected by national policies to control costs. Wage and price controls under Nixon did work to slow health expenditure growth. Even the threat of mandatory controls under the Carter administration substantially slowed growth. The removal of controls, however, or the threat of controls was followed by a marked acceleration in costs.

An accumulation of evidence also suggests that state-level all-payer hospital systems have been effective in slowing the growth in hospital costs. Maryland is the only state currently with an all-payer hospital payment system that includes a Medicare waiver. During the 1980s, however, Massachusetts (fiscal years 1983–1985), New York (1983–1985), and New Jersey (1981–1988) also operated all-payer systems.

Several studies have analyzed the effects of state all-payer regulation of hospital expenses, after accounting for such other factors that may affect costs such as wage levels, case-mix, and population characteristics. Using data for the 1982–1986 period, Robinson and Luft (1988) found, for example, that growth in hospital costs per admission was reduced in all-payer states, compared with other states. Compared with an adjusted growth rate of 58 percent over the period from 1982 to 1986 in all other states, the growth rate was 47 percent in Massachusetts and Maryland, 52 percent in New York, and 56 percent in New Jersey. Schramm, Renn, and Biles (1986) found that between 1976 and 1984 the rate of increase in hospital expenses per adjusted admission was 87 percent less in rate-setting states than in nonregulated states.

All-payer systems appear to be more effective in controlling costs than partial-payer systems. Thorpe and Phelps (1990), for example, found that New York's all-payer regulation reduced inflation in costs substantially, when compared with the partial-payer system that preceded it. Preliminary evidence also suggests that costs have accelerated in those states that changed from an all-payer system to a partial-payer system in the late 1980s.

Maryland is the only state to maintain an all-payer hospital system over the 1980s. Maryland experienced an increase of 134 percent in hospital expenditures per admission over the period from 1979 to 1989, compared with 216 percent for the United States as a whole (author's calculations based on AHA data). On a per capita basis, Maryland's rate of increase was 139 percent over the period from 1979 to 1989, compared with 216 percent nationally.

Trends in National and Medicare Physician Expenditures. The Congressional Budget Office has also analyzed trends in real physician expenditures over the period from 1970 to 1989. Unlike the case of hospital expenditures, outlays for physician services have continued to accelerate in the 1980s. As shown in figure 10–1, real national physician expenditures increased at an annual rate of 5.4 percent from 1970 to 1980, increased to 6.3 percent from 1980 to 1985, and further accelerated to 8.3 percent from 1985 to 1989.

Growth in real Medicare physician expenditures over this period exceeded national trends, although the differential narrowed. In the period from 1970 to 1980, Medicare physician expenditures increased at 10.6 percent, slowing slightly to 10.0 percent from 1980 to 1985, and to 9.3 percent from 1985 to 1989.

On a per person basis, real physician expenditures per capita accelerated from 4.5 annual percent increases in the 1970s to 5.3 percent in the first half of the 1980s and 7.2 percent in the second half. Real Medicare physician expenditures per beneficiary increased at an annual rate of 7.0 percent in the 1970s, 8.1 percent in the first half of the 1980s, and 7.2 percent, or the same as the national per capita average, in the period from 1985 to 1989.

While controlling hospital costs has been the primary focus of policy attention in the past two decades, it is clear that the 1990s will focus greater attention on the far more rapid increases in physician expenditures. Comprehensive Medicare physician payment legislation was enacted and began in January 1992. The new Medicare physician payment system has three major features: a Medicare fee schedule with resource-based relative values; a limit on actual charges by physicians to Medicare patients, eventually not to exceed the fee schedule by more than 15 percent; and a Volume Performance Standard, or expenditure target, which bases increases in fees for future years on performance in meeting prospective expenditure targets. This system should provide incentives for lower cost primary care. By basing prices of physician services on resource costs, inappropriate incentives for costly specialized care should be greatly reduced. In addition, the system for the first time provides a mechanism for limiting total Medicare physician outlays.

Physician expenditure targets, while new to the United States, have been tried in other countries. Germany had a physician expenditure target system in place from 1977 to 1985, followed by mandatory physician expenditure ceilings. Several Canadian provinces have also instituted physician expenditure targets or ceilings. Experience, while preliminary, suggests that such systems have been effective in slowing expenditure growth (Rice and Bernstein 1990; Kirkman-Liff, 1990).

Universal Health Insurance and All-Payer Provider Payment Reform

While the Medicare hospital and physician prospective payment systems show considerable promise of constraining expenditure growth under Medicare, a partial-payer approach to controlling health care costs is unlikely to be as effective as an all-payer provider payment system. The United States is the only major industrialized nation without a single system for paying hospitals and physicians. In a partial-payer system, costs can be shifted to other payers, or access to care for Medicare beneficiaries may become restricted.

Evidence also suggests that attempts to control health care costs without ensuring universal coverage can lead to reduced access to care for the uninsured (Davis et al. 1990; Rowland 1987). As hospital revenues from Medicare and Medicaid have been restrained in the 1980s, hospitals have reduced their willingness to take uninsured patients, and some hospitals have also tightened access to care for Medicaid beneficiaries. The unfortunate side effect of partial-payer cost controls, therefore, is to squeeze out of the health care system those who are low-income and uninsured.

More than two dozen legislative proposals for health system reform have been introduced in the 102nd Congress (Congressional Research Service 1991). These include proposals to provide tax incentives for the purchase of private health insurance, relying primarily on market incentives to control costs. Other proposals would establish a single public plan covering the entire population, with global budgets or other mechanisms to establish limits on total health spending. Some proposals would put state governments in a lead role in controlling costs; others would rely on a federally administered system. Some proposals would simply extend the current Medicare program to the entire population, along with its methods of provider payment.

In the middle are employment-based universal health insurance proposals that would provide employers with a choice of covering workers under private health plans or paying a payroll tax to cover workers and dependents under a public plan. Mechanisms for controlling costs include using Medicare provider payment systems as a basis for all-payer provider payment, or establishing a mechanism for negotiation of such systems along with expenditure targets or ceilings. The ways in which the provider payment rates would be set under these proposals are described in more detail below.

HealthAmerica—Affordable Health Care for All Americans Act. HealthAmerica: Affordable Health Care for All Americans Act, S. 1227, sponsored by Senator George Mitchell, Democrat of Maine, and other Democratic senators, would create a Federal Health Expenditure Board to establish national, state, and regional goals for health care expenditures for each year. The board would be charged with overseeing negotiations between purchasers and providers of care to develop payment rates to achieve expenditure goals. If agreement were reached, these rates would be binding on all parties. If no agreement were reached, the board would issue nonbinding advisory rates. States could establish their own alternative payment systems, rates, and methods for achieving the national goals.

Medicaid acute care benefits would be replaced by a new public plan, AmeriCare, which would also cover workers and dependents in those firms where employers chose to pay the payroll tax rather than obtain private coverage. AmeriCare would use Medicare payment methods and rates. Medicaid payment rates would be replaced and phased up to Medicare rates over time. In addition, businesses with fewer than 100 employees that did not provide coverage before enactment could buy private health insurance coverage from a private insurer under which providers of care would be paid on the basis of Medicare rates for up to five years.

Senator Paul Simon, Democrat of Illinois, has introduced a bill (S.1669) that would amend S. 1227 to make the Health Expenditure Board–determined rates mandatory if negotiators did not agree. In addition, his plan would permit states to opt out of the employment-based system if they adopted a single-payer plan.

Pepper Commission Health Care Access and Reform Act of 1991. The Pepper Commission Health Care Access and Reform Act of 1991, H.R. 2535 and S. 1177, is sponsored by Congressman Henry Waxman, Democrat of California, and Senator Jay Rockefeller, Democrat of West Virginia. Like HealthAmerica, it is an employment-based universal health insurance plan, in which employers have a choice between covering workers and dependents under private plans or under a new public plan. Medicaid acute-care benefits would be replaced by the new public plan.

Payments to providers for all beneficiaries in the new public plan would be made according to Medicare's payment rules. Small-employer plans would have the option of having payment for basic health care services at rates no higher than those under the public plan. Providers participating in the public plan could not charge enrollees under such small-employer plans more than the balance bills allowed under the public plan. Medicaid payments would be replaced by Medicare payment rates for hospital, physician, and other acute-care services covered by the plan. States could establish all-payer systems for one or more services that would apply to private plans, Medicare, and the new public plan.

Health Insurance Coverage and Cost-Containment Act of 1991. Congressman Dan Rostenkowski, Democrat of Illinois, has introduced the Health Insurance Coverage and Cost-Containment Act of 1991, H.R. 3205. Like the Mitchell and Rockefeller-Waxman plans, H.R. 3205 gives employers a choice of covering workers and dependents under private plans or a new public plan. The bill calls for the establishment of a Health Care Cost-Containment Commission with eleven members appointed by the president and confirmed by the Senate. It establishes a limit on total health care spending, linked to the growth in gross national product. By the year 2000, health care outlays would increase each year at the same rate as the gross national product. Each year the commission would allocate the total health care spending limit across covered services after conducting negotiations with professional and other associations representing health care providers. The secretary of Health and Human Services would establish payment rates for covered services that would result in total expenditures consistent with these expenditure limits, by type of service. The commission would review and approve such payment rates if it found that such rates were consistent with its allocations.

Provider payment rates are to be based on payment methodologies currently used by Medicare, including inpatient hospital payment per patient based on diagnosis-related groups, and payment for physicians' services based on a resource-based, relative-value scale. Physicians and hospitals would be paid the same, regardless of whether a beneficiary were covered under the new public plan, Medicare, or private plans.

Medicare as a Basis for an All-Payer Provider Payment System with Expenditure Targets

These legislative proposals, particularly the Rostenkowski proposal, suggest how Medicare could be used as the basis for an all-payer-provider payment system. Hospitals would be paid a prospective payment rate per patient, based on the diagnosis-related group of the patient for the care of all patients—whether covered under a public plan or a private plan. Physicians would be paid on a fee-for-service basis, according to the resource-based, relative-value schedule used by Medicare for the care of all patients—both publicly insured and privately insured. Under the Medicare payment system, physicians are permitted to charge patients fees up to 15 percent above the fee schedule. Hospitals are not permitted to balance-bill patients under the Medicare program, and payment is considered payment in full.

The level of approved payment rates under the all-payer system could be established initially on a system-wide, revenue-neutral basis—that is, in the aggregate, payments to hospitals and physicians would be the same as under the current health system. For any given type of patient, however, this payment rate could be less or more than under the current system. In general, physicians and hospitals would receive higher payment rates for care of the uninsured and Medicaid beneficiaries relative to current practice, and lower payment rates from privately insured patients. Over time the level of payment rates would depend on expenditure goals by service and experience with increases in the volume of services provided.

Research Implications. Although it is conceptually straightforward, considerable research and analysis would be needed to develop and implement such an all-payer system. Currently no data system exists for assessing the level of physician expenditures nationally or by geographic area, such as by state. Very little is known about how different providers with different patient mixes by source of insurance coverage would be affected by such a system, or how long a transition would be required to avoid major disruptions in the system. Further, Medicare's prospective payment systems have been designed for an elderly and disabled patient population. Modification may also be needed of the values assigned to hospital inpatient diagnostic groups for nonelderly patients, to reflect the resource cost of younger patients, as well as some further refinement of the physician resource-based, relative-value scale for a younger population.

Impact of an All-Payer System. Six advantages of this system are outlined below.

Equitable access to care. An all-payer system with expenditure targets has considerable appeal. It would reduce the discrimination against patients for whom providers now receive lower payment rates—the poor, the uninsured, and Medicaid beneficiaries. It would guarantee that no patient is denied access to care based on the source of his insurance coverage.

Administrative simplicity. Establishment of a single system for the payment of hospitals and physicians should also reduce the administrative burden on providers from the currently mixed, public-private health financing system. A uniform claim form and a uniform method of billing for care rendered should eliminate the confusion and complexity of the current system. Providers would know with certainty the price they would receive for any given service.

Effective cost controls. An all-payer system embodied in expenditure targets also has the greatest potential for effective cost controls (Reischauer 1991). Total expenditure limits can be reached either by adjusting payment rates concurrently to stay within the preset limit or by setting payment rates in subsequent years to reflect any deviation from actual expenditures from preset limits.

Consistency with competitive approaches. An all-payer provider payment system is compatible with other efforts to control health care costs through competitive mechanisms. Persons covered under both private plans and public plans could be given the choice of enrolling in health maintenance organizations or other managed care options, and financial incentives could be built in for those selecting lower-cost, capitated options. Preferred provider plans (PPOs) could still exist, although providers would be paid at the same rate under all plans. PPOs could attract enrollees either through lower costs, as the result of better utilization performance of preferred providers, or by agreeing not to balance-bill patients.

Quality of care. One concern that has been raised about all-payer payment systems is the possible adverse effect on quality of care. If payment rates, for example, are set at quite low levels either by very tight expenditure targets or by continued rapid growth in the volume of services, then the quality of care might be adversely affected. Although this objection is theoretically valid, the United States starts at a very high level of expenditures. Physician fees and incomes are considerably higher in the United States than in other countries. Hospital costs per day and staffing ratios are considerably higher than in other countries. The United States spends more than 40 percent more per capita on health care than does the next closest country. An extensive research literature suggests that unnecessary or medically inappropriate care is common. As more health outcomes-and-effectiveness research is conducted, there should be an opportunity to reduce costs that are now in the base.

Concern has also been expressed that such a system would discourage physicians from entering medical practice or would cause them to abandon practice. This has not been a problem in other industrialized nations with government-established fee schedules. Rather a physician surplus—not a lack of physicians—is more typical. Given the growing supply of physicians in the United States, it seems extremely unlikely that availability of health care services will become a serious problem.

Innovation and technological change. A closely related concern is that a universal health insurance system with a uniform system of paying health care providers will deter innovation and technological change. Again, while in theory this possibility exists, the United States starts with a very advanced, high-technology health system. Proposals such as the Rostenkowski one would permit further increases in health spending as a percentage of gross national product for the next decade, after which health expenditures would be stabilized in relation to gross national product. Expenditure limits, in fact, might well be a stimulus to innovation and technological change. The experience of other sectors of the economy is that international competition has led to restructuring, cost reductions, and improved productivity and efficiency. With budgetary constraints in the health system, cost-reducing technological change would become a priority.

Summary

The United States has left the control of health care costs to market forces for decades. In the 1980s a competitive approach to controlling rising health care costs was tried by private insurers and employers—without noticeable effect. The consequence has been a steady climb in the share of the nation's economic resources going to health care. Continued inaction and the absence of a national policy to reform the health system to achieve both universal coverage and effective cost controls are no longer tolerable.

The Medicare program has led the way in reforming provider payment for both hospitals and physicians. New prospective payment systems give health care providers an incentive to provide care more efficiently and give government the mechanism for controlling outlays for Medicare beneficiaries. Medicare hospital-expenditure growth has slowed remarkably since the introduction of the prospective payment system in late 1983. The new system of paying physicians according to a resource-based, relative-value fee schedule subject to expenditure targets should be equally effective.

The next step is extension of these prospective payment systems to the care of all patients. This would ensure that providers do not shift the cost of lost revenue from publicly financed beneficiaries to privately insured patients. Universal health insurance coverage would also ensure that no one is squeezed out of the system, as cost controls are tightened. An all-payer provider payment system would ensure equitable access to health care services for all patients and would greatly simplify the administration of claims. It would permit a negotiated or political determination of total health spending—permitting trade-offs between the use of social resources for health care and other important national priorities.

This rationalization of the health system is urgently needed. As a nation we stand alone among industrialized countries, both in failing to ensure access to health care for all our citizens and in failing to use the power of government to ensure that health care services are provided at a reasonable rate. To continue to avoid comprehensive reform while placing faith in market forces will simply extend the current, unacceptably high rates of health-expenditure growth well into the next century. In the meantime, millions of Americans go without needed health care, and billions of dollars are wasted in a health system unchecked by market or regulatory forces.

References

Congressional Research Service. *Health Insurance Legislation in the 102nd Congress.* Report prepared by Beth C. Fuchs, Janet Lundy, and Joan Sokolovsky. Washington, D.C., July 1, 1991.

Davis, Karen, Gerard Anderson, Diane Rowland, and Earl Steinberg. *Health Care Cost Containment.* Baltimore, Md.: The Johns Hopkins

University Press, 1990.

Kirkman-Liff, B.L. "Physician Payment and Cost-containment Strategies in West Germany: Suggestions for Medicare Reform." *Journal of Health Politics, Policy, and Law* 15 (1990): 69–100.

Reischauer, Robert D. Testimony before the Subcommittee on Health, Committee on Ways and Means. U.S. House of Representatives, July 11, 1991.

Rice, Thomas, and Jill Bernstein. "Volume Performance Standards: Can They Control Growth in Medicare Services?" *The Milbank Quarterly* 68 (1990): 295–319.

Robinson, James C., and Harold S. Luft. "Competition, Regulation, and Hospital Costs, 1982 to 1986," *Journal of the American Medical Association* 260 (1988): 2676–81.

Rowland, Diane. *Hospital Care for the Poor and Uninsured.* Doctoral dissertation, Johns Hopkins School of Hygiene and Public Health. Baltimore, Md., 1987.

Schieber, George, and J. P. Poullier. "International Health Expenditures," *Health Affairs* (1991).

Schramm, Carl J., Steven C. Renn, and Brian Biles. "Controlling Hospital Cost Inflation: New Perspectives on State Rate Setting," *Health Affairs* (1986): 22–33.

Thorpe, Kenneth E., and Charles E. Phelps. "Regulatory Intensity and Hospital Cost Growth," *Journal of Health Economics* 9 (1990): 143–166.

11

The Five W's of Utilization Review

David Dranove

Health insurers routinely perform some kind of utilization review (UR) before authorizing payment for health services. UR takes many forms. According to A. Foster Higgins & Co. (1991), 81 percent of all insurance plans require "preadmission certification," while 65 percent require "concurrent review," and 73 percent require a second opinion for surgery. UR is also required for Medicare and many state Medicaid plans. The widespread use of UR is relatively new; just ten years ago few public or private insurers performed UR (Wickizer 1990).

Advocates claim that UR can eliminate unnecessary utilization and move service delivery to low-cost settings. Offsetting these benefits are the costs to the insurer and provider of administering UR as well as the costs to patients of inappropriately forgoing care. Given the widespread use of UR, one might imagine that there is a consensus that its benefits exceed its costs. No such consensus appears to exist. A survey of 2,000 large employers, for example, revealed that although 93 percent used UR, 64 percent did not know if UR contained utilization (Blue Cross-Blue Shield 1991). Many believe that UR cannot achieve cost savings without "far more stringent and intrusive micromanagement" than currently exists (Grumbach et al. 1991). The value of UR will be a key policy question in the 1990s.

Many national health insurance proposals promote UR either directly or indirectly. Private insurers must evaluate whether it is worth their while to remain on the UR bandwagon. This chapter explores the so-called five W's of UR: who, what, when, where, and especially why. The chapter also discusses how well. UR is compared with other cost-containment schemes such as increased patient cost sharing and changes in compensating providers. While the schemes for changing the compensation of providers work to eliminate "systematic" overconsumption of health care services, UR works to eliminate "mistakes" in consumption. Unfortunately, evaluations of UR to date have focused on levels of utilization rather than on its appropriateness. Thus it is difficult to determine if UR is fulfilling its promise.

Who?

The idea of reviewing utilization to identify questionable practices originated with medical care providers. Some hospitals have had internal utilization review committees for decades. These follow in the tradition of peer review as practiced in many professions. Since the reputation of an entire medical staff may be tarnished when one of its own members provides inappropriate care, it is in the staff's interest to conduct UR to maintain its quality.

External UR emerged in the early 1970s in conjunction with the Medicare program. Professional standards review organizations (PSROs) were established in each state to assess the appropriateness of care provided to Medicare patients. PSROs established criteria for hospitalization and length of stay based on the patient's condition. PSROs could (but rarely did) reprimand or deny payment to physicians whose treatments of Medicare or Medicaid patients deviated substantially from protocols.

Although PSROs died out, the notion of external UR did not. Upon the introduction of the Medicare Prospective Payment System in 1983, many PSROs were resurrected into peer review organizations (PROs). At the same time hundreds of private UR service agencies have emerged. The majority of hospitalizations today are subject to some kind of UR.

What, When, and Where?

There is no well-accepted definition of UR. The U.S. Institute of Medicine (IOM) considers UR to be "a set of techniques used by or on behalf of purchasers of health benefits to manage health care costs by influencing patient care decision making through case-by-case assessments of the appropriateness of care prior to its provision" (IOM 1989). The "influencing" of the decision making mentioned by the IOM usually involves denial of payment for nonapproved treatment. Patients presumably refuse to purchase treatments no longer covered by their insurer.

The UR process is straightforward. Each case under review passes through a series of screens. In the case of preadmission review, the admitting physician (or an admitting nurse) first telephones the appropriate UR service agency and reports the patient's diagnosis, vital signs, and any relevant laboratory results. A UR service agency employee records the information and, with the help of computer software, is able to issue an approval within a few minutes. If the vital signs are not acceptable, the case may be reviewed in more detail by a professional reviewer, usually a registered nurse with advanced clinical and academic training. If necessary, the UR service agency will contact the admitting physician for further justification of the admission. If the case fails all of these screens, the UR service agency will deny approval for admission. In some cases the treatment may be approved but only in a nonhospital setting (for example, in an outpatient surgicenter). The cost of adding UR to a basic insurance package is about $1.50 to $2.50 per employee per month (Vibbert 1990).

A good example of a utilization review program is the Severity of Illness/Intensity of Service (SI/IS) system pioneered by Interqual. This is the system of choice for Medicare UR. IS criteria include "diagnostic and therapeutic services generally requiring hospitalization," whereas SI criteria include "objective, clinical parameters reflecting the need for hospitalization" (Interqual 1989). According to Interqual,

> Any patient admitted to the hospital must meet either one SI or one IS criterion on admission and must have met both an SI and an IS criterion by the first review following the completion of 24 hours in the hospital.

Interqual provides to UR service agencies specific IS and SI criteria for different medical conditions, as well as a flowchart to help the UR practitioner determine when to apply the various criteria for admission, subsequent review, and discharge.

Why?

In recent years insurers have taken a number of steps to eliminate wasteful medical care expenditures. These steps include the introduction of UR, increases in patient cost sharing, and changes in provider incentives. This section presents a very simple model to explain the motivation behind each of these insurer initiatives. The model considers individuals with a common illness determining whether or not to purchase treatment. In this model, individuals differ according to their perceptions of how sick they are (for example, patients may make mistakes) and their own idiosyncratic evaluations of the value of care (some patients like their medicine and others do not). The decision by an individual to purchase or forgo care involves an assessment of benefits and costs, which can be affected by physician treatment recommendations as well as by insurer cost-containment activities.

Consider a group of individuals with the same underlying medical condition. Let V_a denote the *average* amount that fully informed patients are willing to pay for a sure-fire cure. The amount that any given individual is willing to pay may differ from the average because his income, taste for treatment, threshold for pain, and the like may not be average. This amount is $V = V_a + V_i$, where V_i is the individual's

FIGURE 11–1
WHICH INDIVIDUALS SHOULD BUY MEDICAL TREATMENT?

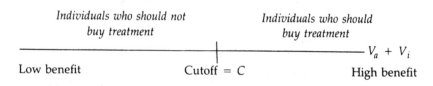

NOTE: V_a is the average amount that fully informed patients are willing to pay for a certain cure. V_i is the individual patient's idiosyncratic value of treatment.
SOURCE: Author.

"idiosyncratic" value of the treatment, and may be positive or negative.

Let C denote the cost of treatment.[1] If treatments are allocated optimally, then a given patient would purchase treatment if and only if

$$V_a + V_i > C \tag{11.1}$$

Figure 11–1 illustrates decision condition (11.1). Imagine that patients are arrayed according to the benefits of care, $V_a + V_i$. There is some cutoff patient for whom the benefits are sufficiently large to justify the cost (that is, for this patient $V_a + V_i = C$). If treatments are allocated optimally, then all patients with higher benefits should receive treatment, and all patients with lower benefits should not.

For a number of reasons patients may not line up in their proper places on either side of the cutoff in figure 11–1. Decision rules for patients may diverge from the optimal decision rule for a number of reasons: first, the patient may have insurance; second, the patient's information about the value of treatment may be imperfect; and third, the patient's physician may try to mislead him about the value of treatment ("induce demand"). Each of these is modeled below.

Insurance. Most individuals are insured for a substantial fraction of the costs of treatment. Let λ denote the fraction of the total cost paid for by patients (that is, the patient pays λC.) A fully informed patient will tend to overconsume care whenever $\lambda < 1$. This is the familiar problem of moral hazard.

---

1. I do not consider substitute treatments. I also assume that cost and price are identical. This avoids issues of wealth distribution and monopoly dead-weight loss.

242

Imperfect Information. Most patients cannot determine with certainty how much a particular treatment is likely to improve their health. We can model this information imperfection by assuming that each patient imprecisely estimates the value of treatment. Suppose that in the absence of any information from physicians, patients estimate the value of treatment to equal $V_a + V_i + V_e$, where V_e denotes the error in the patient's estimate.

For illustrative purposes, suppose that V_e is normally distributed in the population with mean μ_e and standard deviation σ_e. If $\mu_e > 0$, then patients systematically overestimate the value of treatment. If $\mu_e < 0$, then patients systematically underestimate the value of treatment. Even if patients do not systematically over- or underestimate V_a, some patients will make "mistakes." The larger is σ_e, the noisier are the patients' estimates of the true value.

Physician Influence. Suppose that physicians can bias or confound the patient's estimate of the value of care. In particular, suppose that once the physician provides information about the value of treatment, the patient estimates that the value of care is $V_a + V_i + V_e + V_d$, where V_d denotes the effect of information imparted by the physician. Let V_d be normally distributed with mean μ_d and standard deviation σ_d. If $\mu_d > 0$, then physicians are systematically "inducing demand." That is, they are providing information that leads the patient systematically to overestimate the value of treatment. If $\mu_d < 0$, then physicians are systematically underprescribing treatment.

Even if physicians do not systematically try to over- or underprescribe care, their recommendations can lead to inappropriate use. This is captured in the model by σ_d, which measures the variation in treatment recommendations from one physician to the next. In this model I am assuming that such variation around the mean represents mistakes; that is, all physicians should make the same recommendation for a given patient. This assumption is generally too restrictive. If physicians have different skills, then it may be optimal for them to make different recommendations.

Let $V_x = V_o + V_i + V_e + V_d$, where V_x is the patient's noisy and possibly biased estimate of the value of treatment. The patient will purchase treatment if:

$$Vx > \lambda C \tag{11.2}$$

A comparison of equation (11.1) and equation (11.2) shows that an individual will overconsume (that is, purchase care even though equation (11.1) is not satisfied) whenever

FIGURE 11–2

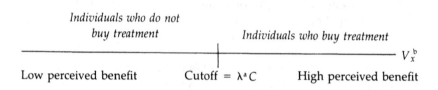

Individuals who do not buy treatment. Individuals who buy treatment. Low perceived benefit. Cutoff = λᵃC. High perceived benefit.

a. Fraction of total cost paid for by the patient.
b. Patient's estimate of the value of treatment.
SOURCE: Author.

$$Ve + Vd > -(1-\lambda)C \qquad (11.3)$$

Thus, an individual inappropriately purchases a service whenever his belief about the value of the service exceeds the true value or whenever he has insurance. If the inequality in equation (11.3) is reversed, the individual inappropriately forgoes care.

To better understand condition equation (11.3), consider arraying a group of patients according to their perceived benefits, Vx. Figure 11–2 depicts such an array. For the "cutoff" patient, who is indifferent about receiving treatment, the perceived benefits equal the after-insurance cost, λC. Patients with higher perceived benefits purchase treatment; those with lower perceived benefits do not.

The patients on each side of the cutoff in figure 11–2 may not be the same as the patients on each side of the cutoff in figure 11–1. Thus, many patients may make inappropriate purchase decisions. According to the model, patients may come to make inappropriate purchase decisions in two distinct ways.

Purchase decisions can be inappropriate if individuals *systematically* over- or underconsume. When mistakes are systematic, the ordering of the patients in the two figures is identical. The patient with the highest true benefit, for example, also has the highest perceived benefit. The position of the marginal patient changes, however, so that a different number of patients receive care from what is optimal. Systematic overconsumption occurs if $\mu_e + \mu_d > -(1-\lambda)C$. Systematic underconsumption occurs if $\mu_e + \mu_d < -(1-\lambda)C$.

Purchase decisions can be inappropriate if consumers make *noisy* estimates of the value of service. Estimates are noisy if $\sigma_e > 0$ or $\sigma_d > 0$. If this is the case, then the ordering of the patients in the two figures may differ. Some patients who are to the right of the cutoff in figure 11–1 will be on the left in figure 11–2, and vice versa. An important distinction between systematic errors and noisy errors is that the systematic ones can be corrected by shifting the cutoff, whereas the noisy ones cannot. A corollary to this is that some cost-containment strategies work by shifting the cutoff, while others work by reducing noise.

It is presumed in this analysis that all individuals at the time they choose their health insurance plan would prefer that treatments were allocated according to the condition equation (11.1). This would offer the maximum expected benefits net of costs. Insurers can therefore offer a more competitive product by correcting mistakes.

Evidence on the Two Types of Mistakes. Based on empirical studies, it is possible to guess at the magnitude of systematic and noisy mistakes. Since most patients have insurance, for example, one expects some systematic overconsumption due to moral hazard. The Rand national health insurance experiment offers evidence on how large moral hazard consumption is likely to be (Manning et al. 1984). Rand finds modest price responsiveness when consumers switch from free care to low coinsurance rates and very little price responsiveness in the face of additional cost sharing. (Price elasticities of demand for many medical services are in the range of −.2 to −.3). The Rand findings suggest that moral hazard is likely to be a serious problem only when insurance requires no cost sharing.

Patients may also systematically overconsume because of biased perceptions of the value of care. Biases may result from incorrect patient evaluation or demand inducement. Evidence on demand inducement is decidedly mixed. Studies linking physician density to demand report weak inducement effects at best (see Cromwell and Mitchell 1986). Studies linking ownership of diagnostic equipment to high incidence of its use suggest a stronger inducement effect but fail to account for endogeneity of physician ownership. That is, physicians predisposed to use equipment are more likely to own it. Studies regarding possible persistent biases in patient perceptions of the value of specific treatments have been difficult to identify.

Undoubtedly, patients and physicians have noisy estimates of the value of care. Individuals possess varying degrees of medical expertise. Kenkel (1991) finds, for example, a great dispersion in individual knowledge about the health consequences of drinking and exercise. Physicians also vary widely in their perceptions about how best to treat different conditions. So-called "small-area variations" reveal large practice differences among physicians that surely cannot be attributed to differences in patient conditions or patient preferences (see Tedeschi, et al. 1990). Assuming some treatment standard for a given patient, then the existence of small-area variations suggests that recommendations by physicians vary substantially around the standard.[2]

Insurer Strategies to Promote Appropriate Consumption. Insurers have available to them a number of strategies to change purchase decisions. In its 1990 report to its board of directors, the Health Insurance Association of America identified a few, including consumer cost sharing, use of financial incentives in HMOs and PPOs, and use of practice protocols and guidelines, that is, utilization review. This section discusses these strategies, as well as rationing, which is receiving more attention in light of Oregon's efforts to reduce Medicaid expenses through a rationing program.

Raise copayments. Insurers increasingly require some copayments from their enrollees (Blue Cross 1990). In terms of the model, this requirement shifts the cutoff in figure 11-2 to the right, without affecting the estimated values of care. Thus, fewer individuals purchase care.

Shifting the financial burden toward patients at the time of purchase will probably have limited effectiveness as a cost-containment mechanism, for two reasons. On the one hand, increasing copayments slightly will deter only a small percentage of patients from purchasing care. On the other hand, raising copayments by a large amount exposes patients to financial risk. This approach inherently limits the degree to which cost sharing can be used to reduce utilization.

Cost sharing may be more effective if it encourages patients to choose a less costly delivery site. This way may be a more desirable use of cost sharing because the price elasticity of demand for treatment at a particular site is undoubtedly larger than the elasticity for treatment anywhere.

Change provider incentives. The theory of demand inducement suggests that providers who are reimbursed fee-for-service have incentives to overstate the value of services systematically. This practice can lead to overconsumption. An obvious solution would be to pay providers in some other fashion. In the past decades insurers have experimented with a number of different payment mechanisms, including salarying physicians, setting prospective fees per admission to hospitals, and

---

2. If physicians possess different skills, then a uniform standard could be undesirable. For example it may be appropriate for a patient to receive bypass surgery if a highly skilled surgeon is available but to receive medicinal treatment if only average surgeons are available.

providing annual capitated payments to medical groups.

In terms of the model, these changes in provider payments have the primary effect of reducing μ_d. In figure 11–2, this would decrease the perceived value of care, without affecting the cutoff value. Thus, fewer individuals purchase care. Numerous studies suggest that paying physicians a fixed amount does lead to systematic reductions in utilization (see Manning et al. 1984). At the same time there is abundant evidence that hospital prospective payment leads to reductions in inpatient utilization (see Long et al. 1990; Custer 1991).

Rationing. A central planner allocates a limited number of treatments using some nonprice allocation mechanism. The ordering of values in figure 11–2 is relevant only to the extent that individuals with high perceived values will likely have higher places in the rationing queue.

Ideally the central planner bases the allocation of services on a comparison of V and C; that is, the central planner follows the condition in equation (11.1). At best, one's place in the rationing queue will likely be based on V_a rather than V. This is acceptable if there is little idiosyncratic variation in the value of care. At worst, the central planner may be unable to assess V_a accurately, with the result that patient and physician errors are replaced by central planner errors. This argument has been made in critiques of Oregon's proposed Medicaid rationing plan.

Utilization review. UR is a rationing scheme. It offers two potential advantages over centralized rationing: first, UR agencies compete to offer the "best" rationing scheme; and second, individuals can obtain otherwise rationed services by paying the full price. It is plausible to believe that UR agencies can take advantage of scale economies to become expert on cost effectiveness. They can then use this knowledge to eliminate inappropriate utilization. This view of UR, incorporated directly into the definition by the Institute of Medicine, is embodied in the "principle of UR" that appears in the 1990 report of the Health Insurance Association of America to its board of directors:

> In order to improve quality and reduce the cost of care, health plans should cover and reimburse for the cost of services that have been demonstrated to be medically necessary, medically effective and cost-effective.

A similar view of UR is expressed by the founders of the UR service agency Interqual: "UR serves to provide information (to patients and physicians) and to compare the suggested treatment against generally accepted medical norms" (Jacobs and Lamprey 1991).

These views reflect the role of UR that was developed in my model.

Yet consider other ways to view UR:

- "Few disagree that utilization review has evolved into a means of saving money and little more" (Zusman 1990).
- "Utilization management functions as a stand alone cost-containment program" (Kelch 1991).
- "Many employers are using UR to control costs" (Vibbert 1990).

It is troubling to hear UR described in these terms. A UR program can easily reduce cost without addressing appropriateness—the UR agency could randomly reject requests for treatment authorization. Alternatively, the UR agency could harass providers so that obtaining UR approval works like a tax, thus shifting the cutoff in figure 11–2. But unlike most taxes, there would be no associated tax revenue, only dead-weight loss. UR does not make sense as a pure cost-containment mechanism. The effectiveness of UR depends on its ability to eliminate mistakes.

The next section reviews the literature on UR effectiveness. The literature to date suggests that UR does contain costs to a limited extent. Unfortunately, the literature offers no insight into whether UR is eliminating noisy mistakes.

How Well?

A report by the Institute of Medicine (1989) and a review article by Wickizer (1990) summarize the literature evaluating UR. In this section I will discuss the highlights of the IOM and Wickizer reports.

Wickizer distinguishes between public and private UR. He thoroughly reviews studies of PSROs and similar public UR programs in place during the 1970s and early 1980s. These studies generally compare actual utilization with predicted utilization where predictions are based on experiences in other regions without UR or with patients not covered by UR. The most comprehensive studies cited by Wickizer were HCFA evaluations of PSROs. Two different HCFA studies reached the same conclusion that PSROs produced only very small reductions in utilization and generated benefits that were no larger than the costs of implementation. Wickizer also discusses several studies of Medicaid UR programs. Again, the evidence that UR affects utilization is weak to nonexistent.

Wickizer's review of the literature evaluating private sector UR programs is terse. He disparages this literature, stating that most studies of private UR programs are "little more than anecdotal assessments." The notable exception is his review of his own research (Feldstein et al. 1988; Wickizer et al. 1989). These studies evaluated the effectiveness of UR programs operated by CNA Insurance Companies of Chicago during the period 1984–1986 and report significant reductions in inpatient

248

utilization among the populations subject to UR.

A 1989 report by the Institute of Medicine reviews eight separate studies of private UR programs. All eight studies compare utilization by patients under UR with utilization by a comparison group. Five studies also examine medical care expenditures. All eight studies report significant reductions in inpatient utilization associated with UR. Four of five studies report decreased hospital expenditures associated with UR.

The IOM criticizes these studies for having a number of methodological weaknesses. None of the studies use randomized design. Only one study considers outpatient utilization, and no study considers nonhospital utilization. None of the studies consider the costs to providers of complying with UR requirements. Finally, none of the studies consider whether UR eliminates utilization mistakes. The IOM relates this weakness to quality of care: "Most importantly, all of the studies reviewed confine their focus to utilization patterns and costs to the purchaser. The committee found no empirical research on quality of care" (IOM 1989).

Yardsticks for Evaluating UR. All recent studies of UR identified by Wickizer and the IOM focus on levels of utilization and cost—the same yardsticks as are used to evaluate other cost-containment schemes. The model developed in this chapter suggests that it is inappropriate to rely solely on these yardsticks. To see why, let us reconsider the theoretic rationales for adopting cost-containment strategies.

Consider first the effect of strategies such as raising copayments and changing provider incentives. Recall from the model that these strategies have the effect of reducing purchases either by raising the cutoff value or lowering the perceived value of care. If in the status quo there is systematic overconsumption of care, then it is easily shown that patients who forgo care must have had true values that were, on average, less than the full cost of care. Thus, marginal utilization reductions from these cost containment schemes are welcome.[3]

There is no similar theoretical rationale for welcoming utilization reductions from UR. How then can a purchaser of UR services determine if the advertised cost reductions are desirable? One possibility is to examine UR screening criteria. UR service agencies will not readily divulge this information, however, because it is the industry's chief competitive tool. In the absence of any systematic evidence on appropriateness of care, purchasers must rely on anecdotal evidence from

---

3. This is certainly true for initial cost reductions, assuming that there is systematic overconsumption. One can, of course, restrain consumption too much.

employees. Purchasers of UR services, then, will be somewhat well informed about the full price of the service (that is, the administrative charge less the medical expenditure savings) but poorly informed about the quality (that is, the appropriateness of care).

How might the market for UR services function under these circumstances? The model of Dranove and Satterthwaite (1992) offers some insight. They show that when consumers are well informed about price and poorly informed about quality, then sellers will maintain low prices and low quality. They demonstrate further that when information about price improves but information about quality does not, prices and quality both decrease. They construct examples in which the welfare costs of the quality reductions vastly exceed the welfare benefits of the reductions in price, so that total surplus in equilibrium is lower.

The implication of the Dranove and Satterthwaite analysis for the UR services market is as follows. As purchasers of UR services become better informed about the prices and cost savings afforded by various UR service agencies, the agencies will be forced either to lower their prices or to provide more utilization savings. Either way, the incentives for UR service agencies to make the expenditures necessary to ensure appropriateness may be reduced. Purchasers may well be made worse off by the continuing focus on cost savings.

Whither UR?

The largest potential obstacle to the success of UR appears to be the need for good cost-effectiveness research. As the Health Insurance Association of America (1990) reports:

> In many instances the kind of rigorous research that is required to determine what is necessary and effective has not been done. New technologies and procedures are introduced and become widely adopted before there is sound evidence about their effectiveness. Even the most conscientious physician may have difficulty determining the best medical practice.

There appear to be several barriers to successful cost-effectiveness research and implementation:

- equating different outcomes
- physician-specific effects
- proper measurement of costs
- measuring systemwide outcomes

Equating Different Outcomes. Alternative treatments may not produce easily comparable results. Coronary bypass surgery, for example, generally offers the patient the possibility of extended life expectancy with minimal discomfort at the slight risk of immediate death (during or just after the operation). Alternative medicinal treatment may offer a life expectancy similar to surgery. The trade-off is that medicinal treatment is often associated with moderate discomfort but poses little risk of immediate death. It is difficult to see how a UR service agency can balance these competing health risks. There has been some progress in trying to "score" different types of illnesses on a cardinal scale, the Quality Adjusted Life Years (QALYs) scale being the best known example (see Torrance 1986). Researchers do not agree on the validity of such approaches. Even if a consensus were reached, the UR service agency would still have to calculate a dollar equivalent for each QALYs score.

Given reasonable estimates of the value of a life, a costly treatment can probably be justified even with only a small chance that it will improve outcomes. The well-publicized comparison of the blood clot dissolvers streptokinase and TPA offers a case in point. TPA costs over $2,000 per dose, whereas streptokinase costs less than $100. The cost difference is small when compared with the value of health improvements afforded by the drugs. Thus, TPA needs to offer only a slightly higher efficacy to justify its cost. So far, although clinical trials have been unable to detect any difference in efficacy, the studies to date lack the sensitivity necessary to reject the use of TPA conclusively.

Physician-Specific Differences. The model presented above abstracted from differences in the skills of physicians. In reality large differences may exist in these skills. Luft et al. (1987), for example, identify substantial differences in the outcomes from surgery apparently based on the experience of the surgical team. Thus, a UR recommendation appropriate for one physician may be inappropriate for another. The importance of learning in medicine makes UR especially problematic. Learning is often a "public good." The mistakes of physicians in the early stages of developing a new treatment often lead to the successes of many physicians later on. If UR service agencies ignore learning, then the rate of adoption of new treatments will be less than optimal.

Measuring Costs. UR dogma appears to hold that home care is cheaper than institutional care and that hospital care is more expensive than nonhospital settings. Interqual, for example, promotes its UR product by citing an instance in which it uncovered tens of thousands of acute care days that could have been shifted to other settings. The "fact" that this saves money is assumed to be self-evident. As the following example suggests, however, the savings can be illusory.

Consider a patient who is scheduled for same-day surgery on a Friday but wishes to enter the hospital on Thursday evening. He will consume "hotel" services only overnight. Although the true marginal cost of that overnight stay may be very low, the UR panel will almost surely deny the stay on the grounds that the "cost" exceeds the benefits. The reason is that the UR service agency bases its estimate of costs on the hospital's per diem, which reflects average cost rather than marginal cost.[4]

One cannot fully fault UR companies for their unsophisticated treatment of hospital costs. Hospitals generally fail to adjust their bills to account for differences in patient costs within the same cost center; UR companies correctly respond in kind. The UR service agency saves dollars for its client even if society's resources are not conserved.

Measuring Systemwide Outcomes. The literature on UR effectiveness generally focuses too narrowly on inpatient hospital costs. Recent studies appear to be broadening the focus to include at least outpatient costs (see Bergman et al. 1990; Custer 1991). This is a step in the right direction.

My own study of the costs of caring for ventilator-assisted children (VAC) in alternative settings (Dranove 1989) points out the importance of proper cost measurement and adopting a systemwide perspective. Conventional wisdom holds that hospitalization in an intensive care unit is much more costly than home care. This is certainly true if one simply compares medical bills. Several states have attempted to reduce expenditures by promoting early discharge of VAC.

The policy of early discharge for VAC turns out to be somewhat questionable if one takes a systemwide perspective. The cost of hospital care for VAC turns out to be much lower than naive analysis would suggest because most VAC require minimal nursing attention even in intensive care. As a result, the hospital bill (often over $1,000 per day in room charges alone) drastically overstates resource use. At the same time the costs of home care are far higher than indicated by medical bills, because parental nursing substitutes for professional nursing. Once these factors are accounted for, the costs of home care are seen to be comparable to the costs of hospital care.

Conclusion

Amid widespread calls for reform, the U.S. health care system is evolving on its own. The past decade has seen the emergence of vertically

---

4. I am indebted to Burt Weisbrod for this example.

integrated managed-care systems, which rely heavily on UR and changes in provider incentives to package a more cost-effective health care product.

Most "procompetitive" health insurance reform proposals stress the continued growth of such systems. These proposals concentrate on reforming the system of financing the purchase of health insurance through one of these systems (see Kronick and Enthoven 1991). Skeptics respond that even if consumers make cost-conscious choices between systems, the systems themselves will be unable to improve the health care product (Grumbach et al. 1991).

Those skeptical about the ability of managed-care systems to improve the health care product may have a point. With only weak evidence on UR, competitive forces may drive UR service agencies to focus on cost savings at the expense of appropriateness. The same arguments about the short-comings of UR, however, may be used to assess the alternatives offered by the skeptics. Grumbach et al. (1991), for example, offer a national health insurance proposal featuring a combination of changed provider incentives, rationing of hi-tech capital equipment, and possible rationing of costly services. In their proposal the states in negotiation with doctors and hospitals would set the incentives and rationing limits. For all the difficulties that employers may have in measuring the appropriateness of rationing activities, it is difficult to imagine that states would be even more responsive to appropriateness.

Cost cutting through UR is easy. Improving the health care product through UR has thus far proven to be difficult. As the UR industry matures, we can hope that its product improves as well. UR is uniquely capable of eliminating unnecessary health care services while simultaneously ensuring the consumption of necessary ones.

References

A. Foster Higgins & Co. Inc. *Health Care Benefits Survey 1987–1991.* Princeton, N.J.

Bergman, A., et al. "Technology and Outpatient Review: A Preliminary Evaluation." *Quality Review Bulletin* (June 1990): 234–39.

Blue Cross-Blue Shield Association. "Environmental Analysis—1990." Internal Report.

———. *Environmental Analysis.* Chicago, Ill.: 1991.

Cromwell, J., and J. Mitchell. "Physician-induced Demand for Surgery." *Journal of Health Economics* (1986): 293–313.

Custer, W. "Employer Health Care Plan Design and Plan Cost: Analysis of Claims Data from Employers in the Los Angeles Area." EBRI Special Report SR-12 (1991).

Dranove, D. "The Cost of Caring for VAC." In *Pediatric Home Care: Results of a National Evaluation of Programs for Ventilator Assisted Children*, by L. Aday et al. Chicago: Pluribus Press, 1988.

Dranove, D., and M. Satterthwaite. "Monopolistic Competition When Price and Quality Are Not Perfectly Observable." *Rand Journal of Economics* 1992 (forthcoming).

Feldstein, R., et al. "Private Cost Containment: The Effects of Utilization Review Programs on Health Care Use and Expenditures." *New England Journal of Medicine* (May 19, 1988): 1310–14.

Grumbach, K., et al. "Liberal Benefits, Conservative Spending." *New England Journal of Medicine* (May 15, 1991): 2549–54.

Health Insurance Association of America. "The Health Insurance Industry Strategy for Containing Health Care Costs." *Report to the Board of Directors* (February 1990).

Interqual. *The ISD—A Review System with Adult Criteria*. 1989.

Jacobs, C., and J. Lamprey. "Emerging Trends in Utilization Review and Management." *Journal of the American Association of Preferred Provider Organizations* (April–May 1991): 15–22.

Kelch, B. "Utilization Management—Caveat Emptor." *Journal of the American Association of Preferred Provider Organizations* (April–May 1991): 26–27.

Kenkel, D. "Health Behavior, Health Knowledge and Schooling." *Journal of Political Economy* (April 1991): 287–305.

Kronick, R., and A. Enthoven. "Universal Health Insurance through Incentives Reforms." *JAMA* (May 15, 1991): 2532–36.

Long, M., et al. "A Reassessment of Hospital Product and Productivity Changes over Time." *Health Care Financing Review* (Summer 1990): 69–77.

Luft, H., et al. "The Volume Outcome Relationship in Surgery: Selective Referral Patterns or Practice Makes Perfect." *Health Services Research* (June 1987).

Manning, W., et al. "A Controlled Trial of the Effect of a Prepaid Group Practice on Use of Services." *New England Journal of Medicine* 310 (1984): 1505–10.

National Institute of Medicine. *Controlling Costs and Changing Patient Care? The Role of Utilization Review*. Washington, D.C.: National Academy Press, 1989.

Tedeschi, P., et al. "Micro-area Variation in Hospital Use." *Health Services Research* (February 1990): 729–40.

Torrance, G. "Measurement of Health State Utilities for Economic Appraisal: A Review." *Journal of Health Economics* (May 1986): 1–30.

Vibbert, S. "Utilization Review: A Report Card." *Business and Health* (February 1990): 37–46.

Wickizer, T. "The Effect of Utilization Review on Hospital Use and Expenditures." *Medical Care Review* (Fall 1990): 327–63.

Wickizer, T., et al. "Does Utilization Review Reduce Unnecessary Care and Contain Costs?" *Medical Care* (June 1989): 632–46.

Zusman, J. "Utilization Review: Theory, Practice and Issues." *Hospital and Community Psychiatry* (May 1990): 531–36.

12

The Hidden Costs of Budget-constrained Health Insurance Systems

Patricia M. Danzon

A number of recent studies have compared health care spending in the United States with that in budget-constrained health care systems such as Canada's and noted that the measured costs are lower in Canada.[1] The conclusion is then drawn that a public monopoly insurer that imposes budget constraints on providers is more efficient at delivering insured medical care than competitive private insurance markets. This conclusion implicitly assumes that the benefits are similar and that measured costs accurately reflect real social costs. A more careful analysis of how private and public insurers operate, however, concludes that there are hidden benefits in private insurance and hidden costs in public monopoly systems. Accurate comparison of total costs and benefits of private and public insurance systems raises important conceptual and measurement questions that this chapter can only begin to answer. The main purpose here is to lay out a more appropriate conceptual framework for defining overhead costs and to point out why existing comparisons are grossly misleading.

Framework for Comparison

Much of the criticism of private insurance focuses on its allegedly higher overhead costs. Estimates of the overhead costs of private insurers in the United States range from 11.9 to 33.5 percent of benefit payments, compared with roughly 1.0 percent for public insurance in Canada. In addition, dealing with many diverse plans is said to add wasteful

---

1. I would like to thank Ted Frech, Sharon Tennyson, and Roger Feldman for comments on an earlier draft and Mark Pauly for many helpful discussions. Any remaining errors are mine.

expense for physicians, hospitals, and patients. Woolhandler and Himmelstein (1991) estimate that overhead and billing expenses accounted for 25–48 percent of expenditure on physicians' services in the United States in 1987, compared with 18–34 percent in Canada; hospital administration was 20.2 percent of hospital costs in the United States in contrast with 9.0 percent in Canada.

These accounting measures are misleading and partial estimates of the full overhead costs of delivering insured medical services through private or public insurance. Any insurer, private or public, must perform three functions: collect premiums, monitor and pay for services (control of insurance-induced overuse or "moral hazard"), and bear the risk that is not eliminated by the law of large numbers. In private insurance markets, the cost of performing these functions is largely monetized and appears as accounting overhead of premium collection, claims administration, and return on capital.

The methods used by public insurers to perform these same functions generate lower observable accounting cost but much higher hidden costs. Partly this result reflects the government's use of fiat to force people to pay taxes, accept prices and restrictions on services, and bear risk, whereas private insurers must induce voluntary participation of consumers, providers, and risk-bearing capital. A full analysis of why governments tend to choose mechanisms that result in hidden rather than explicit costs is beyond the scope of this chapter—the quick answer is that these mechanisms reduce line-item budget costs of the program because hidden costs are off budget. This chapter's objective is to point out the hidden costs imposed by public insurers that are the analogue of the overhead costs incurred under private insurance and to present a more accurate though still rough estimate of the true overhead costs of the Canadian system relative to private insurance in the United States.

A prior question is, What systems should be compared? Existing empirical studies compare Canada with private insurance as it currently operates in the United States. This is the basis for numerical estimates in this chapter, since empirical evidence necessarily pertains to existing systems. But for the debate about national health insurance in the United States, the relevant comparison is between a public monopoly system and a well-designed but practical, competitive private insurance system. A reformed private insurance system would eliminate wasteful distortions of the current U.S. system but include provisions to ensure that coverage is universal and affordable to all. We have described such a system elsewhere, but to estimate its overhead costs would be speculative (Pauly, Danzon, Feldstein, and Hoff 1991). While the conceptual discussion here compares overhead costs under monopoly public insurance and competitive private insurance markets in general, it draws on actual experience in Canada and the United States for empirical evidence. Since this chapter focuses on overhead costs, I do not attempt to measure all the inefficiencies in the United States that result from tax and regulatory policies that are neither essential nor desirable features of a well-designed private insurance system. In particular, this chapter is not concerned with the hidden costs of the tax subsidy to employer contributions as they affect the price, quantity, and quality of medical care (Feldstein 1973; Newhouse 1986; Manning et al. 1987); I also do not attempt to measure the losses from nonoptimal coverage of the uninsured. In discussing the empirical estimates of overhead costs of private insurance in the United States, however, I point out (without attempting to quantify) where current tax and regulatory policy result in higher overhead costs than would occur in a well-designed private insurance market.

This chapter first identifies some inaccuracies in widely cited measures of overhead costs in the United States, presents corrected measures, and then addresses the question of how much of this is pure waste. The chapter then identifies the analogous costs of public monopoly insurers and presents rough empirical estimates of major components of hidden costs usually omitted from calculations of overhead costs in Canada. It also discusses free riding by public insurers on foreign research and development. The concluding section summarizes the conceptual framework and the empirical estimates.

Overhead of Private Insurers in the United States

Biases in Measures of Private Insurer Overhead. Woolhandler and Himmelstein (1991) and others following them first estimate overhead as a percentage of benefit payments in both countries and then convert this to a measure of overhead dollars per capita. This method biases the comparison against the country with higher benefit payments per capita: the same overhead *percentage* applied to larger benefits per capita yields higher overhead *dollars per capita,* simply reflecting the fact that delivering additional benefits entails some additional overhead cost. To avoid this bias, comparisons here are stated as a percentage of either premiums or benefit payments, not dollars per capita.

A second fallacy is to use the expense ratio (ratio of expenses to claim payments) reported by private insurers as an estimate of the overhead costs of private insurance. In *Premiums without Benefits: Waste and Inefficiency in the Commercial Health Insurance Industry,* for example, the Citizen's Fund reports that administrative, marketing, and other overhead expenses of commercial insurance accounted for $14.9 billion in 1988, compared with $44.5 billion of claim payments. The resulting expense-to-claims ratio of 33.5 percent is interpreted as a measure of insurer inefficiency.

Use of this accounting measure fails to recognize the administrative functions that commercial insurers perform for self-insured employer plans. By 1990, 59 percent of employers funded their group health plans themselves, including 37 percent of firms with under 500 employees (Business Insurance 1991). These firms typically employ a third-party administrator to handle benefit payments, under minimum premium, and administrative services only plans. Commercial insurers that provide administrative services necessarily have a high reported expense-to-claims ratio because claim payments corresponding to the expenses do not appear as a cost on the balance sheet of the insurer but of the self-insured firms.[2]

Overhead Expense of Private Insurers in the United States. The national health accounts estimate the overhead of private insurance as 10.5 percent of premiums, or 11.7 percent of benefit payments for 1987. Overhead of public insurers in Canada is 0.9 percent of total spending or roughly 1 percent of benefit payments (Woolhandler and Himmelstein, 1991).

Overhead for private insurers in the United States is estimated as the difference between premium payments and benefit payments, adjusted for dividends and other retroactive premium adjustments.[3] This difference includes premium taxes (roughly 2.3 percent for commercial insurers and some Blue Cross–Blue Shield plans), return on capital (roughly 3.5 percent), and investment income (1.5 percent) for commercial insurers and Blue Cross–Blue Shield plans (see table 12-1). These components should be netted out for purposes of fair comparison with the overhead of a public insurer (see appendix 12–A). Premium taxes are a pure transfer to state government. Investment income is a return to policy holders for advance payment of premium. Return on capital is netted out here because of the difficulty of estimating the analogous cost of public insurers.[4]

---

2. For example, for Aetna Life and Casualty, 65 percent of its business on a claims-paid basis was administrative services only, 28 percent under minimum premium plan arrangements, and only 7 percent was conventionally insured. *Business Insurance,* January 28, 1991, p. 12.

3. Premiums and benefits estimates are separately derived from a variety of sources, including commercial insurers, Blue Cross–Blue Shield, surveys of HMOs and self-insured firms, and provider surveys for estimates of benefit payments. K. Levitt, personal communication.

4. All insurers incur risk; however, only private insurers report that cost as an

TABLE 12–1

BREAKDOWN OF ADMINISTRATIVE EXPENSES FOR CONVENTIONALLY INSURED
HEALTH PLANS, AS PERCENTAGE OF INCURRED CLAIMS, 1988

Number of Employees	Claims Admin- istration	General Admin- istration	Interest Credit	Risk and Profit	Com- missions	Pre- mium Taxes	Total
1 to 4	9.3	12.5	−1.5	8.5	8.4	2.8	40.0
5 to 9	8.6	11.2	−1.5	8.0	6.0	2.7	35.0
10 to 19	7.2	9.2	−1.5	7.5	5.0	2.6	30.0
20 to 49	6.3	7.6	−1.5	6.8	3.3	2.5	25.0
50 to 99	4.3	4.8	−1.5	6.0	2.0	2.4	18.0
100 to 499	4.1	4.0	−1.5	5.5	1.6	2.3	16.0
500 to 2,499	3.9	3.2	−1.5	3.5	0.7	2.2	12.0
2,500 to 9,999	3.8	1.4	−1.5	1.8	0.3	2.2	8.0
10,000 plus	3.0	0.7	−1.5	1.1	0.1	2.1	5.5

SOURCE: U.S. Library of Congress, Congressional Research Service; estimates by
Hay/Huggins Company based on underwriting practices of major insurers.

With these adjustments, private insurance in the United States,
including commercial insurers, Blue Cross–Blue Shield, other plans, and
self-insurers, entails an overhead rate of roughly 7.6 percent of benefit
payments, net of premium taxes, return on capital, and investment
income (see appendix 12–A). Although this percentage exceeds the
reported overhead rate of 0.9 percent for Canada, this ordering changes
if one adjusts for major hidden costs in Canada.

How Much Is Waste? The view that overhead expenditures of insurers
are pure waste would be correct in a world of perfect information and
costless transactions. But in the real world where obtaining information,
negotiating, and enforcing contracts are costly, such expenditures can
serve a useful function. In competitive markets, private insurers incur
overhead costs only to avoid other, even larger costs to policy holders.
A more careful analysis reveals that relatively little of private insurers'
overhead is waste and that most has offsetting benefits. Public insurers
spend less to perform the same functions, but corresponding costs that
do not appear in national health accounts are larger.

---

accounting return on capital. Ideally, one should estimate and include the hidden
cost of risk bearing for self-insured plans in the United States and for the public
monopoly insurer in Canada. Since the necessary data are not available, the
alternative adopted here is to net out the cost of capital for private insurers, to
achieve comparability, even if it results in an understatement of true costs for all
insurers.

Underwriting expense. Although medical underwriting is one of the most frequently criticized features of competitive private insurance markets, it accounts for less than 2 percent of claim costs. Neither self-insured firms nor experience-rated firms, which cover the majority of privately insured individuals, use medical underwriting.[5] It is more common in the nongroup and small-group market, which accounts for only about 20 percent of all privately insured individuals.[6] Moreover, the view that medical underwriting is pure waste from a social perspective is overstated. To the extent that risk rating of premiums discourages risky or unhealthy lifestyles, there is an allocative benefit, although this may be small, given all the other pecuniary and nonpecuniary costs associated with poor health.

Medical underwriting and risk rating of premiums need not violate social equity goals, since other policy tools are available to achieve desired distributional purposes. Eliminating medical underwriting implies cross-subsidies from the healthy and others with low use of medical care to heavy users of medical care, not all of whom are in poor health or have low income. Even if the social objective is greater equality of incomes *net* of expenditures on health insurance, this end can be achieved by subsidizing the cost of health insurance for high risks through general revenues. This approach may have more desirable distributional and allocative effects than arbitrary cross-subsidies to high risks from the low risks that happen to be a community-rated insurance pool (see Pauly et al. 1991). Thus objections to medical underwriting under the status quo reflect more on the failure of other government policies to make coverage affordable to the poor and high risks rather than a waste intrinsic to private insurance.

Claims administration. Claims administration is the largest overhead component, accounting for 3–4 percent of benefit payments. It reflects the costs of monitoring and paying claims in fee-for-service plans, the costs of information systems to monitor patient and provider utilization under managed-care plans, and the costs of implementing provider-targeted incentive systems in health maintenance organizations (HMOs).

---

5. U.S. GAO (1991, 9) reports that 56 percent of employees are in self-insured firms. The percentage of all privately insured individuals would be larger because large firms are more likely to self-insure and they cover a larger fraction of dependents.

6. Although the cost of medical underwriting is small in the aggregate, it may cause significant hardship for some individuals and undermines the ability to insure against the possibility of becoming high risk. These concerns, however, can be addressed by risk-rated subsidies (Pauly et al. 1991). It does not require a public monopoly insurer or mandatory community rating.

Expenses stemming from claims administration are often erroneously viewed as pure waste, since they involve denying coverage and impose costs on patients and providers. This view ignores the real benefits of controlling patients' and providers' incentives to overuse medical care when the patient is insured—that is, moral hazard. Insurance, whether private or public, provides financial protection by reducing point-of-purchase prices of medical care to patients. Patients thus have incentives to use services that are worth less than their full cost, and providers tend to be willing to comply, since increased utilization serves the interest of the individual patient in the short run and, in conventional insurance, also benefits the provider financially. Because premiums for the group must cover the full cost, however, in the long run consumers benefit if insurers limit the use of care that is not worth its cost.

Private insurers compete by devising ways to control moral hazard in more cost-effective ways, including structured copayments, utilization review, case management, selective contracting with preferred providers, and provider-targeted financial incentives, such as capitation and other risk-sharing forms of prospective reimbursement. The costs of implementing these strategies appear as claims administration costs to insurers, providers, and patients. The increase in overhead expense during the 1980s noted by Woolhandler and Himmelstein (1991) is not surprising, since it was a time of intense innovation in strategies to control moral hazard. This was made possible in part by development in computer technologies that permit the development of information systems that would previously have been prohibitively costly.

The offsetting benefit of expenditure to control moral hazard, though, is the reduction in dead-weight loss—that is, the difference between premium cost and the value of benefits—that occurs if use is unconstrained. Competition leads insurers to incur the costs to control moral hazard only as long as they gain at least the equivalent savings from control of overuse. From the patient's perspective, the total overhead cost of insurance includes not only the measured overhead but also the dead-weight loss from use of care worth less than its cost. Effectively, the dead-weight loss from negative net benefit care becomes an additional loading charge of insurance.[7]

---

7. The after-tax gross price of insured medical benefits B is:

$P = B(1+m)(1-t)$, where m is the administrative load and t is the marginal tax rate. The value, in terms of after tax dollars, is $V = B(1-g)(1-t)$ where g is the dead-weight loss discount. The net price is:

$$N = P-V = B(1-t)[(1+m) - (1-g)] = B(1-t)(m+g)$$

The competitive firm would set m to minimize N, which implies $\frac{\partial g}{\partial m} = -1$.

Competition creates incentives for insurers to minimize the sum of these two components of overhead. There is no reason to believe that the resulting costs would be socially excessive, in the absence of other distortions. The current tax subsidy to employer contributions, however, subsidizes spending on insurance overhead as well as on medical services. Spending on claims administration under the status quo is therefore likely to be excessive and higher than it would be if open-ended tax subsidies were eliminated.

With this caveat on account of the tax subsidy, the emerging dominance of hybrid, point-of-service plans (where the copayment varies according to the consumer's choice of provider) indicates that consumers differ in their willingness to accept copayment or limited choice of provider, that their willingness varies with the type of medical service, and that many consumers are willing to pay the slightly higher administrative costs of these hybrid plans.

Do Private Insurers Impose Excessive Burdens on Providers and Patients? Because operating a system of diverse, complex insurance plans also costs more in overhead for providers and consumers than would a single uniform system, some have viewed these costs as an additional source of waste. The magnitude of these costs has been exaggerated, however, and the offsetting benefits have been ignored. Woolhandler and Himmelstein (1991) estimate that physician and clerical staff time accounts for 25–48 percent of physicians' total billings in the United States, compared with 18–34 percent in Canada.

The higher estimate for the United States assigns all the difference in physician overhead except medical liability to excess administrative costs and is almost certainly too high, as Woolhandler and Himmelstein acknowledge. A significant fraction of the difference reflects the lower use of nonphysician medical inputs in Canada, partly because the Canadian fee schedule discourages the performance of procedures in physicians' offices. Physicians can bill only for evaluating procedures, not for the "technical" component that covers input costs other than the physician's time (Evans 1989), to discourage the physicians from acquiring capital equipment to perform in-office procedures. By contrast, the U.S. reimbursement system permits fees that cover the cost of nonphysician personnel, capital, and supplies required to perform in-office procedures, and this is reflected in higher total overhead for U.S. office-based physicians. Thus the lower figure of 25 percent is probably a more accurate measure of insurance-related costs for U.S. physicians, which may be compared with 18 percent for Canada.

It seems plausible, regardless of the empirical estimates, that insurance that controls moral hazard through prices and information-

263

based strategies will entail higher reported administrative costs for providers than insurance that relies on patient time and other nonprice forms of rationing. These provider overhead costs may also increase with the diversity of insurance plans. But there is little reason to believe that the complexity and diversity of coverages that emerge in competitive insurance markets generate excessive costs, that is, costs that exceed the offsetting benefits. Contractual forms of moral hazard control require the time and effort of patients and providers to fill in forms and prove that the services were medically justified, appropriately priced, and covered by the terms of the insurance contract. But insurers cannot ignore these costs and treat the time of providers and patients as a free resource. On the contrary, competition forces insurers to internalize the costs that they impose on patients and providers, and these costs influence the types of plans that survive in the marketplace.

In the case of patients, if plan A requires more complex forms, delay, and other inconveniences to obtain reimbursement or get approval for services than does plan B, patients would enroll in plan B, unless plan A's premium is sufficiently lower or plan A has other offsetting advantages, such as more freedom of choice. Thus costs, such as time, imposed on patients by an insurer's moral hazard control strategies are internalized to insurers through patients' choice of plans and the premiums that they are willing to pay. In group plans these signals are channeled through the choices of benefits managers, who have strong incentives to satisfy the preferences of employees.

Similarly, the level of reimbursement that a provider requires to accept insurer A's patients depends on the costs associated with billing, utilization review, and financial risk (if the plan has capitation features). Thus the terms on which providers are willing to serve an insurer's patients—or contract directly with the insurer, in the case of an HMO or preferred provider organization (PPO)—cause the paperwork and time costs that the plan imposes on the provider to be internalized by the insurer. A physician intolerant of paperwork, for example, would require a higher hourly wage to participate in a point-of-service plan than in a salaried staff model HMO—other things being equal.

Thus the diversity of insurance plans that emerges in competitive insurance markets reflects, on the demand side of the market, the diversity of patients' preferences between premiums, copayments, paperwork, and restrictions on freedom of choice. It reflects on the supply side the willingness of providers to trade off between higher reimbursement, freedom of practice style, and administrative expense. The more homogeneous are patient preferences, the more uniform is the equilibrium range of plans and the more likely that a provider can achieve his desired patient load with only one type of plan. Some providers may prefer to diversify and serve multiple plans. If capitation plans, for example, require more nondiversifiable financial risk but fee-for-service plans entail more paperwork, then a risk-averse physician may prefer a mix of capitated and fee-for-service patients.

Excessive diversity and excessive costs for providers, patients, and insurers can arise if insurance markets are imperfectly competitive, for example, because consumers and providers are imperfectly informed about each plan's true "quality." If plan B's utilization review, for instance, requires procedures different from plan A's but is operationally equivalent, there is no allocative benefit in adding plan B, and any additional cost from adding plan B is waste. But competitive pressures tend to reduce waste from excessive diversity. A "me-too" plan B that entered the market would minimize costs and be more attractive to providers if it simply copied plan A's forms and strategies. The remaining diversity costs are further reduced by intermediaries that consolidate forms and utilize review programs if differences are truly spurious. Since the technologies of moral hazard control are still evolving, the existing diversity of plans may create higher costs than will survive in long-run equilibrium. But this is no different from the life cycle of any new technology—initial prototypes are simple; competition to develop more cost-effective models continues until a long-run equilibrium is reached with a mixture of products and prices that corresponds to the diversity of consumer preferences.

The potential for excessive diversity exists in all markets but is not usually considered a reason for preferring a public monopoly. The propensity for excessive entry is directly related to the potential monopoly profits. This is not significant in health insurance, however, because regulatory barriers to entry are generally low and self-insurance is a feasible option even for medium-sized employers. Prior consumer information may be imperfect, but this problem is reduced by the role of benefits managers, agents, and experience. Indeed, consumers gain information from experience much more rapidly with health insurance than with other forms of insurance, where claims are less frequent. Product proliferation and the existence of intermediaries as consolidators, both present in many financial services markets, do not show that a government monopoly would improve efficiency. Health insurance markets are not intrinsically different.

Two features of the status quo in the United States, however, distinguish between health insurance markets and increase the likelihood of excessive diversity. First, because the tax subsidy to employer contributions subsidizes insurance overhead as well as insured medical services, excessive diversity may result.

Second, state regulation of commercial insurers, together with the Employee Retirement Income Security Act (ERISA) exemption, has contributed to the proliferation of separate plans, as more employers self-insure to avoid the costs of state-mandated benefits, high risk pools, free choice laws, and other regulatory constraints on PPOs and utilization review.[8] The number of plans and total system-wide costs may therefore be excessive, if each plan entails some fixed costs. Since costs imposed on providers, however, are internalized to employer-sponsored plans, excessive proliferation of distinct types of plans should not occur. In fact, many use standard plans.

The benefits of markets that offer choices among plans offset the higher overhead costs to providers and patients because diverse consumer preferences are better satisfied by choice than by a uniform public plan. Diversity is probably excessive, and some overhead may be wasteful in current U.S. private health insurance markets. But these inefficiencies are caused largely by tax and regulatory distortions. Excessive diversity is not intrinsic to private insurance markets, since the costs to providers and patients are internalized by insurers through input and product prices. Without these distortions, there is no more reason to expect excessive diversity in health insurance than in other financial services markets.

The presumption that insurers internalize the paperwork costs imposed on patients and providers and therefore have appropriate incentives (without the tax subsidy and ERISA) does not apply to Medicare and Medicaid. Costs that these programs impose on providers may therefore be excessive. Because these costs cannot be factored out from accounting statements, the overhead costs reported by providers in the United States overstate the costs attributable to private insurance.

Risk and Profit. The risks and profits of private insurer overhead reflect the return on capital that buffers unanticipated shocks to aggregate losses. Unanticipated increases in medical input prices, changes in technologies, and other economy-wide factors that affect all insured in the risk pool are not diversified by increasing the number in the pool. Insurers therefore hold buffer funds—capital and surplus—and the adequacy of these reserves relative to liabilities is a widely used measure of the quality of the insurer. The return on capital is thus a cost of supplying reliable insurance in a world of uncertain macroeconomic factors.

While public insurers face similar risks, most public programs do not hold adequate buffer funds. Unanticipated shocks to the loss distribution are either shifted to taxpayers through tax increases or

---

8. In some states the deficit of the high risk pool is recouped from commercial insurers that must participate in the pool. This cost must ultimately be passed on as a cost of commercial insurance. Self-insured firms are exempt from the pools.

reductions in other government programs, or borne by patients or providers through limits on service or delays in reimbursement. In the United States, the increase in tax rates to shore up the Medicare health insurance trust fund illustrates risk shifting to taxpayers; Medicaid budget caps that result in delayed or partial reimbursement of providers shift risk to providers and to patients, to the extent that providers are less willing to take Medicaid patients.

In Canada, provincial governments have absorbed deficits of hospitals that are unwilling or unable to stay within their budgets (Evans et al. 1989), thereby shifting costs to either taxpayers or other program beneficiaries, depending on how the provincial budget is balanced. If physicians work fewer hours as expenditure ceilings are approached, their expenditure targets shift risk to providers and to patients. The reported overhead of public insurers does not reflect these risk-bearing costs that are shifted to taxpayers, providers, or patients.

A public monopoly system does eliminate the firm-specific risk related to market share and risk selection. The risk related to macro-factors, however, remains and is shifted to individuals who do not specialize in risk bearing, in contrast with private insurers who diversify through capital markets. Indeed, risk bearing in public systems is particularly inefficient to the extent that risk is shifted to patients and providers who incur other losses that are positively correlated with the shock to the public medical system. An economic downturn, for example, may leave a patient unemployed and unable to find a doctor if public deficits have stalled reimbursement through public programs. The real social cost of risk may therefore be higher in public systems.

The more common argument, that monopoly insurers have lower costs of risk and of other functions because of the larger risk pool, is inconsistent with the "survivor" evidence. In any competitive market with significant economies of scale, large firms tend to drive out smaller firms over time. The cosurvival of small and large insurers indicates that scale economies from risk pooling are eliminated at a fairly small scale or can be achieved through reinsurance. For the critical insurance functions of claims administration and control of moral hazard, scale economies are probably exhausted at quite small scale. The costs of provider-specific information, for example, tend to increase with geo-graphic distance. That Medicare contracts out its claims administration to local intermediaries and is attempting to enroll beneficiaries in private HMOs rather than develop its own HMO is further evidence that national insurers do not have significant scale advantage over local insurers.[9]

---

9. Several studies of economies of scale in insurance have concluded that returns to scale are constant over a very large range; see Doherty (1981) and Geehan

Overhead Costs of Public Monopoly Insurers

A public monopoly insurer must perform the same basic functions as a private insurer: collect premiums, pay providers, control moral hazard, and adjust to nondiversifiable risks. But the full costs of performing these functions are understated in reported measures of overhead. Omitted as well are dead-weight costs (forgone net benefits) from forcing on everyone the same level and type of insurance, and other production and consumption distortions, which should be viewed as overhead costs of the health insurance system.

Hidden Costs of Nonprice, Noninformation-based Rationing. Public insurers use a more limited range of strategies to pay providers and control moral hazard. These cost-control mechanisms are strikingly similar in Canada, Germany, and Japan, where physicians remain independent private contractors and hospitals are quasi-private and not for profit.[10] All three countries pay physicians according to a fee schedule that has not kept pace with inflation; patient copayment is minimal—zero in Canada; and very little use is made of information-based systems, utilization review, managed care, or provider risk sharing. Physician expenditure targets have been added in some Canadian provinces and in Germany to control unbundling and increases in service volume in response to low fees. Canada controls hospital expenditures by annual budget caps for operating revenues and direct control over capital acquisition. By using uniform, province-wide fee schedules with no patient copayments and no provider or patient-specific information systems, Canada has achieved lower reported insurer and provider overhead costs than have private insurers in the United States.

The public insurer, however, imposes the hidden costs of moral hazard control on patients—costs analogous to those of private sector claims administration. These hidden costs include excessive time costs for patients that result from proliferation of multiple short visits in response to controls on physicians' fees; forgone productivity and quality of life from delay or total nonavailability of surgical procedures; and loss of productivity (producer surplus) through underemployment of some medical inputs. Rough estimates suggest that these hidden

---

(1977). Because it is impossible to measure a homogeneous unit of insurance output, however, estimates of scale economies that are based on accounting data are less reliable than the evidence from survival of small and large firms.

10. It may reflect the greater influence of provider organizations in public monopoly systems.

overhead costs of public insurers exceed the measured overhead costs under private insurance. This conclusion is not surprising, since public insurers that are both monopolists and monopsonists have weaker incentives than private insurers to minimize overhead borne by patients and providers.[11]

Patient time costs. In Canada and Japan the fee schedules of physicians have not kept pace with inflation. Not surprisingly, physicians have responded by unbundling (subdividing services into multiple small units) and upcoding (reporting more comprehensive services, in order to qualify for a higher fee), and by reducing their own time and other inputs per billable unit. Patients must therefore make multiple visits to receive the services previously provided in a single visit. This reduction in real services per visit ("quality"), the increase in number of visits, and the resulting increase in patient time costs are the mechanisms used to ration the excess demand created by making care free to patients.

The scant evidence from Canada confirms this hypothesis of reduction in input of physician time per billable unit, decrease in convenience for patients, and increase in patient time costs. In Quebec, in the two years immediately after the introduction of universal health insurance, home visits dropped by 63 percent, telephone consultations fell by 41 percent, physician time spent per office visit declined by 16 percent, and office visits rose by 32 percent (Enterline et al. 1973, 1975). Nevertheless, physicians' relative net income increased over 30 percent in the same period (Comanor 1980).[12] In Japan the increase in patient time costs is more dramatic because fee controls have been more stringent. The average length of visit is roughly five minutes, and the Japanese on average make twelve visits per year to a physician, or roughly three times as many as Americans, where the average visit length is fifteen to twenty minutes.

Fuchs and Hahn (1990) report that real resources per physician visit were 34–36 percent lower in Canada than in the United States and that Canadians made more visits per capita. They conclude that Canadians

---

11. Of course copayments and utilization review entail rationing. But this is efficient, given scarce resources and excess demand induced by moral hazard. Rationing by copayment entails no excess burden (other than the administrative costs already discussed); it also need not violate equity concerns, given appropriate income-targeted subsidies to ensure that insurance is universally affordable. Information-based UR also entails no excess burden (other than the administrative cost already discussed) if it eliminates care that would cost more than it is worth.
12. I am indebted to Ted Frech for drawing this evidence to my attention.

receive more physicians' services and that the services are produced more efficiently. An alternative interpretation of these data is that the average duration of visit is shorter in Canada and that medical services are produced with a lower ratio of physician time and other medical inputs relative to patient time, because this is a rational response to constraints on reimbursement for physicians and a zero money price to patients. Unfortunately, these contradictory interpretations of the data cannot be resolved because the average length of the physician-patient encounter is not reported in this study and, fundamentally, the real health benefits per visit cannot be measured.

Thus when public insurers eliminate price and information-based mechanisms to control insurance-induced moral hazard, the main devices that ration excess demand in the physician services market appear to be reduction in "quality" (medical resources per visit) and increase in patient time costs of obtaining medical care. Time costs rise because each visit entails fixed costs of travel and some waiting in the office, regardless of the duration of the visit. These excess patient time costs are excluded from the national health accounts and from public visibility because they appear as innocuous travel time and time in the physician's waiting room or office.

The magnitude of these excess patient time costs depends on the distribution of patients' time costs, relative to marginal benefit from care, and on whether rationing by time price allocates services to those who benefit most. In general, the dead-weight loss from excess patient time costs and resource misallocation is equal to (less/greater than) total expenditure on physicians' services, if time costs are uncorrelated (negatively/positively correlated) with money willingness to pay (see appendix 12–B).[13]

Several objections may be raised to the conclusion that the hidden costs of excess patient time and forgone benefits under nonprice rationing may equal or exceed total expenditures on physicians' services. First, shouldn't a fair comparison include patient time costs under private insurance? The answer is no. The measure here is *excess* time costs, over and above the efficient level required to receive medical care in a well-designed competitive private insurance system. Of course, the mix of patient time and physician inputs under current private insurance in the United States is unlikely to conform to this benchmark, because of the tax subsidy and other distortions. But because the tax subsidy applies to medical and insurance inputs but not to patient time, there is more likely to be excessive use of medical inputs relative to patient time in the

---

13. Money willingness to pay is related to expected wealth benefits, given income-related subsidies to make insurance affordable.

United States, and these input costs are already included in the national health accounts. Thus there is no reason to add an estimate of excess patient time costs to the estimate of overhead for the United States under the status quo.

A second objection is that rationing by time rather than by money price is more equitable. The objection to using prices to control overuse, however, is more efficiently addressed with income-related subsidies to ensure that the poor can afford insurance coverage.

In conclusion, public monopoly insurers that tightly control physician fees while charging a zero money price to patients and forgoing information-based rationing incur large hidden costs in patient time and probably additional costs due to displacement of more serious by more trivial medical treatments; they also underuse physicians' time if expenditure constraints are binding. The mix and the magnitude of these hidden costs depend on the ability of physicians to circumvent the fee controls and maintain hourly earnings and on the exact methods for rationing the excess demand when care is free. But under reasonable estimates of demand elasticities, these costs could be at least as large as reasonable estimates of overhead costs of physicians in the United States.

Gains from monopsony power? The evidence from Canada and even more strikingly from Japan, that tight fee schedules lead to reduction in physician time per billable unit and hence excess patient time costs, is also relevant to the claimed advantage of a monopoly public insurer in exercising monopsony power. Monopsony power could yield a distributional gain with no efficiency loss if a monopsony public insurer could control physicians' fees and incomes without any adverse effect on the supply of physician manpower. Evidence cited in support of this view is the fact that average net income of physicians is lower in Canada than in the United States ($82,740 in Canada; $132,300 in the United States in 1987 U.S. dollars). Nevertheless, the number of physicians per capita has increased as fast in Canada as in the United States, and the average number of applicants per medical school opening is 4 in Canada, compared with 1.6 in the United States (U.S. General Accounting Office 1990, 37; 1988–1989 data.)

The relevant measure of physician supply, however, depends on the value added per physician, as well as on the number of physicians. Ineffective use of monopsony power simply distorts the input mix and leads to excessive patient time costs. Exploitation of monopsony power tends to reduce hours of work per physician, resulting in a loss of productivity due to the underuse of physician manpower. This loss from exercise of monopsony power can be avoided *only* if either physicians' hours are totally inelastic in response to reduction in revenue per hour or if a public monopsony insurer can devise a system of reimbursement that extracts any monopoly rent *without* affecting marginal incentives. Both of these conditions seem unlikely. Even if physicians earn monopoly rents in competitive private insurance markets, it is extremely hard to design reimbursement systems that tax away these rents without reducing incentives to work. Low fee schedules and expenditure targets do not do it.[14]

The evidence that lower monetary incomes have apparently not adversely affected applications to medical schools in Canada relative to the United States does not prove that low fees have extracted monopoly rents without affecting productivity per physician. The income measure relevant to the decision to apply to medical school is the expected lifetime (utility) return on the investment in medical training, relative to other career alternatives. This relative return may be higher in Canada for several reasons: costs of medical training are more heavily subsidized in Canada than in the United States; expected hours of work may be shorter (Enterline 1973, 1975); the disutility from expected medical liability is probably lower, since the rate of malpractice suits is five times higher in the United States than in Canada (Danzon 1990); and expected returns and risk on other careers may differ. The relevant question is whether a given level of physician effort can be obtained at lower social cost in a monopsony public insurer regime or in a system that relies on (undistorted) competitive private insurance markets, holding constant the liability regime and opportunities in other careers. A simple comparison of average annual incomes and number of applicants to medical schools in Canada and the United States cannot answer this question.[15]

Hidden costs of rationing hospital care. In Canada each hospital negotiates an annual global operating budget with the provincial government. Although capital expenditures are funded from a variety of sources, approval is required from the same provincial agency that also contributes a major share of the funding.

These expenditure controls have resulted in a much slower growth

---

14. It is sometimes argued that even if low fee schedules lead to a reduction in physicians' hours of work, the result is minimal if any net social loss because much care provided by physicians has little real benefit. But if the net patient benefit of physicians' time is zero or negative at the margin, the efficient solution is to train fewer physicians, not to subsidize medical training and then use reimbursement constraints to discourage their work effort.

15. Carr and Mathewson (1991) suggest that the Canadian system has increased the real incomes of physicians, particularly specialists, in Canada relative to the United States. This finding is consistent with the earlier evidence reported in Comanor (1980).

of capital and labor inputs per hospital day ("service intensity") in Canada than in the United States, reflecting nursing hours, use of operating rooms, magnetic resonance imaging, and other capital-embodied technologies. Total hospital costs per capita are lower in Canada, although the number of admissions per capita and length of stay are 5.2 percent and 52 percent higher, respectively, in Canada than in the United States (Neuschler 1990).

Access to acute care services, however, is more limited in Canada. A larger fraction of hospital beds in Canada are occupied by elderly patients with an average length of stay of over sixty days, despite waiting lists for acute care admissions. This situation is in part a predictable response to the incentives facing hospital administrators and employees under fixed budget constraints. If they perform more surgical procedures, they receive no more revenue with which to purchase additional supplies or nursing time. Thus, increasing medical procedures, given the fixed budget, simply adds to the stress and workload of existing staff. Conversely, hospital administrators and nonphysician personnel suffer no revenue loss (except to the extent that next year's budget is related to this year's admissions) and can enjoy an easier life if they keep the hospital beds full with long-term patients whose daily requirements are relatively low or prolong the length of stay for acute care patients. This example again illustrates how the costs of patient time relative to medical inputs are a logical response to tight limits on provider reimbursement.

Evans et al. (1989) tend to dismiss the increasing "rhetoric of underfunding, shortages, excessive waiting lists, and so on" as

> part of the process by which providers negotiate their share of public resources—including their own incomes. . . . Since the boy always cries wolf (and must do so, given the political system of funding), one does not know if the wolf is really there. The political dramatics should not lead external observers into believing that the wolf is always at hand.

Survey evidence reported in Globerman and Hoye (1990), however, tends to confirm that the average wait and the number of people waiting have increased and that this represents a real social cost. Their results are based on a survey of a random sample of specialists in British Columbia for six common procedures performed by each specialty. They find that while the average wait for some procedures such as mastectomy is as short as two weeks, most procedures require waits of at least three months and some require up to ten months. This survey overwhelmingly refuted the common allegation that waiting lists are artificially inflated by duplicative bookings or voluntary waiting.

This evidence may be upward biased because the survey occurred roughly six months after a nurses' strike. A "significant percentage but well less than the majority" of respondents cited the nurses' strike in British Columbia as a factor. The estimates may be downward biased for Canada as a whole, though, for several reasons. First, British Columbia has a higher ratio of physicians per capita than other provinces, and each physician is therefore likely to have a shorter queue. Second, surveys derived from physicians or hospitals cannot reflect those patients who are discouraged by the wait or by their general practitioner from seeking specialist care, a bias likely to be more serious in rural areas. Third, random sampling of physicians, without stratification to reflect regional differences in physician-population density, will probably oversample physicians in areas of high physician-population density, where waits per capita are likely to be relatively short.

Globerman and Hoye estimate the "income loss" associated with queues by multiplying the estimated total weeks waiting by the percentage of patients in each specialty who were "experiencing difficulty in carrying on their work or daily duties as a result of their medical condition."[16] This product is then multiplied by the average weekly industrial earnings for 1989. The resulting estimate is $132 million or 0.2 percent of provincial gross domestic product (GDP) for that year, which they note is roughly equal to the total wages and salaries lost through strikes and lockouts in that year.

This measure of lost income understates the real economic costs of involuntary waiting for hospital procedures. A more complete measure would include all loss of market and nonmarket productivity, reduction in "quality of life," including physical and psychological pain and suffering and increased use of other inputs—for example, the additional time of other family members in caring for an elderly person who cannot get a hip replacement.[17]

---

16. This question was asked of the physician respondents. The average reported percentage varied from 88 percent for cardiovascular surgeons to 14 percent for gynecologists (p.26).

17. Globerman and Hoye's income loss estimate assigns zero value to loss of productivity for hours beyond the normal working hours (as reflected in average weekly earnings) and zero loss of real income for those patients who were not experiencing difficulty in working or other daily duties, as reported by physicians. Omitting these losses in nonmarket productivity is partially offset by assuming loss of total weekly earnings for those experiencing significant difficulties. The use of average provincial weekly wage for retirees and children as well as adults may also entail bias, as the authors note. Ideally, losses should of course be measured relative to expected productivity and well-being after surgery.

Globerman and Hoye's conservative estimate implies that waiting for surgery accounts for 0.2 percent of GDP in British Columbia. If hospital expenditures are roughly 3 percent of GDP, this represents 7 percent of hospital expenditures. A more complete measure could be as great as Woolhandler and Himmelstein's (1991) estimated difference in overhead costs (9.0 percent in Canada as opposed to 20.2 percent in the United States). Since some U.S. hospitals' expenditures on information systems surely improves patient care (and a significant part is related to Medicare), these very rough numbers suggest that Canada's methods of rationing result in hidden costs that could be at least as great as the more visible costs of billing, utilization review, and the like adopted by private insurers in the United States.

It may be objected that these forgone benefits are simply the result of lower resource allocation to acute care hospital services in Canada and that this should not be counted as overhead. But to the extent that people are denied access to services that would be covered if they were free to choose their own form of insurance, these forgone benefits are a real cost of the imposed uniformity of a monopoly system.

Moreover, for any given level of resources allocated to hospital care, rationing through waiting is likely to lead to a less efficient use of the scarce facilities than rationing through price and information-based systems. A reimbursement system that offers no reward to providers for additional effort is also unlikely to lead to maximum output from the fixed resources. Thus it is highly likely that the limited number of beds and the capital equipment are not being used to yield the maximum value to patients. These forgone benefits are reflected in the waiting lists. Of course, while longer hospital stays have some benefits to patients, they also have real costs. The willingness of patients in the United States to accept health insurance plans with utilization review and managed care, in return for lower premiums or better coverage of other medical services, suggests that for many the longer stays are not worth their cost.

Forgone benefits are not the only hidden cost of rationing in budget-constrained hospital systems. In Japan, low fees for hospital services have resulted in such low staffing levels of nurses that patients often rely on family members for meals and other "hotel" services while in the hospital. These time costs are omitted from the national income accounts, as are "gifts" to physicians (roughly $3,000 for significant surgery by a well-established physician), which provide an informal system of rationing access to the most sought-after physicians.

In some countries the demand for supplementary insurance provides a rough measure of the extent to which the public system constrains services below the level that people are willing to pay for. Canada does not permit private insurance of services that are covered under provincial

275

plans and heavily penalizes physicians who serve privately insured patients. Therefore, although supplementary insurance is widely purchased in Canada, it covers only services and amenities not covered under the public system so is not a reliable indicator of dissatisfaction with public provision of those services. But in the United Kingdom and New Zealand, where budget constraints on the public system have been tighter, the growth in private insurance to cover services in private hospitals is a rough measure of willingness to pay for more prompt access, free choice of doctor, nicer amenities, and other services not provided by the public system. In New Zealand over 45 percent of the population has private coverage.[18] But supplementary private insurance is a mixed blessing as an add-on to a public monopoly system. Private insurance does reduce the real social costs caused when a public insurer provides less access to services than people are willing to pay for. But as actually implemented in the United Kingdom and New Zealand, supplementary insurance tends to distort production within the public system.

The Hidden Costs of Tax-based Financing. Using the tax system to collect premiums is said to be a major advantage of public monopoly insurers. Although the administrative cost of financing health insurance by raising tax rates is small, the hidden costs are large. These hidden costs ("excess burden") are the production and consumption losses that occur because people change their labor supply and their saving and consumption patterns to avoid taxed activities. These costs are greater, the higher the existing tax rate is when marginal rates are increased. For the United States the excess burden of raising $1 of federal general tax revenue has been estimated between seventeen and fifty cents (Ballard et al. 1985). Other studies have yielded both higher and lower estimates. Even the lower estimate of 17 percent of revenue raised still significantly exceeds the costs of premium collection under private insurance.

The excess burden of raising taxes would not arise if the public system were financed by a social insurance premium or head tax. Indeed, if rated on the basis of risk class, it could have the same positive incentive effects for health lifestyles as risk-rated private insurance premiums. The

---

18. Expenditures on supplementary insurance are not an unbiased measure of the value of additional services, amenities, and financial protection, to the extent that coverage of copayments induces greater use of the free public system and these costs are not reflected in private insurance premiums. In contrast, to the extent that privately insured patients substitute private for public services, the reduction in expected benefits from the public system is like a tax on the purchase of private insurance that is not reflected in premium payments.

administrative costs of financing through risk-rated head taxes, how-ever, would be much higher than existing income and payroll tax systems. Head taxes are also generally considered distributionally unacceptable.

The excess burden from financing national health insurance in Canada may actually have been less than implied by assuming an increase in marginal tax rates, to the extent that the new program was financed by reducing other programs rather than by raising new tax revenues. Lindsay et al. (1978, 38) conclude that

> both the hospital and medical parts of the program have been financed by displacement in the budgets of other social welfare spending categories. . . . Sixty cents of every dollar spent on these combined programs is taken from cutbacks in funds for aid to the blind and disabled, workman's compensation and family allowances.

Similarly, if the United States were to adopt a Canadian-style monopoly public insurance program within the Gramm-Rudman-Hollings constraints, the net increase in excess burden of tax-based financing would be less than (at least) 17 percent of the gross cost of the program. Obviously, there would be an offset for existing expenditures on Medicare, Medicaid, public hospitals, and other tax-financed pro-grams that could be discontinued. The efficiency losses associated with the tax subsidy to employer contributions would also be eliminated. If the net new tax needs, after netting out these savings, were financed by cutbacks in other programs, the marginal excess burden would be reduced. But if the eliminated programs were targeted at the poor, as in Canada, the net benefit to the poor from introducing national health insurance would be questionable.[19]

Providing universal coverage through private insurance would also entail some excess burden of raising tax revenues to ensure that coverage is affordable. But these costs would be much lower than under a public monopoly system because subsidies would be limited to the poor and near poor. If, for example, subsidies equivalent to the cost of coverage for one-third of the population were paid, the excess burden of tax financing would be one-third as high as under a public monopoly system.

---

19. The current appeal of national health insurance proposals founded on mandatory employment-based coverage is consistent with the hypothesis underlying Lindsay et al.'s analysis that political pressures tend to result in programs that redistribute resources away from the tails of the income distribution toward the middle classes.

Free Riding on Foreign Research and Development

Another distortion in the comparison of costs of the U.S. health care system relative to Canada and some other public monopoly systems is that the public systems free ride on R&D expenditures in the United States. This is most obvious in the case of pharmaceuticals but also applies to other medical technologies and information systems generally. R&D in all these areas entails joint costs that benefit all consumers worldwide. If costs are truly joint, then global welfare maximization would set prices proportional to marginal benefits, as reflected in demand elasticities (Ramsey pricing). Unfortunately, "true" marginal benefits for drugs are not revealed by observed demand, because patients may imperfectly understand true benefits, distorting effects of insurance and incentives of physicians. But if willingness to pay is roughly related to income, then clearly the United States pays more than its "fair" share of pharmaceutical R&D, because the difference in drug prices exceeds the difference in income.

The pricing of drugs in Canada may also induce allocative waste. Canada has reduced drug prices below prices in the United States and below the average of the countries in the Organization for Economic Cooperation and Development, by compulsory licensing of drugs while still under patent and aggressive generic substitution laws. To the extent that compulsory licensing results in a redistribution of monopoly profits from the patentee to the domestic generic manufacturer, it induces waste by distorting resource allocation based on comparative advantage.

Some of the international benefits of U.S. R&D spending for some drugs and other medical technologies may be small or even negative, but on balance benefits are surely positive. To the extent that benefits of R&D accrue to other countries that do not pay a fair share of the joint costs, the hidden benefits should be credited against health care costs in the United States in any comparison of real costs and benefits.

Other Hidden Time Costs

The Government Accounting Office reports that 14 percent of the differential in per capita health care spending between the United States and Canada goes for the services of professionals other than medical doctors, including physiotherapists, podiatrists, psychologists, and the like. These services have benefits that are not captured in standard morbidity and mortality statistics, and they reduce the hidden inputs of patient's time to the production of health. Most countries, including the United States, have a high income elasticity of demand for goods and services that improve the quality of life or economize on consumers'

TABLE 12–2
COSTS OF PUBLIC AND PRIVATE INSURERS, AS PERCENTAGE OF CLAIM PAYMENTS

Function	Private Insurance	Public Insurance
Premium collection	Commissions: 1%	Dead-weight costs of taxing: $\geq 17\%$
Control of moral hazard	Prices, information systems, provider incentives: 4%	*Physicians* $\lessgtr 100+ \%$ (excess patient, time costs, etc.) *Hospitals* >7% (forgone patient benefits)
General administration	3–4%	1%
Medical underwriting	<1%	0
Total (net)	7.6%[a]	>45%[b]
Risk bearing	Return on capital, 4.5%	Uncertainty for patients, providers, taxpayers, > 4%
Investment income	–1.5%	0
Premium taxes	(2.2%)[c]	0

a. Net of premium taxes, return on capital, and investment income.
b. Assumes physicians' expenditures, 30 percent; hospitals, 40 percent of total expenditures; excess time cost, 60 percent of physicians' expenditure.
c. Transfer to state government.
SOURCE: Author.

time. Health care has both these characteristics. As any graduate of Economics 1 knows, if a bachelor marries his housekeeper, gross national product goes down. Conversely, if an American visits the physiotherapist, whereas a Canadian spends more time at home doing exercises or cuts back on tennis, health care spending in the United States increases but does not in Canada. Omitting the costs of patients' time understates the real resources devoted to health in Canada and underestimates the benefits of higher spending in the United States.

Conclusions

Table 12–2 summarizes the rough estimates of a comparison between overhead costs of private insurance in the United States and the public system in Canada, adjusted to include some of the hidden costs of the

Canadian system. These estimates indicate that costs associated with tax-based financing and rationing by nonprice, non-information-based methods may be at least as great as the parallel costs of premium collection and claims administration incurred by private insurers.

Costs of risk bearing are almost certainly no higher under private insurance, with risk diversification through capital markets, than under public insurance that shifts risk to patients, providers, and taxpayers. Rather than attempt to estimate the hidden cost of risk bearing in Canada, however, this component has been excluded from the total for both countries. Omitted too from the Canadian total are the losses to Canadians from being forced to consume a uniform level of insurance and medical care, which for many may differ from their preferred level. These losses are partially but not fully reflected in the excess costs of patients' time and forgone benefits. Table 12–2 does not include the higher overhead costs borne by providers and patients in the United States, under the assumption that there are at least equivalent offsetting benefits in satisfying diverse preferences.

How might the costs of private insurance overhead change if coverage were mandatory and a system of refundable tax credits to ensure affordability replaced the current tax subsidy to employer contributions (Pauly et al. 1991)? Assuming tax financing of subsidies equal to one-third of the cost of coverage, premium collection costs would increase to roughly 6 percent. There would also be some costs of enforcement that should be small because enforcement would be through existing tax and welfare systems. Medical underwriting expense might also increase, but this rise too should be small, since most people would probably obtain coverage through employment or other groups. Elimination of the tax subsidy and regulatory distortions, however, would probably lead to some reduction in claims administration and general administration costs since policy holders would face the full marginal cost of these expenses.

The empirical estimates in table 12–2 are necessarily very rough. Their main purpose is to illustrate the thesis of this chapter, that the widely discussed comparisons of overhead costs of alternative health care systems are based on a flawed conceptual framework. A simple comparison of accounting costs can be grossly misleading. The true "overhead" of a health insurance system also includes all the hidden costs associated with financing and operating the insurance and with insurance-induced distortions in the production and consumption of medical care. Simple theory suggests that these costs would be lower in competitive private insurance markets than under a monopoly public insurer, because the public insurer has much weaker incentives than private insurers do to take into account all the costs imposed on patients and providers. The rough empirical evidence tends to confirm that overhead costs in Canada, adjusted to include some of the most significant hidden costs, are indeed higher than under private insurance in the United States. Although there may well be waste in U.S. private insurance markets at present, this waste is attributable primarily to tax and regulatory factors and is not intrinsic to private health insurance.

Appendix 12–A: Calculation of Private Insurance Overhead

The decomposition of overhead for commercial insurers is shown in table 12–1, which reports the components of overhead, expressed as a percentage of incurred claims, as estimated by Hay/Huggins Company, based on underwriting practices of major insurers (Congressional Research Service 1988). Because these data are for conventionally insured plans written by commercial insurers, they are not representative of the range of coverages or insurers in the markets. Blue Cross plans in some states and all self-insured firms are exempt from premium taxes.[20] Self-insurers do not prepay premiums so would not accrue investment income. Their premium-minus-benefit differential would probably also not include a return on capital.

Based on figures for the 100–499 size class, overhead net of premium taxes and return on capital was 8.2 percent of claims for commercial insurers; they made 43 percent of claim payments.[21] The same overhead percentage is assumed for Blue Cross and Blue Shield plans that made 28 percent of claim payments. For self-insured and HMO plans, which paid 29 percent of claims, I use the 500–2,499 size class, which implies a 6.3 percent overhead rate on claims. Taking the weighted average yields 7.6 percent as the average overhead rate on claims, net of premium taxes, return on capital, and investment income for private insurance in the United States.

20. Blue Cross–Blue Shield plans and self-insured plus HMO plans account for 32.0 and 34.0 percent of total private insurance claims payments respectively (HIAA, 1989).
21. Based on the May 1988 Current Population Survey, EBRI (1991, 181) reports that 49 percent of workers whose employers offered plans were in firms of 250 or more. Since large employers are more likely to offer dependent coverage, it is reasonable to assume a larger size class as representative for insured employees and their dependents in total. Since large firms, however, are more likely to self-insure, I use the 100–499 size class for commercially insured firms and the 500–2,499 size class for self-insured firms. Ideally, a weighted average should be used.

FIGURE 12–A1
WELFARE COSTS OF TIME RATIONING

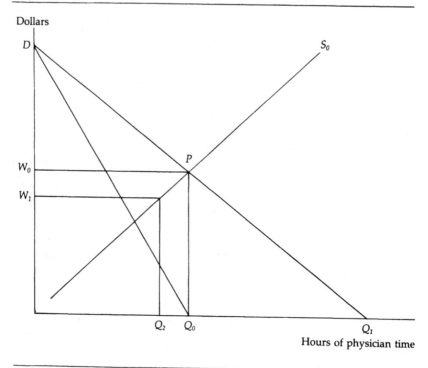

SOURCE: Author.

Appendix 12–B: Costs of Nonprice Rationing of Physicians' Services

Figure 12–A1 represents the market demand for and supply of hours by physicians. Consider first a system of universal coverage delivered through competing private health insurers, with income-targeted subsidies to achieve social goals with respect to universal access and affordability. In Figure 12–A1, the demand curve DPQ_1 is assumed to represent marginal benefits to patients[22]; the supply curve is S_0. Physi-

---

22. This assumes that distributional concerns have been addressed through subsidies to purchase insurance (for example, as in Pauly et al. 1991). It also requires that patients have unbiased (but not necessarily perfect) information about the value of medical services. Even if expectations are not unbiased, the analysis still estimates the difference in welfare cost generated by the form of

cians receive an hourly wage of W_0.[23] Quantity of hours supplied is Q_0. Since the user price to insured patients is less than P_0, quantity demanded would exceed Q_0. But assume that quantity demanded is restrained to Q_0 by some combination of copayments, information-based rationing, and provider incentives, hereafter "managed care."

With a zero copayment, consumer surplus S_0 is equal to the area under the demand curve $1/2(D - W_0)Q_0 + W_0Q_0$, and the costs of time rationing can be measured relative to this benchmark. With a positive copayment, consumer surplus is S_0 minus total copayment, and this must be netted out to yield the net excess cost of time rationing relative to price and information-based rationing.

In competitive private insurance markets, patients incur some time costs for travel, waiting, and receiving treatment. But since physicians in competitive markets have incentives to internalize patients' time costs, care is produced with the efficient mixture of patients' time, physicians' time, and other resources. The demand curve DPQ_1 reflects patients' willingness to pay for services, assuming this optimized resource intensity and patient time per visit.

Now assume that the competitive private insurance system is replaced by a public monopoly national health insurance (NHI) scheme. Physicians' fees are initially regulated at a level consistent with $W_{0,}$ and all copayments, information-based rationing, and managed care are eliminated. When patients face a zero money price and no other constraints on demand, the quantity demanded at the pre-NHI time cost would be Q_1. But since only Q_0 physician hours are supplied, there is excess demand that must somehow be rationed.

If physicians are perfect agents, they would allocate the Q_0 hours to the patients who would have received care under price and information-based rationing, since by assumption these patients receive the highest value from the services. Thus with perfect agency—defined as providing services only as long as marginal benefit is at least equal to marginal social cost—the NHI could save the costs of administering copayments and managed care insured by private insurers. Since resources are optimally allocated with perfect agency, there are no dead-weight costs of excess patient time or misallocation of patient resources. This is the ideal envisioned by those who argue that rationing should be delegated

---

rationing, as long as public insurance does not systematically improve patients' information. This is unlikely, since physicians have less incentive to spend time providing information when fees are low and regulated.

23. Although insurers may use different reimbursement systems, including fee-for-service, capitation, and others, they can be converted to an effective risk-adjusted hourly wage.

to medical providers, since they have better information.

But the propensity of physicians to be good agents for patients is presumably independent of the form of insurance. Thus the extent that physicians eliminate low-benefit care without third-party controls is reflected in lower administrative costs under private insurance and lower time costs under public insurance than if physicians have no agency concerns. The demand curve in figure 12–A1 is assumed to reflect the same agency propensities under private and public insurance and can be used to measure incremental losses from time rationing.

Time Costs of Rationing. Assume that the excess demand $Q_1 - Q_0$ under NHI is rationed solely by increasing patients' time per unit of medical care. This increase in time could result from a reduction in inputs of physicians' time or other ancillary resources per visit (unbundling).[24] Both imply an increase in patient time per unit of real medical care, since more visits and therefore more travel and waiting-room time are required to obtain a given real amount of medical care.

Rationing by time can entail dead-weight loss from two sources: the opportunity cost of additional patients' time spent to obtain care and, in some circumstances, a resource misallocation cost or loss in consumer surplus if medical services are not allocated to their highest-valued use. The magnitude of these costs depends on the distribution of willingness to pay in time and the correlation between time and money willingness to pay.

Assume the consumer has a utility function that is additively separable in income (a proxy for other goods and services) and health:

$$V = U(Y - pq - wtq) + H(q) \tag{12.1}$$

where $t = f + k + h$, V = total utility, U = utility of income, Y = gross income, q = units of medical care, or visits under competitive insurance, p = price per unit of medical care, t = total time per visit, f = travel time, k = waiting room time, h = duration of visit, w = opportunity cost per unit of time, and H = utility of health.

The functions U and H are assumed continuous and twice differentiable. Subscripts $_m$ and t denote values under money and time rationing, respectively, V, U, H, Y, q, f, and w may differ across consumers. Subscripts to denote individual consumers are suppressed for simplicity.

---

24. Some reduction in resources per visit is likely since this increases net revenue for the physician, whereas longer waiting room time is costly to patients and, by itself, does not increase revenue for physicians.

Maximizing equation 12.1 with respect to q yields:

$$p + w_t = H' / U' = MRS$$

At the margin, the total price, including money and time, that the consumer is willing to pay is equal to the marginal rate of substitution between health and wealth.

Price rationing. Under price rationing, the maximum price P_m that the consumer would pay, conditional on t_m, is

$$P_m = H' / U' - wt_m$$

Assume that waiting room time k and visit duration h are uniform across patients. Then money willingness to pay P_m is positively related to marginal valuation of health relative to wealth and negatively related to travel time f and cost of time w. The distribution of P_m over consumers defines the money willingness to pay demand curve DPQ_1 in figure 12–A1.

Time rationing. If consumers pay zero money price and services are rationed solely by time, then the money-equivalent willingness to pay Pt is

$$Pt = H' / U' - wt_t$$

where t_t, total time per unit of medical care, embeds the market-clearing conditions for h and k.

The difference between money and time willingness to pay is:

$$P_m - Pt = H' / U'_m - H' / Ut + w(t_t - t_m)$$

Thus if income effects are zero, the demand curve (or net benefits curve) shifts down by the increase in time cost per unit of care $w(t_t - t_m)$. If income effects due to the elimination of copayments are positive ($U'_t < U'_m$), it is possible that $Pt > P_m$, particularly if w is very low. The ith individual has zero net benefit and drops out of the market if $H' / U'_t < wt_t$.

Dead-weight loss under time rationing. Several types of dead-weight losses occur when health care is rationed by time.

• *Homogeneous* P_t *across consumers.* If all of the consumers are homogeneous with respect to net benefits P_t, then the condition for market clearing is:

$$Pt = H' / U'_t - wt_t = 0, \text{ or}$$

$$t_t = H' / U'_t w \text{ for all consumers}$$

Since all Q_1 consumers must be served but only Q_0 units are supplied, each consumer receives Q_0/Q_1 units.[25] Total consumer surplus S_1 is zero. Total costs of rationing are $Q_0 w t_t$. This dead-weight loss is at least equal to total consumer surplus S_0 under competitive insurance; the loss could exceed Q_0 if income effects are positive. Thus the maximum dead-weight loss from time rationing occurs when consumers are homogenous and income effects from eliminating the copayments are positive.[26] Although homogeneity of time willingness to pay P_t (and hence total elimination of surplus) seems unlikely if money willingness to pay is heterogeneous, it is not impossible. It could occur if change in marginal rates of substitution $H'/U'_t - H'/U'_m$, due to income effects of eliminating price rationing, are positively correlated with the difference in time costs with $w(t_t - t_m)$.

- *Homogeneous time costs or* wt_t *and* P_m *uncorrelated.* If wt_t is either uniform across consumers or uncorrelated with P_m and there are no income effects, market clearing requires that for the marginal consumer $H'/U'_t = wt_t = W_0$. This is also the time cost for all consumers under uniformity. If time costs differ but are uncorrelated with P_m, the net benefit curve is parallel to the money demand curve but is shifted down by wt_t; some inframarginal consumers retain some surplus, but this is offset by the resource misallocation cost of displacing some relatively high-valued users by lower-valued users who have relatively low time costs. The loss in surplus is equal to $W_0 Q_0$, or 100 percent of total expenditures, if income effects are zero. If income effects are positive, the market-clearing time t_t must be higher, and the loss of surplus is greater.

- *Positive correlation between* wt_t *and* P_m. If time costs are positively correlated with P_m, the net benefit curve rotates around Q_1 if w is zero for the last consumer; it also shifts down and reduces the horizontal intercept if w is positive for the last consumer. Since positive correlation between P_m and wt_t increases the homogeneity of P_t across consumers, total time and resource misallocation costs are higher and hence loss of surplus is higher than when time costs and P_m are uncorrelated. If in addition some income effects are negatively correlated with P_m, homogeneity increases, and the loss of surplus could equal or exceed S_0.

- *Negative correlation between* w *and* P_m. If income effects are zero and

---

25. If each one of N consumers would have demanded $q_1 > 1$ visits under the money willingness to pay demand curve, where $Q_1 = Nq_1$, under time rationing each consumer receives q_0/q_1 visits.

26. Suen (1989) concludes that the maximum dead-weight loss is S_0 because he ignores income effects. He also concludes that homogeneity of consumers results in the maximum loss of surplus.

$t_t - t_m$ is uniform for all consumers, the downward shift of the demand curve is proportional to w. If w is perfectly negatively correlated with P_m and is zero for the first consumer, the demand curve rotates inward around D, to DQ_0. The dead-weight loss is DPQ_0, which is equal to $1/2W_0Q_0$. If $w > 0$ for the first consumer, the vertical intercept shifts down and the loss in surplus exceeds $1/2W_0Q_0$.

- *Perfect positive correlation between P_m and P_t.* If willingness to pay in time and money is perfectly correlated and equal, then the net benefit curve under time rationing is identical to DPQ_1. The Q_0 services are rationed to the highest-valued users, but there is a dead-weight loss from excess time costs equal to the rectangle W_0Q_0, or 100 percent of total expenditures. The total surplus retained by inframarginal users is $S_1 = 1/2(D - W_0)Q_0$. Perfect correlation between P_t and P_m is unlikely, however. If t_t is either uniform or uncorrelated with w and H'/U', then perfect positive correlation between P_m and P_t requires a positive correlation between w and the positive income effect, $H'/U'_t - H'/U'_m$, such that the increase in time costs is just offset by income effect that increases gross willingness to pay.

Conclusions Emerging from This Analysis. First, the dead-weight loss is likely to be at least $1/2W_0Q_0$ and could equal or even exceed total surplus $S_0 = 1/2(D - W)Q_0 + W_0Q_0$ if consumers' willingness to pay under time rationing is homogeneous. If wt_t and P_m are uncorrelated and there are no income effects, the loss in surplus is W_0Q_0. In general, the loss is less than W_0Q_0 if P_m and w are negatively correlated and exceeds W_0Q_0 if P_m and w are positively correlated, since this tends to increase homogeneity across consumers. Positive correlation between P_m and w is more likely for those services for which income elasticities of demand are high; however, this may be mitigated if poor health and hence high H' are associated with low w, or if t_m under price rationing is sufficiently high to reduce P_m for those with high w. The dead-weight loss is larger if there are positive income effects due to elimination of price rationing, since this increases demand and hence increases the market-clearing time price. Positive income effects from eliminating price rationing are unlikely, however, since by assumption the private insurance system is designed to include universal coverage with copayments inversely related to income. Moreover, since the NHI must be paid for, income effects cannot be positive systemwide.

This analysis suggests that a reasonable middle ground estimate is that the dead-weight loss under time rationing is equal to total expenditures on the rationed services. This is the loss relative to private insurance if private insurers control moral hazard perfectly by managed care. To the extent that private insurers use copayments, or some dead-weight loss remains because of imperfect control of moral hazard, total surplus under private insurance is less than S_0. Copayments on physicians' services under private insurance in the United States are typically 20 percent after a deductible under major medical plans, less in PPO and HMO plans. Copayments also reduce welfare because of lower financial protection, although this is small under plans with a reasonable stop loss. With these adjustments for copayment, a reasonable assumption is that surplus under price and managed-care rationing is $S'_0 = 1/2(D - W)Q_0 + .6Q_0 W_0$, surplus with time rationing S_1 is $1/2(D - W)Q_0$. Thus the loss of surplus under time rationing relative to price and managed-care rationing is $.6W_0Q_0$.

Random Rationing. Random rationing is an alternative to time or money rationing. It does not entail the real resource costs of time rationing. Random rationing, for example, by drawing numbers for a limited number of tickets, is explicitly used in the allocation of tickets for concerts or sporting events. In health care systems that forgo price and informa-tion rationing, personal connections may ensure prompt access or a longer, more careful visit. Connections may be largely random relative to marginal value. Similarly, geographic or interspecialty differences in supply of services relative to demand, due to bureaucratic lags or relative power of different medical specialties in allocating public funds, could imply partially random rationing relative to marginal value.

The effects of random rationing are illustrated in figure 12–A2. As before, assume that with elimination of price and information rationing, the quantity demanded is Q_1, Q_0 units are supplied, and $Q_0 = \alpha Q_1$. Each consumer has a $(1-\alpha)$ chance of receiving services. One representation of random rationing is that the expected value of services to the ith consumer is $(1-\alpha)P^i_m$, where P^i_m is the marginal value or money willingness to pay of the ith consumer. The expected net benefits curve rotates downward to EQ_1, where $E = \alpha D$. The net dead-weight loss from resource misallocation is the trapezoid $EDVT$ (the loss in surplus to inframarginal consumers) minus the triangle TQ_0Q_1, which is the gain to extramarginal consumers who receive a fractional allocation of the services under random rationing, whereas they would have been priced out of the market under price rationing. The opportunity cost of serving extramarginal consumers is the value of the services to the inframarginal consumers.

An alternative representation of random rationing is illustrated by the demand curve DQ_0. The interpretation is that all consumers receive a fraction $\alpha = Q_0/Q_1$ of the total services they would have demanded at that price. The total surplus is ODQ_0. Thus, the loss in surplus is the triangle DVQ_0, which is equal to $1/2W_0Q_0$. This reflects the loss to

FIGURE 12–A2
WELFARE COSTS OF RANDOM RATIONING

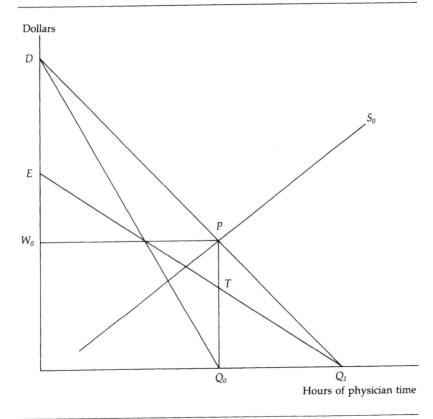

SOURCE: Author.

inframarginal consumers minus the gain to extramarginal consumers who now receive a pro rata allocation. In the case of linear demand, the net welfare loss is the same under these two representations of random rationing, but this need not hold under more general demand assumptions. The loss under random rationing is equal to one-half of total expenditures under price and managed-care rationing and is thus generally less than under time rationing. This is not surprising since random rationing entails no excess time costs. Random rationing is likely to entail a higher resource misallocation cost than time rationing, however, because preferences have some influence under time rationing, but have no effect under random rationing.

Loss in Producer Surplus. The measures of dead-weight loss from time or random rationing discussed so far assume that the hourly wage to physicians remains at W_0 and hence that hours supplied remain at Q_0. If low fee schedules cannot be offset by reduction in cost per visit and increase in visits, because of restrictions on unbundling or expenditure caps, effective hourly wage falls, say to W_1, and hours supplied fall to S_2. The time costs of rationing and the loss in consumer surplus increase, and there is a loss of producer surplus.

A reduction in total physician hours supplied is particularly likely in areas that physicians consider "undesirable." Since fees and monetary incomes cannot rise in these areas to compensate for undesirable amenities, physicians will tend to locate in more desirable areas. Conversely, the influx of physicians to more desirable areas implies that waits will be shorter, visits longer, and more trivial medical conditions will be treated than in less desirable areas. Lindsay et al. (1978) report evidence that the physician-to-population ratio has increased more rapidly in urban areas since the introduction of national health insurance in Canada.[27] This observation is consistent with the prediction that the discrepancy in access to medical care between desirable and undesirable areas increases with uniform fee schedules.

---

27. A similar pattern in the United States can be explained largely by the increase in the ratio of specialists to generalists in the physician population in the United States (Newhouse et al. 1986). This explanation is less plausible in Canada, where the ratio of specialists to GPs is much lower. Fuchs and Hahn (1990) report a ratio of specialists to GPs and FPs of 6.54 for the United States and 1.28 for Canada in 1985. This is later than the period of the Lindsay et al. study, but it is an indication of the general policy of the Canadian government of using both training allocations and fee schedules to discourage specialists.

References

Ballard, C. L., J. B. Shoven and J. Whalley. "General Equilibrium Computations of the Marginal Welfare Costs of Taxes in the U.S." *American Economic Review* 75 (1985): 128–38.

Business Insurance. "Spotlight Report: Self-Insurance." January 28, 1991: 3–14.

Carr, J. and F. Mathewson. "The Effects of Regulation: Incentives and Health Insurance." Institute for Policy Analysis, University of Toronto. Mimeo. 1991.

Citizens Fund. *Premiums without Benefits: Waste and Inefficiency in the Commercial Health Insurance Industry.* Washington D.C., 1990.

Comanor, William S. *National Health Insurance in Ontario: The Effects of a Policy of Cost Control.* Washington, D.C.: American Enterprise Institute, 1980.

Congressional Research Service. "Costs and Effects of Extending Health Insurance Coverage." Report prepared for the House Committee on Education, Labor, and Energy and Commerce and the Senate Special Committee on Aging, 1988.

Danzon, Patricia. "The 'Crisis' in Medical Malpractice: A Comparison of Trends in the U.S., Canada, the U.K. and Australia." *Law, Medicine and Health Care* 18 (1990): 48–58.

———. "The Hidden Costs of Budget-Constrained Health Care Systems." Paper presented at the American Enterprise Institute Conference on Health Policy Reform, Washington, D.C., October, 1991.

Doherty, N. "The Measurement of Output and Economies of Scale in Property Liability Insurance." *Journal of Risk and Insurance* 48 (1981): 390.

Employee Benefit Research Institute (EBRI). *Databook on Employee Benefits.* 1990. Washington, D.C.

Enterline, P., et al. "Effects of 'Free' Medical Care on Medical Practice—the Quebec Experience." *New England Journal of Medicine* 288 (1973): 1152–55.

———. "Physicians' Working Hours and Patients Seen before and after National Health Insurance." *Medical Care* 13 (1975): 95–103.

Evans, R. G. "The Canadian Health Care System: The Other Part of North America Is Rather Different." Paper presented at the International Symposium on Health Care Systems, Taipei, 1989.

Evans, R. G., J. Lomas, M. Barer, R. Labelle, C. Fooks, G. Stoddart, G. Anderson, D. Feeny, A. Gafni, G. Torrance, and W. Tholl. "Controlling Health Expenditures: The Canadian Reality." *New England Journal of Medicine* 320 (1989): 571–77.

Frech, H. E. III, and W. C. Lee. "The Welfare Costs of Rationing by Queuing across Markets: Theory and Estimates from the U.S. Gasoline Crisis." *Quarterly Journal of Economics* 102 (1987): 97–108.

Fuchs, V., and J. Hahn. "How Does Canada Do It? A Comparison of Expenditures for Physicians' Services in the United States and Canada." *New England Journal of Medicine* 323 (1990): 884–90.

Geehan. "Returns to Scale in the Life Insurance Industry." *Bell Journal of Economics* (1977): 497.

Globerman, S., with L. Hoye. "Waiting Your Turn: Hospital Waiting Lists in Canada." Vancouver: Fraser Institute, 1990.

Health Insurance Association of America. "Source Book of Health Insurance Data." Washington D.C., 1989.

Lindsay, C., S. Honda, and B. Zycher. "Canadian National Health Insurance: Lessons for the United States." Roche Laboratories, 1978.

Manning et al. "Health Insurance and the Demand for Medical Care: Evidence from a Randomized Experiment." *American Economic Review* (June 1987): 251–77.

Neuschler, E. *Canadian Health Insurance: The Implications of Public Health Insurance.* Health Insurance Association of America, 1990.

291

Newhouse, J.P., A.P. Williams, B.W. Bennett, and W. B. Schwartz. "Does the Geographical Distribution of Physicians Reflect Market Failure?" *Bell Journal* 13 (Autumn 1982): 493–505.

Office of National Cost Estimates. "National Health Expenditures, 1988." *Health Care Financing Review* 11 (Summer 1990): 1–41.

Pauly, Mark, Patricia Danzon, Paul Feldstein, and John Hoff. "A Plan for Responsible National Health Insurance." *Health Affairs* (Spring 1991): 1–25.

Suen, Wing. "Rationing and Rent Dissipation in the Presence of Heterogeneous Individuals." *Journal of Political Economy* 97 (1989): 1384–94.

U.S. General Accounting Office. "Canadian Health Insurance: Lessons for the United States." GAO/HRD-91-90. Washington, D.C., 1990.

———. "Private Health Insurance: Problems Caused by a Segmented Market." GAO/HRD-91-114. Washington, D.C., 1991.

Woolhandler, S., and D. U. Himmelstein. "The Deteriorating Administrative Efficiency of the U.S. Health Care System." *New England Journal of Medicine* 324 (1991): 1253–58.

Commentary on Part Three

Robert M. Crane

The health care challenge discussed in these chapters reminds me of a story. Two cows are grazing in a pasture. Along a little country road comes a huge milk truck, with large red lettering on its side—pasteurized, homogenized, vitamin D added. One cow stops chewing, looks at the other, and says, "Makes you feel kind of inadequate, doesn't it?"

Although I am not an economist, I will speak from an operations perspective on how health care reform can promote cost containment. I believe that a pluralistic system is preferable to a government-run system. I base this view on points made by other contributors and on substantial personal experiences in both systems, including a stint as the chief regulator in New York state, where I oversaw the operation of an all-payer system that Karen Davis describes. This experience has made me less sanguine than I once was about government's ability to manage this piece of the cost equation.

Competition among prepaid, organized systems of health care that are committed to quality has the best long-run potential to moderate health care costs. Note I did not say managed-care plans. As is pointed out in other chapters, all managed care is not created equal. Managed care is a term that covers diverse plans, some that have good cost-containing features and some that do not.

This view of prepaid organized systems is based on a belief that high-quality care is cost-effective care, that the fee-for-service system is inherently inflationary, and that competition among plans can improve quality and moderate cost. The cost management of these systems comes from their ability, either real or potential, to follow natural incentives to deliver care in the most cost-effective setting. There are systems that can organize care more efficiently and use improvement tools, such as total quality management or continuous quality improvement, to reduce the cost of poor quality, to improve performance, and to make it more cost effective. They can carry out outcomes research to improve the product of health care; using an enrolled population, they can develop explicit evidence about what works and what does not work, leading to clinical guidelines and to more cost-effective care. Finally, large systems can take advantage of size and diversity to innovate, to carry out operations research, and to learn more about clinical effectiveness and better ways of delivering care.

Richard Kronick indicates that effective competition among health plans or systems requires rules. Alain Enthoven is perhaps the leading theoretician on that point of view with his plan, "Managed or Regulated Competition." Plans should compete on the basis of quality of care, service, and price. Plans should be paid for the risks they enroll and not benefit by enrolling only those who do not need or use health care services, as Harold Luft has suggested.

Much of the competition in health care in the United States has been among physicians and hospitals for patients, which has fueled cost increases, rather than among prepaid systems on the basis of quality and service.

How can public policy and other initiatives encourage the development of cost containment and of more organized systems? First, the growth and development of organized or prepaid integrated health care systems could be better encouraged by public policy. The promotion of HMOs in the 1970s and 1980s has been largely replaced by a more neutral and, some would say negative, federal policy. If competition in health care has not occurred in the right way, then setting some basic rules about how it should be carried out will allow better-organized systems to excel. This effort is worth undertaking.

Second, under public programs prepaid, organized systems could be paid at least as much as the fragmented fee-for-service system is. Medicare, for example, is willing to pay prepaid, organized systems only 95 percent as much as the fee-for-service providers. Such a policy has encouraged little growth of those systems in serving the Medicare beneficiary.

The additional payment can be used to add benefits or to finance systems improvement and more aggressive research about clinical effectiveness.

Third, capitation and other prepaid arrangements could be used to organize care effectively across a spectrum of settings. Most of the current proposals—certainly the one built into Karen Davis's chapter—continue paying hospitals out of this bucket and physicians out of that bucket. That method does not encourage either the integration of care or the movement of care from inpatient to outpatient settings; nor does it discourage increased utilization within our current systems. Similar notions can be applied to long-term care, the social HMO, and other settings.

Fourth, individuals could be better rewarded for selecting cost-effective plans than they are now in many multiple-choice settings. Both Alain Enthoven and Mark Pauly propose using the tax system to achieve this goal. Tax benefits could be limited to the cost of the most efficiently run system within a geographic area. That would be difficult under our tax system, but it should be considered.

Fifth, government and employers can use their purchasing power to reward better organization of health care services. Hal Luft and Rick Kronick suggested one such example: a pooled employee model in which a sponsor purchases prudently on behalf of multiple small groups. These rewards can encourage movement down the managed care continuum from managed indemnity to more effective managed care systems such as group and staff model HMOs.

Systems in which physicians are more directly committed to a given health care plan can also be encouraged. So much of our managed care today has physicians participating in almost any plan, without a substantial commitment to the success of that plan. Both the government and private employers can encourage enrollees or employees to join plans in which a majority of the physicians' patients are already enrolled. This step will also deal with plans that are getting an artificial economic advantage by contracting with discounts or contracting at the margin.

These five initiatives can help achieve reform. It is equally important that we recognize that there are a wide variety of providers and that we may not want to treat all of them the same way. We may have to consider regulatory approaches to better structure competition among plans. In the cost-containment debate, there has been too much discussion about overlaying controls on a nonsystem with perverse incentives, and not enough about creating systems that have the kind of incentives we want.

Michael D. Bromberg

Some of the chapters have tried to differentiate between unnecessary, ineffective, or inappropriate care on the one hand and medically necessary services on the other. I reject a regulatory approach to health care because it is obviously incapable of such distinctions and hope to find some other approach that could. I am open to suggestions and can probably support almost any proposal—and there is a growing list of them—that directly addresses ways of eliminating or reducing unnecessary, ineffective, or inappropriate care.

Patricia Danzon's chapter makes a highly innovative and interesting addition to the academic literature. I think policy makers should be especially mindful of Patricia Danzon's counterintuitive bottom line: "Rough numbers suggest that Canada's method of rationing results in hidden costs that are *at least as great as* [emphasis added] the more visible costs . . . [incurred] by private insurers in the United States."

Karen Davis claims in her chapter that "we tried competition in the 1980s and it did not work." As a true believer in the market, however, I would argue that we have never tried competition because we have never tried to make the marketplace for health care a normal one.

In a recent article in the *Atlantic Monthly*, Regina Herzlinger writes,

> Imagine the effect on the automobile industry if American car purchases were insured and employers paid for automobiles. Pretty soon the cars of yesteryear would reappear, loaded with options that people often don't choose when they have to pay for them. The absence of vigilance in the health care system has created the health care equivalent of the 17-foot car—overlarge and numerous hospitals loaded with redundant technology.

My example is different. Suppose tomorrow we had a law that gave us an unlimited, open-ended tax subsidy for food. Does anyone doubt not only that the price and, more important, the volume of food consumed would increase but that we would now be reading proposals for a DRG system for food? It would have to come to that, because we could not afford the rising costs. We ought to try to make a marketplace first before we say it does not work. Without some change in the tax law and a number of other things to remove barriers to competition and cost containment, we have perverse incentives in the health care marketplace: that is the problem.

Regarding David Dranove's chapter on utilization review, I was struck by his comments that cost cutting through utilization review is easy. UR is important, but it is unwise to rely solely on looking for flaws, cracks, and faults retroactively. An army of second-guessers cannot be the only way to find value in health care.

Probably the single most innovative thing that managed care has done is to switch from its early days of reliance on utilization review to selective contracting, which is prechoosing the doctors and hospitals that will provide high-quality care at a competitive price. With a Mayo Clinic model, a Kaiser model, or an innovative type of managed care, the need for utilization review diminishes. UR occurs through a different approach, the selection of a health plan.

Karen Davis's graphs and charts, while accurate, are missing some important data. First, we have no evidence that the Medicare DRG system was the sole or even the primary reason that hospital expenditures have been controlled. I think technology had much to do with it. The shift to outpatient procedures had a lot to do with technology. The critics of DRGs predicted that short-stay admissions to hospitals would increase to maximize profits. That did not happen, probably for a lot of reasons other than the DRGs.

Second, hospital spending in this country as a percentage of GNP has been between 4.1 and 4.3 percent for the past eight years. It has been static, while health care as a percentage of the GNP has gone from 9 to 12.2. I do not understand why she would single us out for a DRG-type system.

Third, there was no mention in the chapter of demand, an issue that must be addressed. The rate-setting data were absolutely accurate but incomplete in the chapter. Rate-setting states have slowed the growth of spending, but the growth of spending still exceeds the national average, especially in the competitive states with a high concentration of HMOs, such as California. We have no evidence that rate setting has worked. It has created in the providers a beat-the-regulator mindset, rather than a be-innovative-with-managed-care mindset. This leads to the last point, which pertains to the increasingly popular argument that rate setting and more innovative delivery systems are compatible. They are not. When one is in a survival mode and gets propped up with a utility rate, why bother taking risk? I have my own definition of what the underlying reasons for costs are and some comments about what I would do about them. First of all, I see six underlying reasons for high costs:

- unrestrained demand, which is a problem of volume
- lack of price competition
- market failure, best illustrated by the small employer insurance debates, state coverage mandates, and state anti–managed-care laws
- the cost shift from inadequate government programs to the private sector
- defensive medicine, including malpractice laws
- lack of medical treatment protocols that can be used to differentiate between necessary and unnecessary care

Of the proposals that address these reasons behind costs, the one I am most wedded to is the tax cap, because I see it as the one with the most immediate short-term effect. But many others would accelerate the managed-care movement and do other desirable things as well.

Incremental reforms, as they are sometimes called, are disparaged by proponents of national health insurance and rate controls. They claim that the problems call for radical, comprehensive reform because we cannot just tinker with these incremental changes.

I am trying to devise a third category called "major incremental reforms," which falls between simple small-employer market reform and the Senate Democrats' HealthAmerica bill. We should remember that Medicare, Medicaid, child care, the Rockefeller Child Commission proposals, and all these other things that have passed or have been proposed are also incremental reforms. We might get much further toward action if we had a little more bipartisan concern for addressing the underlying factors.

All four chapters add to the health care reform debate, but I think we should focus on the differentiation between needed and unneeded services. There are big savings to be made through tax, regulatory, and legal reforms, which collectively create strong incentives to minimize inappropriate care. This approach creates enduring cost containment, and unlike national health insurance plans does not put at risk innovations designed to improve value to the consumer.

H. E. Frech III

I would like to describe two meetings I attended a month apart in 1989. The first meeting, held at the University of Pennsylvania, dealt with cost containment in Medicare. This meeting's ambience can be described only as funereal. People seemed to be saying, "There's no possibility of meaningful reform; copayments aren't going to be able to be raised; we're not going to be able to tax or prohibit the Medigap insurance that's so destructive; we're not going to be able to use HMOs and PPOs." Although the participants expected the resource-based relative value scale would succeed politically, they did not believe it would help.

The next meeting, held at the University of Arizona, was on private managed care. The difference could not have been greater. There was a feeling of excitement—this meeting was upbeat. Clearly, things were going in a very good direction in private health insurance, and new possibilities were opening up day by day. Copayments were increasing everywhere, which is a very good thing. Managed-care combinations of all kinds were being tried and discussed. Participants were explicitly concerned with the tastes and values of different employee groups, referring to the problems of this company versus that company in a very specific way.

This leads to my particular interest: how do we compare single-payer, monopolistic systems with multiple-payer competing systems? First, in some of the chapters there has been confusion of competition at two distinct levels. The first level is competition among insurers to be chosen by a company, by an employer, or, in Richard Kronick's terms, by a sponsor. The second level is competition within the limited menu presented to the employees or group members. We have had too much stress on the second. The more important arena of competition in today's market is for choice by the employer or by the group.

Several authors have claimed that since there is some competition on selection, insurers are not competing on cost containment. This view is very strange. It is like saying that because automakers compete on the styling of their cars, they do not compete on performance. Wouldn't they be competing on both, just as insurers compete on both selection and cost containment?

Another claim made earlier was that independent practice associations (IPAs) do not really compete and thus will be ineffective. This asssertion seems incorrect as a matter of economic theory. Moreover, the empirical work of Harold Luft and comments by Robert O'Brien indicate that some of these IPAs have been very effective. It is interesting to note that IPAs and related preferred provider organizations (PPOs) are the fastest-growing insurers.

Now I want to turn to Patricia Danzon's chapter on the hidden costs of centralized, nonprice rationing. This exciting chapter opens new vistas and contributes to our understanding of nonprice rationing. It outlines the correct conceptual framework for comparing very different health care systems. It also provides a direction for future research into the costs and consequences of different types of nonprice rationing, within both market systems (competing nonprice rationers, like competing HMOs) and centralized, nonprice rationing systems.

Patricia Danzon's message is that the costs of nonmarket, monopoly, single-payer, nonprice rationing are large and well concealed. I agree. This view is apparently shared by policy makers in many countries who are moving away from single-payer monopolistic systems—most radically the Dutch, the New Zealanders, and even the British.

At a more detailed level I find Danzon to be too harsh on medical underwriting and too favorable toward community rating. Mark Pauly's classic demonstration that community rating is inefficient and his argument that it is unfair need more attention.

Insofar as one takes Patricia Danzon's chapter as more than a framework but a comparsion of the actual U.S. with actual Canadian costs, it is important to note that the U.S. system is not an equilibrium. Many changes and innovations are going on. It is a time of great trial and experimentation, as insurers and others grope for ways to manage care that are sensitive to the tastes of providers and especially to the tastes of consumers in a decentralized, competitive setting. If we take a snapshot right now, we would see a system that is not as efficient at rationing as it will be and is not as sensitive to consumers as it will be. The future U.S. system may have far lower administrative and rationing costs. A monopoly single payer has weaker incentives to fine-tune nonprice and price rationing to different tastes and to allow choice. And a monopoly system would have less incentive to avoid imposing red tape on people.

One of Patricia Danzon's insights is that the centrally organized system rations by waiting in a disguised way, in particular by short doctor visits, requiring patients to come back more often. This is a brilliant idea: the system forces rationing by waiting, but no one sees people waiting very much. What clears the market is that patients make extra trips. Superficially, this looks like reasonable, productive behavior, but it is really not so.

To the extent that single-payer systems use rationing by waiting, one can refer to some simple models developed by Barzel (1974), by Deacon and Sonstelie (1991), and by Bill Lee and me (1987) to get estimates of the magnitudes of the losses. The welfare losses are large. And to the extent that rationing is done by these short but frequent visits, the losses are hidden very nicely.

In sum, Patricia Danzon has produced a chapter that provides an excellent framework for understanding and comparing centralized single-payer systems with decentralized, market-oriented ones.

Karen Davis's chapter supports the single-payer approach: particularly the resource-based relative value scale. This enthusiasm is far from universal among economists. Several authors in a recent AEI book, including Mark Pauly and Joseph Newhouse, stress that a resource-based relative value scale can cause volume to go either up or down. It may lead to more primary care, less surgery, or the opposite. The proponents of this system believe that somehow it will lead to more primary care, which they think is good, and to less surgery, which they think is bad. In addition, the limits on balance billing, which are very strict, are likely to cause access problems and disguised nonprice rationing. After Patricia Danzon's chapter we should be sensitive to these problems.

I want to mention briefly the idea of the expenditure targets, where the government reduces the payment to the physicians based on what their expenditure growth is. This is not a new idea. In a rough and ready way, the history of Medicare for the past ten years can be interpreted as an expenditure target policy. Because expenditures went up fast, Medicare froze fees, not allowing the full usual, customary, and reasonable updates. In fact, Medicare drifted away from the UCR system a long time ago. This approach in the past has been a complete failure. It has also been tried in Medicaid, variously by different states. Most states have held physician prices very low, causing tremendous access problems.

Karen Davis's chapter also claims that if there is one payer, no one is rationed out or squeezed out, and there is no access problem. This is a misunderstanding. If there is only one payer and that payer restricts prices enough to cause nonprice rationing, everyone gets squeezed out. We cannot point to one group, for example, those on Medicaid or

Medicare, and declare they were squeezed out and that others were not: everyone gets squeezed out. The main effect of squeezing out everyone is to hide the nonprice rationing. This is particularly true if the controls are tightened gradually as in Canada.

Let us consider the long sweep of history of Medicare expenditures. As Karen Davis noted, Medicare's record in the past few years in slowing the growth of dollar expenditures is good, but over the long sweep, Medicare's cost-containment record is the worst in the United States. Medicare is hardly a good model for a new system. In this connection, Karen Davis claims that market reforms have not worked. I would disagree. There is a lot of evidence that large savings are available from health maintenance organizations, preferred provider organizations, copayment, and even the simplest kind of utilization review. These are not merely one-time savings. Burton Weisbrod has recently argued that tightening insurance reimbursement has already changed the direction of research, development, and innovation. One would expect this trend to continue.

Regarding Jack Meyer's chapter, I wish to stress the impediments to progressive insurance innovations. In the past, the main impediment has been organized medicine and hospitals, often in collusion with Blue Cross–Blue Shield. Over the years, as Blue Cross–Blue Shield has become weaker and antitrust has weakened organized medicine, provider opposition has greatly declined. That decline explains why we are getting the aggressive managed care now that we did not twenty years ago. Apparently, however, physicians and hospital interest groups have succeeded alarmingly well in getting all kinds of anticompetitive, anti–managed-care state laws. Examples include mandated benefits and constraints on cost-sharing incentives for preferred provider organizations. These state rules are a very serious problem. Like others, Jack Meyer seems to be overly concerned with avoiding experience rating and to think too favorably of community rating.

Last, I want to turn to David Dranove's chapter, which is the most narrowly focused one. It highlights the difficulty of tailoring utilization review to consumers' tastes. I believe David Dranove underrates moral hazard. The RAND experiment showed a large difference between 100 percent insurance and a little bit of copayment (Manning et al. 1987). It is important to remember that despite recent progress, there are still many people in this country with essentially 100 percent coverage. Most people in Medicare with Medigap insurance have 100 percent, first-dollar coverage, as do most people with Medicaid and many with Blue Cross–Blue Shield coverage, especially in the Northeast. The Rand study also ignored the norms effect: changing the copayment systemwide would have a greater effect than the study showed.

On this point, I agree completely with Karen Davis. There is a strong presumption that health care in the United States is overdone greatly in quantity and quality, at least for middle-class people with insurance. We have, then, a big margin for utilization review—even of a fairly crude kind—to improve things. (And some of the early managed-care efforts are quite crude.) And finally, tying into the main theme, David Dranove notes that the incentive and information problems with utilization review apply more strongly to a centralized monopoly system without strong incentives to be sensitive to consumer tastes.

In summary, single-payer systems can reduce dollar outlays if their nonprice rationing is strict enough. But there are many other hidden costs borne by consumers and providers. The mere ability of single-payer systems to reduce dollar outlays does not mean they are good for us.

References

Barzel, Yoram. "A Theory of Rationing by Waiting." *Journal of Law and Economics* 17 (April 1974): 73–96.

Deacon, Robert T., and Jon Sonstelie. "Price Controls and Rent Dissipation with Endogenous Transactions Costs." *American Economic Review* 81 (December 1991): 1361–73.

Frech, H.E. III, and William C. Lee. "The Welfare Cost of Rationing-by-Queueing: Theory and Estimates from the U.S. Gasoline Crises." *Quarterly Journal of Economics* 102 (February 1987): 97–108.

Manning, Willard G., Joseph P. Newhouse, Naihua Duan, Emmit B. Keeler, Arleen Leibowitz, and M. Susan Marquis. "Health Insurance and the Demand for Medical Care: Evidence from a Randomized Experiment." *American Economic Review* 77 (June 1987): 251–77.

Containing Health Care Costs

Discussion of Part Three

ROGER FELDMAN, University of Minnesota: Patricia Danzon, since the private health insurance industry in this country is subsidized to the tune of 25 to 33 percent by the tax system and the tax system involves a 17 percent dead-weight cost, wouldn't you want to add that as a cost on the U.S. side of the ledger? In other words, haven't we imported some of the evils of the Canadian system?

PATRICIA M. DANZON, Wharton School, University of Pennsylvania: Yes. Mine was not by any means a comprehensive calculation of all the dead-weight losses in both systems. I said in my chapter that I would like to compare the dead-weight losses of a Canadian public monopoly system with a well-designed private insurance system, which I assume would not include the tax subsidy. But I emphasized the excessive costs related to administration that are induced by the tax subsidy. What you are saying is that I may have underemphasized those costs. Your point is well-taken.

C. EUGENE STEUERLE, Urban Institute: My first question is to Michael Bromberg. Didn't you go a little too far when you argued that the main way we could save on cost is to eliminate unneeded care? I wonder if that approach doesn't ignore the typical case where we do have positive benefits from care but the benefits are not in excess of the cost. This seems to me to be one of our major problems.

MICHAEL D. BROMBERG, Federation of American Health Systems: I do not think we are ready for the next step of that discussion yet. Even if we had no budget deficit, we still should get rid of ineffective, inappropriate care and seek better value. Even with a budget deficit, though, I do not think that we have reached the limit of our resources. It is ironic to me that the states that are talking about such coverage decisions are states with either a budget surplus, no income tax, or no sales tax—they just want better value.

So, in my view, there is not much on the present political agenda beyond eliminating unnecessary care. The politicians are ready for it because no bill in Congress really gets to the coverage issue. The country is not ready for it yet, and the public opinion polls show that.

MR. STEUERLE: My second question is to Karen Davis. If we suppose that we really had the ability to determine what percentage of GNP to spend on health care and that about one or two percentage points of GNP represent inefficient care, then we might be able to agree that we would not want the percentage of GNP spent today to be any greater than it is already. What happens when the system is thirty or forty years old? What mechanism is there to determine the value of the health care we have and what percentage of GNP we really want to spend on it?

KAREN DAVIS, Commonwealth Fund: For the percentage of GNP, the Rostenkowski proposal gives some sense of how it would work. First of all, it slows the growth in health spending gradually to about the year 2000, by which time we will probably be at about 15 percent of GNP. So that proposal does not hold the line at today's percentage of GNP. We are not talking about 5 percent of GNP. We are not talking about the United Kingdom. We are not talking about rationing, long waits, and the like. We are talking about spending probably more than we are now but really trying to slow the growth over time.

Obviously, in our system it is a political determination of whether society chooses to put more resources into health over time. One can hold it at 15 percent of GNP for 30 years or decide annually to have more health care and less in the way of automobiles, VCRs, or whatever we are buying in the private sector. Or we can decide to have 14 percent of GNP in health care and more education or other goods. It becomes a political determination of what share of the nation's resources we wish to devote to health care. We make those decisions politically and incrementally by sensing what we can gain by devoting more of our resources to education, health, or whatever. So if we have technological change, if there are costly life-saving benefits, one can make those determinations on a collective basis, not necessarily on an individual market basis.

MARK V. PAULY, Wharton School, University of Pennsylvania: At the risk of being accused of piling on, I have two additional hidden costs of the Canadian system. Imagine that there is no rationing. Imagine that when a Canadian calls for an appointment, he is immediately scheduled and there is no waste. Still, a feature of the Canadian system is that everybody gets the same coverage and the same form of cost containment subject to the same budgetary rules in the hospital. If you want to spend less than the Canadians spend on you and you are a Canadian, you cannot do that, at least you will not save any money by doing it. And if you want to spend more than the system will spend, you are not allowed to do so. So to the extent that people have different preferences as to how they want their health care delivered, the enforced uniformity of that system imposes a cost.

And I suppose the Canadians realize that. They do not have a national health care system, but a provincial one, and each province does it differently. Quebec is certainly different from British Columbia, and nobody knows about Newfoundland.

The other hidden cost is one I will illustrate with a somewhat tongue-in-cheek proposal. Let us reduce costs by limiting the rate of growth in wages for nurses and other professional hospital employees. That, after all, is where the money is spent. Employee compensation is the largest share of health care expenditures and the part that has been increasing the most rapidly in the past few years. Why not do it that way if our objective is to reduce costs? Alternatively, we could control the income of physicians instead, because they earn more money and act superior anyway.

The more fundamental point is, if we reduce our share of health care expenditures as a percentage of GNP by reducing wages to nurses or, for that matter, payments to doctors, we have not really reduced health care costs in the economic sense, which is the only real sense that matters. Where cost means the amount of other goods and services that are not available to people in the economy, all we have done is to redistribute those goods and services.

If we are talking about share of GNP and its aggregate macroeconomic consequences, we should not be measuring it as expenditures. We should be measuring it as real opportunity cost, which means that we should take out "monopoly rents"—economic jargon for money a person gets that he does not really deserve—to calculate the real cost of health care. Otherwise, as Victor Fuchs has shown, the reason the Canadians spend less on doctors' services than we do is that they pay their doctors 20 percent less: doctors do not cost anything less than they do here; they just do not do as well relative to the rest of us.

If we continue to be obsessed by health care costs, my plea is that we at least be obsessed by the right sort of bogeyman.

WARREN GREENBERG, George Washington University: I think Patricia Danzon's chapter is very interesting and very welcome. But I would like to emphasize that Patricia Danzon was just comparing the administrative costs of the Canadian system with the administrative cost and overhead in the U.S. system.

305

That, of course, is only half the story . What are the benefits inherent in both systems? I think the benefits in the United States derive from the innovation in choice of plans that Mark Pauly identified and perhaps the diversity of utilization review techniques discussed by David Dranove.

In reference to David Dranove's chapter, what is the role of utilization review when costs are greater than zero but nevertheless we still have some benefits? Here is where I think we have an economic problem.

DAVID DRANOVE, Kellogg Graduate School of Management, Northwestern University: I agree with you. My intention in the chapter was to review who was comparing the full benefits and the full costs. What is interesting in practice is that utilization review agencies are essentially ignoring costs. The hospital service will either help the patient or not help the patient. If an agency cannot find evidence that the service will help the patient, it refuses it. If the agency finds some reason to believe it will help the patient, it approves the treatment, without regard to costs.

WILLIAM J. DENNIS, JR., NFIB Foundation: Jack Meyer, what do you think is the appropriate role for the consumer or patient in controlling costs? I get the distinct impression that the only alternative we have before us in the discussion so far is whether we use a large public bureaucracy or whether we use a large private bureaucracy. Are those the only alternatives?

JACK A. MEYER, New Directions for Policy: I think that patients have two major responsibilities. First is to behave in a socially responsible way and stop contributing to the destruction of their own bodies. This point rarely comes up in discussions about health care. We are all human and do not have to be perfect, but I think that it is up to society to reward healthy behavior through incentives and to penalize poor behavior.

Second, patients have a responsibility to try to choose health plans responsibly. We have made it very difficult for them to distinguish between the health plan that does a good job of managing resources and controlling costs and one that does not. In fact, I would argue that we have actually made it in their interest to take the higher-cost plan. Although we have not given patients much incentive to be responsible in either of those two ways, we could change that.

That is why I agree with Ted Frech, if I understood his point correctly. The more important choice that businesses make is in managing the selection of the health care plan, as opposed to trying to reduce costs once the employees are in it. While I believe that cost sharing is beneficial, I do not think we should try to operate on the consumer by raising cost sharing through the ceiling to the point where consumers give up necessary and valuable services. Cost sharing has a role, but it should be kept within limits. The consumer should be brought more into the picture, but not just by paying more of the total cost.

HAROLD S. LUFT, University of California, San Francisco: I would encourage Patricia Danzon to include in her analysis some of the administrative costs in the United States so that she is not comparing Canada with an ideal United States, but Canada with the real United States. Part of the concern that I hear from physicians and hospitals is the enormous number of different claims they must deal with. The paperwork is very complex—it is a little bit like having a MasterCard and Visa system where each retailer has to send each chit to a different bank rather than to a single clearinghouse. The time that patients spend filling out reimbursement forms is a major exercise, at least when I have done it. The fact that experience-rating drives many people, particularly in the small employer market, to change insurance among carriers offering nearly identical products is probably a dead-weight loss. It is not clear that we are gaining much from these changes. Having some copayments, having a reasonable number of providers to offer choices, and sensitivity to the market are major gains, but I think we can certainly do better than what we have without imitating Canada.

MS. DANZON: My point about patient time costs and physician billing costs was that in a competitive private insurance market private insurers have an incentive to take into account the costs they are imposing on patients. When patients choose among alternative plans, they are less likely to choose a plan—other things equal—that imposes a lot of billing hassles. They are less likely to choose a plan that entails—other things equal—long waits for visits. Therefore, when consumers choose among plans, they are taking into account the hassle factors as well as the cost of the plan and the expected quality and so forth. Private insurers have an incentive to take those costs into account, while a public insurer does not, if it is a monopoly.

The same thing applies on the provider side. When a private insurer establishes a new plan that imposes hassle costs, billing costs, or risks on physicians or hospitals, that insurer will have to take those into account. Whether physicians or hospitals will be willing to sign up with this plan would depend on their total reimbursement and on the hassle costs.

Therefore, in a well-functioning private market, those costs imposed on providers and patients are internalized to the private insurer through the price that the consumer is willing to pay for the insurance plan or the price that the provider would charge as a condition of participating.

Things are distorted by the tax subsidy, by ERISA, and the incentive to self-insure, which I do believe creates a basis for too many different plans. In competitive private markets, those costs are internalized to the companies designing the insurance plans. In a monopoly, as with a public insurer, there is no incentive to take into account the costs imposed on patients or on providers.

JERRY WINKER, Abbott Laboratories: Mark Pauly mentioned that in Canada and the United States we rarely hear about Newfoundland's experiment. I would argue that we rarely hear about Hawaii's experimental approach to addressing the issue of the uninsured. Why is there so little research on Hawaii's system?

MS. DAVIS: Hawaii has had a mandated employer-provided health plan since 1974, when employers were required to cover the worker but not necessarily the dependents, although 90 percent of employers have voluntarily covered dependents. In 1989 Hawaii enacted a state health insurance plan that covered the remaining uninsured under a state-subsidized but privately provided health plan.

An evaluation of that plan is under way by Kaiser Permanente's research staff in Portland. I have been on the advisory committee, and it seems to have been a very successful system, certainly when we consider the economic effects of employer mandates. Hawaii has very low unemployment, and small businesses thrive despite the mandates. Kaiser Permanente is obviously a major option under employer plans as well as under this new state gap-filling health insurance plan. Hawaii has managed to provide universal coverage without major economic disruptions.

It is a model well adapted for the United States, with copayments and a mixture of fee-for-service and capitated providers. I think it is a very interesting model to use.

RICHARD KRONICK, University of California, San Diego: Hawaii's experiment could be instructive in that the small employer has not been forced out of business, one of the concerns raised in the other forty-nine states.

MR. GREENBERG: I was intrigued by Patricia Danzon's observation that a lot more insurance firms were in the marketplace than would be dictated by competition alone, a situation perhaps due to ERISA exemptions. I would also like to suggest that the health insurance industry has something in common with the baseball industry—they both have antitrust exemptions. This loophole allows insurers to join together to look at data and to collude. Small insurers have taken advantage of this exemption and perhaps this is one reason they remain in the marketplace. Otherwise, they would drop out. Perhaps it would be a good idea to examine the McCarran-Ferguson antitrust exemption very closely.

MS. DANZON: Although the McCarran-Ferguson Act does give the insurance industry antitrust immunity, with the ease of entry into insurance, especially through self-insurance, I do not have much concern about collusion.

MR. PAULY: I thought we agreed earlier that it would be good for insurers to collude in the sense of exchanging information on quality providers and so forth. Antitrust laws cut both ways.

MR. MEYER: To return to Mike Bromberg's point, I agree that we have not really tried to create an efficient market. While there is more we could do to create a more efficient health insurance marketplace, still, health care costs are really driven by the explosion of new technology and procedures. We come back to a point Gene Steuerle made earlier: a lot of care does not have zero benefits, and we are learning how to do more medically every day.

For illustration, let's consider two examples, one of routine care and another of more heroic intervention in end-of-life situations. First, the person that comes into a doctor's office with a headache may face only one chance in a thousand that the headache is really an indication of something serious. But, there is every incentive in the current system to perform a brain scan on that person. The incentive to scan that person would remain even if we tinker with the financing system and do better utilization reviews. Our expectations demand them.

The second example involves restarting the heart of a ninety-four-year-old person for the tenth time who we know has only a few weeks at most to live. What should we do? We are making this sort of decision every day. And we seem to want that. We will face more such situations in the future. The aging of the population has not contributed much to health care cost explosion so far.

While I am in favor of reorganizing the way health care is financed and trying to get efficiencies, I think a lot of those efficiencies will lead to one-time savings. But in the long run, we will have to look at whether we want all the fruits of our innovation and who gets them and under what circumstances.

CLARK C. HAVIGHURST, Duke University: The fact is that consumers might be ready, if they were given choices, with price tags attached, to consider giving up some of those marginally beneficial things that Jack Meyer mentioned. The potential savings are very large, but we do not have the tools to realize those savings because consumers are not in a position to agree to limit many of their entitlements under a health plan or to modify their right to sue their doctor by substituting some alternative standard of care for the prevailing professional one.

As some have said, utilization review is essentially an attempt to apply the standard of care that medical professionals agree is appropriate. But those are not the people we should be asking. It is what the consumer wants in the way of care that ought to matter. As things now stand, the consumer cannot authorize the provider to do less than the professional standard demands. He does not have the ability to authorize the payer not to pay for anything that the law deems medically necessary.

Perhaps I am here ten years ahead of my time. Sooner or later, as Jack Meyer says, this issue of allowing aggressive economizing will be before us, and maybe in ten years we will finally be ready to talk about it seriously. But I am disappointed that there is not more urgency about getting on with this now. We do not need an act of Congress to do it, only the willingness of the insurance industry to start offering contracts and litigating their validity. Insurers can start contracting with the providers for a different standard of care, which then becomes a protection in a malpractice suit.

Private payers could begin today to do some exciting things that are both radical and incremental. The traditional vehicle of private contract could give consumers options they never had before. I do not see why people should quarrel with that. If we prepare carefully and well, design our litigation strategy, and educate everyone from judges to consumers, we could make some impressive progress. If all we are trying to do is curtail so-called inappropriate care, however, we are coming close to exhausting our cost-containment possibilities.

MR. FELDMAN: My comment touches on the all-payer proposals discussed by Karen Davis. I do not understand the wisdom of prohibiting price competition. Wouldn't such limits seriously inhibit, possibly destroy the growth of, new and more efficient delivery systems such as HMOs and PPOs? What about a health care plan that develops a better product and wishes to offer that to consumers? Why shouldn't it be allowed to offer a lower price as well as quality or combination of services that consumers want?

That idea is particularly apropos to a city like Minneapolis, where about 40 to 50 percent of the population belongs to HMOs. It is also relevant to the Medicare HMO program. Some of my calculations indicate that about 40 percent of the people covered under that program are enrolled in HMOs that would like to give them a price discount but are prohibited from doing so by federal regulations. Along the same line, Karen Davis's distinction between the all-payer system and international competitive pressure is off base, because in the 1980s foreign producers competed with us very successfully over price and quality.

Ms. DAVIS: Certainly, in my plan, HMOs would be offered as choices to people, whether they are in a public plan like Medicare or in any private plan. Capitated systems could operate side by side, attracting people to enroll. Nothing in what I am talking about would prohibit HMOs from being offered. My proposal would prohibit PPOs from being able to get price-discriminatory advantages. PPOs would have to compete on the basis of better utilization review, not on their ability as a volume buyer to get a better price.

As for the failure of the existing Medicare program to give incentives to beneficiaries to enroll in HMOs, under present law the HMO is required to give the beneficiary any difference between the price that Medicare pays and their price for other business for similarly age-adjusted patients. HMOs are required to plow back to beneficiaries anything above a normal profit in the form of improved benefits or reduced premiums.

MR. FELDMAN: I am referring to the 40 percent of the Medicare HMO beneficiaries who are enrolled in plans that charge no supplementary premium at all. These plans could profitably enroll more people by giving them a premium rebate—that is, giving back part of the government's Adjusted Average Per Capita Cost (AAPCC) payment, but are prohibited from doing so.

MR. DRANOVE: The chief benefit of competition is not to lower the prices that consumers are paying. Indeed, the government has shown that it is very capable of lowering the prices that providers receive. Nor is the chief benefit of competition that consumers can match themselves to the lowest-price providers. Nobel Prizes have been won for demonstrating that the chief benefit of competition is that it promotes innovation. Those who are innovative are able to steal customers away from those who are not, and I think that was Roger Feldman's point. The innovation could take the form of providing insurance, combining insurance and provision of care within the same organization, or, very simply, generating innovations in hospitals that introduce continuous quality improvements to maintain quality at lower cost. If we reduce or eliminate profit incentives, we reduce the long-run opportunity for the single most important benefit of competition.

H. E. FRECH III, University of California, Santa Barbara: In reference to Clark Havighurst's comments, I strongly agree that we should widen the ability of American consumers to contract out of the current legal standard of care. In fact, I think it is a much broader point than medical care but one that applies to the whole tort system, among other things.

But in looking for a formalistic legal contract, Clark Havighurst overlooks the fact that, to a large extent, new standards are already being institutionalized through utilization review and HMOs. When someone signs up with an HMO, he really signs up for a different standard of care. he is much less likely to go to the hospital for the same problem; he is less likely to see the same doctor for a complaint. Thus, to a large and growing extent, the standard of care is changing even without a formal contractual protection.

MR. HAVIGHURST: I see built-in limits to what we can achieve through the HMO, precisely because when a case goes to court, the standard of care applied is the one drawn from fee-for-service practice. So far no HMO has had the courage to write into a contract that it wants to be bound by a different standard. In my chapter I included a draft clause that an HMO might use to try to get out from under this professional standard of resource use. It does not go nearly as far as relying on practice guidelines to specify more particularly what the organization is committing to.

But it is an interesting empirical question, How much is possible under the present system? There is no doubt that a slightly different style of care has emerged, but HMOs remain pretty conventional. I think that proves the limitations of changing standards without being explicit in a contract. HMOs have probably almost exhausted the possibilities of doing it tacitly.

I think it is more legitimate to specify standards in writing than not. But most people seem comfortable with HMOs precisely because they do not acknowledge in writing that their doctors might act differently from the way the profession would dictate. It seems to me we ought to take the next step.

MR. KRONICK: Ted Frech and I have not agreed on much, but we do agree on this point. I do not see how one can successfully specify conditions explicitly while there are still so many uncertainties, so much art, and so little science in medicine today.

MR. HAVIGHURST: We can only do what we can do, but it seems to me we ought to do more exploring.

312

MR. FELDMAN: Let me add a note of empiricism. Although I do not have the exact numbers, in California, Kaiser's Caesarian section rate is just slightly above the public hospitals', around 12 percent. The rate for voluntary and for-profit hospitals is around 20 percent. Kaiser has obviously been able to maintain this lower rate over a long time. A mandatory arbitration clause is contained in the contracts, but I do not think it keeps anyone from suing. But there is an understanding that this is a standard of care, and it is acceptable. Kaiser is probably successful in holding to this standard by monitoring women more carefully. And there is no evidence that the outcomes are any worse.

We have examples showing that HMOs, big and very visible ones, are able to design a different style of care, maintain the same outcomes, and still avoid the malpractice attorneys, who are well-represented in California.

STEPHEN ZUCKERMAN, Urban Institute: I will sound a somewhat pessimistic note about the market approaches for cost containment. Moving toward contracts for different standards of care is far beyond where people have gone so far. Insurers and employers are now trying to introduce products with alternative payment structures, if employees are willing to accept restrictions on the choice of provider.

What we observe in the insurance market, though, is that employees resist restrictions on choice. The plan has to leave in the double and triple options so that the fee-for-service sector stays in play. I think this happens because of a biased selection on the provider's side by PPOs—a random cross-section of physicians within a market area does not agree to give these discounts.

Until consumers really give up the fee-for-service sector, we will not see a great movement toward alternatives. And without the willingness of consumers to change, market competition will not be a very effective cost-containment mechanism.

ROBERT M. CRANE, Kaiser Permanente: I am concerned about Ted Frech's comment on a different level of care in HMOs. There certainly is a different style, as Hal Luft has pointed out. But one could argue—and there is evidence—that patients receive a higher level of care in many HMOs because the care is better organized.

The real focus should be on outcomes. One of the things that Kaiser Permanente has been successful in doing is avoiding Caesarean sections even when one was done on a previous birth. Costs are lower, mothers have been happier, and the quality of care is higher.

On the subject of experimentation around limitations, most health insurance and HMO contracts do contain limitations. These have been very difficult to uphold in court. An obvious limitation is to exclude clearly experimental care. When faced with that issue, courts have ruled that the care must be provided if the experimental procedure is the only way to prevent a premature death.

While I think Clark Havighurst has an interesting idea, it is also important to underscore that it would constitute a significant educational task on all fronts, not least in the judicial system.

MR. BROMBERG: The major difference between the delivery system of the United States and that of other countries is the ratio of specialists to general practitioners. A study of when and where people move outside their managed-care networks and pay out of pocket for health care would be instructive. I am sure it is to see specialists.

I think the way to make managed-care attractive to middle-class, upper-middle-class, and upper-income people would be this point-of-service option, the ability to go to specialists when something really serious happens. Limitations on such consultations are unacceptable to many people.

My outside-the-beltway example is Oregon again. The debate on insurance coverage started years ago over two transplants, a single mother followed by a little boy that needed a liver transplant. One of them died. There was lengthy television coverage, along with private fund raising. I predict that the Oregon plan, whatever happens to it, waived or not waived, will bring us back to the same debate: the media attention will focus on the care denied.

I do not argue that the subject should not be opened up, but it should not be tacked on to the issue of competition and managed care. Such rationing has got to be a government decision on coverage, on technology assessment, and many other things that should not interfere in the debate over competition versus regulation. Those decisions will have to be made, whichever way we go.

PART FOUR

What Are the Choices among Policies to Achieve Reform?

13

Why Is Health Care So Hard to Reform?

Mark V. Pauly

Health care reform has two parts: universal coverage and cost control. Dissatisfaction with the mixed public and private system used in the United States has been commonplace for more than twenty years, and yet the structure of Medicare, Medicaid, and private insurance has changed amazingly little since passage of the two public programs in 1965. Perhaps even more surprisingly, years of debate about national health insurance have produced virtually no action. This essay explores some possible reasons for this inaction. Much of the discussion is an exercise in positive political economy, intended to explain why the 1965 policy equilibrium has proved so durable—even in the face of truly spectacular changes in relative prices, a substantial growth in real income, and a nontrivial shift in the demographic composition of the population. Why has the political demand apparently been unaffected by changes in prices, incomes, demographies, technology, tastes, or any other of the determinants usually invoked to explain why any person or group changes anything?

The normative null hypothesis is that health care reform is not desirable, that the current situation cannot be altered without doing more harm than good to everyone (or almost everyone). I offer some reasons for rejecting this hypothesis, and proposing that, on balance, some desirable changes can be made in the U.S. health care system. Here I interpret "desirable" in the literal economic sense of providing more benefit than cost.

A change (desirable or undesirable) might not happen for three reasons. The first reason is basically distributional: even if benefits exceed costs, perhaps no available method can distribute the net benefits over enough politically decisive people or groups. The second reason relates to program design: design might actually reap the excess of benefits over costs. The third reason relates to the design of the political control system:

voters may feel that once a program is enacted, they may not be able to control how politicians and bureaucrats guide and administer it. I argue that all three of these influences, and especially the third one, have been operating in the United States for the past twenty-five years. The main point of this chapter, then, is to suggest ways of solving these problems.

These reasons concern fundamental questions about objectives, institutional structures, and outcomes. Some less fundamental but still important elements of the discussion of health care reform have also inhibited action. Perhaps the most critical of these impediments has been the lack of distinction, in the political process, between two classes of issues: between ends and means and between desires and achievable reality. I therefore comment on these issues at the outset.

What Is Feasible?

Even to begin to discuss health care reform, we need to avoid some fallacies that often arise and serve to confuse the debate. Two are critical for the following discussion.

1. *Health care costs can be cut or growth reduced without sacrificing anything.* A favorite political slogan is to offer the prospect of holding the line on cost, insurance premiums, or taxes with a simple strategy: just increase efficiency. Here efficiency is interpreted in its common-man sense of figuring out a way to provide exactly the same benefits (or even more) for less money. Concrete steps to pull off this magic usually involve invoking incantations replete with tautologies: we will save money by eliminating "unnecessary surgery," "useless empty hospital beds," or "excessive tests."

One may wish that substantial cuts in the level or rate of growth of cost could be made by eliminating waste. Experts differ on how much waste exists, but no expert has yet proposed a system to eliminate only waste.

2. *Equity demands that every American get the highest possible quality of care.* This is the familiar argument against "two-class" medicine. Undoubtedly we feel uncomfortable limiting anyone's access to effective care, even if the effect is small and the cost large. The Capron commission (The President's Commission for the Study of Ethical Problems in Medicine) was quite explicit in arguing that our public goal is *not* the provision to everyone of the most (effective) care that anyone in society chooses to buy (President's Commission 1983). Instead, the objective is to provide a minimum level of adequate care and insurance, to bring up the bottom of the distribution of use and coverage.

The Efficiency Argument

Because people are heterogeneous, no one insurance scheme is right for everyone. Heterogeneity (at a given set of prices) comes from two sources: differences in income or wealth and differences in taste or value placed on health, hassle, and other goods and services.

We are to a considerable extent schizophrenic when dealing with wealth or income and its relationship to medical care use. After-tax distribution of income in the United States contains a significant amount of inequality. Even more inequality would arise in an unrestricted market; the net effect of taxes and transfers surely evens things considerably, especially in bringing up the levels of consumption (relative to income earned or generated by wealth) of those at the bottom of the income distribution.

Two observations on American attitudes toward this distribution are apparent. First, we do not have unanimous, or anything like unanimous, agreement that this distribution is the most desirable or most pleasing one. Attitudes are rough proxies for political leanings, with Democrats tending to profess favor of more redistribution and Republicans not eager to do so, although the compartments are by no means watertight. Second, we nevertheless do not appear to have a political choice to change the distribution of wealth drastically. That is, while many people surely desire a different amount of redistribution, no subset of the electorate is large enough, given our political rules, to bring about a change. The kinds of recent patterns of distribution appear to represent more unintended consequences of the pursuit of other political objectives, and consequences of exogenous shifts in the structure of the economy, than explicit political choices.

Basically our current income distribution seems a political equilibrium—one that "we" have chosen, given the constitutional rules and procedures that we have selected for making such choices. A perfectly predictable consequence of an unequal distribution of command over resources is an unequal distribution of the consumption that those resources make possible. Further, medical services as well may be distributed unequally. Now the split personality: how can we say that we are unhappy with the distribution of medical care consumption in this country if it is caused by a distribution of income and wealth that we are, at a minimum, willing to accept as tolerable? Those who favor more redistribution of resources for the well-being of the poor would doubtless favor a health care reform that gave care or insurance free or at a reduced price to the poor. But what of those who are indifferent about the distribution of income? Shouldn't they also be indifferent about the distribution of medical care?

Such internal conflict could be resolved by suggesting that people care more about the distribution of some types of consumption than others; they care less about inequity in the consumption of entertainment, recreational travel, or books than of care. We cannot prove this, nor can we offer strong, objective reasons why some types of consumption mean more than others, but we do seem to see, introspectively, that medical care is different in this regard. Economists usually couch these motivations in the language of "altruistic externalities" (Pauly 1971); these provide the economic rationale for the "bring up the bottom" approach discussed earlier. But this approach still allows some substantial inequality in the use of and spending on medical services in a good society. We may feel uncomfortable about the inequality in use between politician and pauper, or between manager and mendicant, even when we help the poor somewhat, but we do not seem disposed to do anything about it. These observations imply that variations in the level of medical care consumption, in the degree of hassle or choice associated with the process of care, and even in final health outcomes are to be encouraged by an efficient medical care delivery system. I do not mean to imply that we ought somehow to encourage inequality; I mean only that we ought to value removal of obstacles to a person's ability to spend income on health care and health insurance as individually decided, even if that choice differs from other citizens'.

The other basis for efficiency of markets arises from variations in taste. If people do place different values on health (and they do), if they place different values on their ability to choose and to switch providers, if they place different values on the presence or absence of hassle in the process of care or care management, they will want to choose different kinds of providers, different amounts of insurance, and different kinds of insurance plans.

Both differences carry a clear message for insurance proposals that involve government's mandating the purchase of a single type of insurance at the market price: the greater the diversity in income or tastes, the less likely such a single coverage plan will be acceptable (Pauly et al. 1991). Indeed, one explanation for the lack of appeal to Americans of uniform national health insurance—a skittishness that appears strange to European commentators—is that, compared with a typical, more homogeneous country of Western Europe, the heterogeneous United States is less well suited to such a policy. The reason is not necessarily a lack of concern for the poor, or even greater skepticism about government management, but rather the realization by the American middle class that a one-size-fits-all insurance policy will not fit all of them. That is, not only do people have different attitudes toward government, as Fuchs (1976) noted; different people *do* potentially have different demands for government-supplied goods.

Complexities increase if the insurance is to be tax-financed; unless a head tax is used, ordinarily people with higher incomes will pay more than others for the same thing. Their higher incomes may make them want more lavish insurance coverage, but the rising tax price may dampen this demand. Dumb luck could lead to a pattern of perfect offsets, so that with the current tax structure everyone would want the same middle-of-the road insurance. But even this scene of amity would be upset by enough variation in tastes (Usher 1977); government, inherently driven toward the uniform level, does not respond properly to people's diverse preferences.

Some empirical facts that could be gathered here could greatly help the debate. Specifically, how diverse are demands for insurance quantity and quality? A uniform NHI policy would make much more sense with slight variability than large. Even so, tax finance may lead to stalemate if the existing level of redistribution is a political equilibrium.

Some variability is evident. Recent research on the relationship between income and the use of medical care, given a uniform illness level and uniform out-of-pocket payment, keeps turning up the surprising result of slight variation with income in quantity of services and total expenditure, although the health levels achieved substantially vary with income. The relationship of income to insurance coverage appears stronger, although disentangling the effect of income per se from the mildly increasing tax subsidy is extremely difficult. Insurance plans that control costs by inconveniencing the insureds—managed-care plans of all sorts—are probably much less popular among the well-to-do. But the state of knowledge on this matter is poor. Better information on variability could change the terms of the political debate.

A second issue associated with efficiency concerns the technique to deal with the uninsured. As noted, for a number of reasons Americans really do want all their fellow citizens to have some insurance coverage, at least basic coverage, although they differ on who should pay how much for it. How do we get people to do more of something (in this case buy health insurance)?

The usual answer to this question is straightforward: we subsidize it. We already provide a subsidy to employment-related health insurance, however, in the form of a tax exclusion. Moreover, the subsidy clearly works; only a tiny minority of Americans, between 12 and 17 percent of the population, are uninsured at any time, although a substantial number of those eventually do obtain coverage.

Why is this minority uninsured? The conventional explanation is that they work for small firms, which are less likely than larger firms to provide part of compensation as health insurance. It is true that the likelihood of being uninsured is higher for persons who work in small firms (fewer than 25 employees) than for persons who work in large firms. The mechanism of action is presumably the higher administrative loading for insurance sold to small firms. This loading can be as high as 40 percent of benefits, although an aggressive employer in a stable economic relationship can frequently get coverage at loadings in the range of 20 percent. A sizable fraction of the uninsured, however, do not work for small firms.

Surveys of employers suggest more to the question than simply firm size and high loading. This group includes contract workers, self-employed, part-time, and unemployed. Many small businesses say that they cannot afford to offer insurance and that even a subsidy to offset the higher loading would not be enough to persuade them to buy. Other employers claim that their employees would not be attracted by health insurance if they had to cut money wages to pay for it. Thus some are uninsured because they have less taste for health insurance than the average person; they are not willing to give up enough money wages to pay for insurance. Moreover, many of the positions in small firms have a high mobility and are available in large firms. In some cases, employees could have taken job with health insurance benefits but chose not to do so. Finally, the loading is high for small groups because the cost is higher for small groups. The underwriting in such groups often adds modestly to administrative expense (perhaps 5 percent of premiums). The rest of the higher cost relates to the expense of selling a particular policy and the cost of keeping coverage paid up. Small firms have many advantages over larger firms, but the administration of group insurance is not one of them.

The final problem is that the uninsured do not differ from the insured in ways that can be categorized. They tend to be somewhat lower income, but most people at those income levels are insured. They tend to work for small firms, but most people who work for such firms are insured. They work in certain industries and occupations, but most people in those industries and occupations are insured. The only category in which the uninsured are a majority is the category "uninsured." The uninsured, in other words, are an atypical minority with special problems—of which being uninsured is only one. General subsidy programs fail to reach them at moderate cost; we are in the range of diminishing returns to a subsidy strategy as a way of dealing with the uninsured. As Patricia Danzon has noted, to affect the few uninsured, one would need to provide a large subsidy to people who would have bought insurance anyway (Danzon 1987). But a subsidy program designed on the basis of being uninsured would create strong incentives for people to change their behavior, become uninsured, and qualify for the subsidy.

The common-sense conclusion is that relying on a subsidy or a tax credit increased from current levels is not effective in insuring the uninsured minority; the subsidy has a relative small yield in increased insurance purchasing per dollar spent. If we increase the subsidy from its current level, we spend more and more to get less and less. There is no stopping short of completely free insurance.

Common sense does conflict with the way economists look at efficiency. Paying a large sum to every person who is already insured to get that one last person to obtain insurance is not inefficient in economic terms since the payment to those who would have bought insurance anyway is only a transfer: it does not cause them to change their behavior. The only undesirable feature is that such ineffective subsidies may involve larger transfers than society wants. And that would be easy to solve: we would just change the general tax structure until we got the desired distribution of after-tax income and transfers.

To reconcile common sense and welfare economic theory, one needs to invent a concept for economics (but not new to common sense or public choice theory): exceedingly complex political arrangements, especially ones involving distribution, redistribution, and re-redistribution, involve a political transaction cost of their own. The corollary of this notion is that simple methods are best. In this case I would embrace the following simple reasoning: we want the uninsured to be insured. The most direct way to accomplish this end is to require the purchase of at least that level of insurance that is regarded (at each income level) as the minimum a "reasonable" person would buy. Persons who buy less are either engaging in strategic behavior, expecting to receive free care in a medical emergency, or are incorrectly perceiving the probability of illness. In either case there is no obvious reason why the distributional consequences of their choices (on insurance premiums paid by them, or cost shifting onto those who are insured) should be tolerated. Therefore, purchase of insurance should be required. The distribution of after-tax, after-premium income should be adjusted to what is regarded as fair.

This is not an airtight argument. Some individuals may truly be risk-loving, deriving pleasure from playing in the high-stakes lottery that might leave them financially wiped out if serious illness strikes. Were it possible for such Evel Knievels of health care costs to sign a binding agreement in which they agree to bear the consequences of their choices, and even forbid other citizens to feel sorry for them or their families—in which they agree to suffer if they cannot afford care because they chose not to insure—we would have a solution that might satisfy the dictates of welfare economists but few normal people.

Compared with most equally productive persons who buy employment-related insurance, those who choose not to buy insurance will pay more income taxes, precisely because they do not benefit from the tax subsidy. This higher tax payment may more than offset any explicit financial cost shifting. I doubt, however, that it offsets the altruistically motivated distress imposed on their fellow citizens, distress felt for family members, if not for the household head.

A fundamental issue here is the freedom of individuals to engage in behavior that their fellow citizens regard as unattractive, even irresponsible. Explicit discussion of this issue, profound as it is, in connection with health insurance is desirable. Ultimately the question cannot be settled by appeal to some principle but only by what citizens choose, particularly in a constitutional sense.

The third broad efficiency issue concerns the level and rate of growth of health care costs. Why should this be a question? Isn't it obvious that the answer is "lower than at present"? The problem with such an answer (given the catalog of fallacies above) is that costs can be lowered only if something of benefit is sacrificed, and the rate of growth in costs can be cut only if some beneficial new technology is curtailed short of maximum health benefits. Building the case for health care reform on the prima facie desirability of constraining costs does not work once one goes beyond the rhetoric and into the details because people come to recognize that they will need to sacrifice something.

The most important issue of political choice, then, is what combination of public and private financing will lead to the closest approximation to the right level and rate of growth in cost, the level that balances benefits and costs. Political choice alone suffers from two problems. One is well-known: political choice requires that benefits be uniform; but if the ideal levels are as diverse as described above, that uniformity in insurance coverage will be excessive. It will be worst if (as in Canada) the politically chosen level cannot be supplemented; it will still be bad if some would be willing to choose less than the group choice. The other problem with political choice is that it need not even settle on the best single level of spending. At this point, governments may spend either too much or too little. Many theories—some based on the comparative numbers of winners and losers—predict which direction mistakes will take. Political choice in medical care spending usually leads to underspending for serious illness, relative to the ideal, even though government may overspend in the aggregate. Care for the seriously ill tends to be constrained, while politicians then blame providers for rationing. The dynamics of the dissemination of political information point in the same direction. Higher taxation to pay for health benefits and costs reduces what people have to spend on other things. The benefits that are lost by benefit cuts (if the program is cleverly designed) are uncertain, diffuse, and in the future. The loss of a benefit can usually be blamed, not on the lower level of resources, but on mismanagement and inefficiency by providers—which coincidentally happen to crop up when resources are constrained.

I do not know whether current health care spending in the United States is too high or too low. At least one reason suggests that spending is too high. The tax subsidy for group insurance purchasers presumably causes their spending to be higher than without the subsidy, to some unknown extent. But basically medical care is expensive and probably will grow in cost at a rapid rate no matter what happens with health care reform.

This discussion has an important implication. The public debate on reform has revolved around the issues of access (for the uninsured) and cost containment. Removal of the tax subsidy would surely help cost containment, although the size of the impact is unknown. Removing this distortion would not, however, guarantee a low rate of growth in cost, a leveling off of the medical expenditures share of GNP in the near future, or less rapid increases in costs of employee benefits. And yet the debate has largely been couched in terms of the unequivocal desire for cost containment. Beyond the tax subsidy distortion, economics has little to add as a legitimate weapon (from a public policy perspective) in the war on skyrocketing medical costs. Health maintenance organizations, research and guidelines on effectiveness, and better information about medical price and quality may all help, but they should be treated neutrally and neither encouraged nor discouraged by specific policy initiatives. Paradoxically, what is efficient to do does not provide strong promise of cost containment, and what seems to work for cost containment (government control of one sort or another) cannot be guaranteed as efficient.

This paradox is at the heart of the confused debate on health care reform. Any reform proposal is first judged, in the typical policy discussion, by whether it will work, by whether it has a good chance of greatly reducing health cost growth. But those plans that work (in this sense) pose a substantial risk of loss of benefits that people value greatly. The cost-containment filter guarantees that proposals will be taken seriously only if they pose the risk of a substantial threat to benefits. Proponents can still pretend that the threat is marginal, or that with good management they and the government can be trusted to make sure that no harm will be done. But their arguments are not credible.

The final efficiency issue, which has not been resolved and has therefore inhibited health care reform, is the employer's role in financing medical services for employees and dependents. As noted some time ago (Pauly 1989), if the bulk of the incidence of employer payments for health insurance does not ultimately fall on workers, then almost all of our capability to understand labor markets will have been lost. The theory

325

in this matter is strong, and some recent empirical studies (Gruber and Krueger 1990) sufficiently encourage the conventional economic view. Moreover, the alternative to employee incidence is forward shifting onto consumers. No serious argument—even from those large firms with vocal benefits managers who think that they pay for employee benefits with what would otherwise be the company's money—supports long-term incidence on employers or stockholders.

Key to understanding the role of employer-paid insurance is understanding who sacrifices real well-being when costs of such insurance rise. Without that understanding, the employer-mandate route first looks deceptively attractive—what could be better than an off-budget cost that nobody is known to pay?—but then becomes a dead end, as participants in the discussion, especially those with some resources (whether stockholders or highly paid worker-consumers) realize that they run a good risk of paying the major share of a cost over which they have little control.

I opt for a financing mechanism that is transparent, is straightforward, and suggests that consumers be required to pay for their own health insurance (Pauly et al. 1991). Subsidies help those who cannot afford the cost. This may appear a hopelessly naive approach to public policy formulation, since it offers few opportunities for slick tricks. And yet this approach is so firmly founded in the normative theory of public choice, the political professionals have been so inept at predicting or selecting political outcomes, and the power of simple ideas (for example, supply-side economics and the virtues of competitive markets) has in the recent past proved so strong that I still hold out hope. Why not try honesty and simplicity for a change?

Distributional Impediments

One impediment to health care reform arises because even good changes are sure to make some worse off. We can hope that the power of improved equity will sweep special interests before it. Sometimes this will work, but sometimes the special interests need to be bought off not only because this is realistic but because sometimes this is right. That is, the long-term presence of a defect, loophole, or privilege sets in place an incentive to people to take advantage of that gain. Eligibility for the break may involve costs; people may willingly absorb those costs as long as they are less than the value of the break. The creation of rents—wealth transfers not based on services rendered—through the political process causes rent-seeking behavior. At the margin, the last person who slips into the privileged class actually gains almost nothing from doing so. Canceling the privileges then leaves that person in a double bind: losing not only the tax break or subsidy break but also all benefit from the costs incurred to qualify for it. One can argue that since the political process set people up for these loopholes, it ought to let them down gradually.

This section considers two types of political rent that should be gradually abolished on the way to health care reform and argues that accomplishment of that reform requires that they be treated carefully. The two important types of rent are (1) the loophole from tax-shielded employer payments for health insurance premiums and (2) payments to medical providers (especially, but not exclusively, physicians) in excess of competitive levels.

Let us first consider closing the exclusion loophole for insurance premiums. Removing the tax subsidy caused by the exclusion of employer-provided premium payments from federal income and pay-roll taxation (and most state and local taxation as well) is the good politician's dream policy: it simultaneously promotes efficiency and equity; it permits government revenues to be expanded in a way that aids rather than harms the private sector. It is, in economic jargon, a financing method with negative excess burden (and two wrongs do make a right).

The efficiency argument for removing the loophole is compelling. At present, every dollar saved on the tax-free costs of health insurance premiums becomes taxable income for someone. If the initial incidence of those premium costs is on workers, the additional money income is taxed at the worker's marginal tax rate, which can easily be above 40 percent if the income tax rate is 32 percent and we take account of the total payroll tax for social security and Medicare. Indeed, in some areas with high state and local taxes, the marginal rate will approach 50 percent. Now consider the trade-off. Suppose workers are considering a new and effective but irritating managed-care option that will allow their money raises for next year to be higher than if they stuck with their usual insurance. With taxation of such wages, workers will be less eager for the managed-care option than if they could keep the full savings. If the marginal tax rate is 50 percent and the option saves one dollar but causes more than 50 cents worth of hassle, employees will turn it down, even though it provides a positive net benefit.

Contrast this decision with the calculus if there were no tax subsidy, if all insurance premium payments, regardless of whether the employer or the employee writes out the check, were treated as part of the employee's taxable income. The person would pay the same income tax regardless of how compensation was split between health insurance and cash; the tax burden would be a given. Saving a dollar on health insurance premiums then would save a dollar in *after-tax* income, income that can be spent, one hundred cents on the dollar, for other items of consumption.

The mildly irritating managed-care plan would then be adopted since—even after deducting the hassle cost—it would still allow more real consumption.

Because the dollar amount of employer-paid health insurance premiums on average rises with income, and because the marginal tax rate rises (mildly) with income, the current loophole provides somewhat larger benefits to higher-income workers. Persons who think it more equable to raise taxes on highly paid workers should therefore favor the redistribution associated with closing the loophole. To be sure, although the value of the loophole rises with income, it does not rise *faster* than income, so that removal of the loophole does not represent as much of a redistribution of income from the rich to the poor as would enactment of a progressive income tax. The net distributional effect depends as well on how the proceeds from closing this loophole are spent (Buchanan and Pauly 1970). If there is a balanced budget adjustment and if the extra taxes are returned on a pro rata basis by income class, the net progressivity across income classes does not change and therefore vertical equity does not change. *Horizontal* equity, however, is definitely served by this change since persons of the same productivity pay the same tax.

The primary argument for closing the loophole is fundamental. I can see no reason why I, a professor at the Wharton School, am able to reduce my taxable income by at least $4,000, while the man who mows my lawn cannot. The inefficiency and unfairness of the tax loophole, however, have not made it a prime candidate for removal. This major loophole survived Ronald Reagan's tax reform and apparently has retained its strong constituency. That constituency seems to be based entirely on the fact that a majority of people benefit from this loophole, while only a minority pay higher taxes than would be the case if it were removed. The pure theoretical arguments for its removal have thus far not been politically effective.

Those arguments should still be made. One process can grease the distributional skids and achieve almost all of the objectives of the tax reform path to health care reform. Such a process involves two elements. First, the tax exclusion must be capped, and capped at no more than the value of the premium for any income level for the lowest-cost reasonable insurance for that level. Second, the exclusion must be extended to all persons at that income level who buy health insurance, regardless of their employment situation.

The exclusion, for instance, might be capped at $2,500 for a family of four with family income of $50,000 and extended to the self-employed and persons with income from property. So long as the cap is kept low enough, relative to the cost of the plan we want people to choose, it does not distort choices of health insurance at the margin. As long as it is available to everyone, the cap does not distort choices about employment status. Indeed, although it may be formally retained as a tax exclusion, for all intents and purposes it is equivalent to an adjustment in the tax structure. The cap is equivalent to changing taxes for all families earning $50,000 by an amount equal to the tax on $2,500; it is equivalent to a tax credit of that amount.

The other distributional issue relates to the distribution of well-being between consumers and producers. Through a combination of government action, private collusion, and past history, some persons who furnish medical services may receive incomes higher than what they would earn in a truly competitive system. Limitation on the number of medical school places has traditionally been viewed by economists as evidence of a cartel-like restriction on supply for the purpose of generating monopoly rents (Friedman and Kuznets 1945). State laws that link exclusive licensure to medical school graduation enforce this set of privileges (Kessell 1958). Some empirical evidence does suggest above-normal average returns to medical education compared with other types of postgraduate education, although the evidence is far from conclusive. The elimination of hospital-based nursing schools by organized nursing likewise limited supply (especially new supply) and may have been a contributor to rapid growth in nurses' wages. Technicians and technologists also have seen rapidly rising wages, although the cause here (as for nurses and physicians) seems to be a mixture of demand-pull and hospital-insurer unwillingness to drive hard bargains.

This chapter does not try to settle the question of the existence of above-normal returns to health professionals. But linking health care reform to efforts (usually barely concealed) to reduce those rents generates opposition by those who receive them. The mere reduction in incomes that providers earn would not be an appropriate goal for health care reform if judged by the canons of welfare economics. The monopoly rents themselves represent only transfers from those who happen to be consumers to those who happen to be producers. Economists oppose monopoly because it makes the prices of services artificially high, thus reducing consumption. This argument, however, is not especially strong for medical care since typical medical insurance also distorts prices but makes them too low (Crew 1969). More generally, if we think too many resources are going into medical care, artificially high prices should be praised rather than blamed.

The real problem from a health care monopoly arises when and if that monopoly inhibits efforts to reduce real costs, the costs of services that use up real resources. Inhibitions to participation in managed care, distortions in the market for nursing and technologist services, and limits

329

on consumers' ability to buy services from providers with less specialized training are the real costs of monopoly.

This analysis sends two important messages, one negative and one positive. The negative message is that a goal of health care reform should not be to force down prices of providers. Doing so would advantage consumers but harm providers; there is no equity rationale for doing so. Paying nurses at service worker wages would make hospital care cheaper, but what principle suggests that doing so is fair? People are usually less squeamish about reducing physician incomes, given the relatively high level of physician income, but even here the equity rationale is weak—and, in any event, net payments to physicians amount only to about 10 percent of all health care spending.

The positive message is that we should pay off providers to get them to participate in health care reform, if necessary. If removal of the consequences of monopoly is efficient, then providers can be compensated and consumers still receive benefits. Moreover, many providers themselves do not earn monopoly rents, simply because of all the cost they incurred to get into and through medical school or to complete a baccalaureate program in nursing. Rent-seeking behavior means that wholesale cuts in provider prices or incomes will disadvantage some people who are barely breaking even.

Controlling the Political System

The final obstruction to health care reform is based on the proposition that voters know that perfect monitoring of politicians and bureaucrats is impossible and take this imperfection into account in deciding which institutional structures to support. In the classic application, Geoffrey Brennan and James Buchanan (1977) explained the use of specific excise taxes as a method by which voters could exert control over the spending level politicians would choose. Victor Fuchs (1976) specifically cites citizen fear of government control over medical services as a deterrent to national health insurance, as does Milton Friedman (1991).

Some strong reasons contend that spending control would be especially difficult for a government health insurance program. Nothing precisely measures what care is effective and what is not, and voters cannot easily tell what benefits they are obtaining relative to cost. Moreover, the line of least resistance for private sector decision makers who have overcommitted to health insurance benefits is often a shift of the obligation (and the blame) for deciding on the quantity of services. Unions and management may want to blame government. Finally, the altruistic motivation that undergirds the case for public intervention has a difficult time being reconciled with differing levels of service in the public and private program.

So far as measuring costs and effects are concerned, voter-taxpayers face a double challenge. They need to determine what benefits are being generated by the program and who is paying how much for them in terms of taxes. The former is difficult because an assessment of benefits requires an assessment of illness levels. The latter is complex because the provision of employer-paid insurance complicates the final incidence of cost.

The task of rationing medical services by refusal to reimburse is distasteful in the extreme since it requires someone to take the responsibility of refusing to pay for unequivocally beneficial services. Union leaders, corporate benefits managers, and politicians who must stand for office are understandably reluctant to do so.

Finally, explicit choice of two-tier medicine is painful since we would like to believe that we really can provide the same quality of care to every citizen as we provide to the president or to a millionaire; we do not want to decide explicitly to give less to some than to others. The recent experience with Oregon Medicaid suggests that such rationing decisions may be possible but an elaborate process is needed to insulate politicians from criticism.

All of these influences indicate a strong temptation for politicians and bureaucrats to overprovide some services, at least at the outset of a national health program. Recognizing the likelihood of overprovision accompanying any change in the level of public activity at all, rational voters may choose to avoid any alteration. The conversion of the modest catastrophic Medicare insurance proposal into a political feeding frenzy that involved drug coverage and serious discussion of (potentially unlimited) coverage of services for chronic illness illustrates this dynamic.

What is the solution to this dilemma? The best approach goes to great pains to make choices explicit. Thus the employer payment option, whose incidence confuses even economists, should be avoided in favor of laying the obligation explicitly on households. The level of coverage or reimbursement should be varied by income level—with the well-to-do permitted to spend more but only if they are spending their own money. Finally, the obligation of choosing one's rationer should explicitly be placed on each person by requiring each person to choose among health plans, or at least to "choose a chooser" in the form of a benefits manager.

Conclusion

The obstacles to health care reform are formidable. This chapter has outlined some methods for overcoming them. The real key to success is the discovery of a way to motivate real world decision makers to make the hard choices needed to achieve this reform—rather than just call for it but then offer no concrete ideas.

Writing about positive political economy in the context of a policy problem always raises a paradox. If one develops a theory to explain the behavior of politicians, bureaucrats, and lobbyists, why should they be expected to take action based on the results? Positive political economy is a low-level version of astronomy; it explains the rotation and movements of some nonheavenly bodies as a function of forces that no person can expect to change. Such a theory gives a prediction, but it does not give policy changes. What can the analyst with some particular policy in mind usefully do?

This essay is intended to achieve two objectives. First, and somewhat inconsistently, not all policy makers really do understand the advantages and disadvantages of all positions; they really do not realize on which side their bread is buttered. Correctly viewed, a market-type arrangement for dealing with the uninsured is better than some of the others, which have been more extensively considered and found wanting. Correct thinking might help to put together a decisive coalition for change.

Second, the analyst, even of the political process, can usefully play the middleman and deal arranger. Especially if people understand what is to their advantage and disadvantage, some modest adjustments in taxes and benefits may describe a change that provides benefits for all (compared with the current situation). I am not overly optimistic here; trying to snatch yet larger gains from trade may lead actors to engage in strategy that confuses the process. Other than pointing out that such zero-sum game playing usually does not lead to permanent advantage for any player but does cause a stalemate, the analyst can do little more before taking a bow and offering hope that the play will go as scripted.

References

Brennan, G., and J. Buchanan. "Towards a Tax Constitution for Leviathan." *Journal of Public Economics* (December 1977): 255–73.

Buchanan, J., and M. Pauly. "On the Incidence of Tax Deductibility." *National Tax Journal* 23 (June 1970): 157–67.

Crew, M. A. "Coinsurance and the Welfare Economics of Medical Care." *American Economic Review* 59 (December 1969): 906–08.

Danzon, P. "Expanding Employment-based Health Insurance." Report to the Program on Access to Care, North Carolina (Duke University, Center on Health Policy, Research, and Education, August 1987).

Friedman, M. "Gammon's Law Points to Health-Care Solution." *Wall Street Journal* (November 12, 1991): 20.

Friedman, M., and S. Kuznets. *Income from Independent Professional*

Practice, New York: National Bureau of Economic Research, 1945.

Fuchs, V. "From Bismark to Woodcock." In *The Health Economy*, edited by V. Fuchs. Cambridge: Harvard University Press, 1986: 257–71.

Gruber, J., and A. Krueger. "The Incidence of Mandated Employer-provided Insurance: Lessons from Worker's Compensation Insurance." NBER Working Paper 3557. Cambridge: 1990.

Kessell, R. A. "Price Discrimination in Medicine." *Journal of Law and Economics* 1 (October 1958): 20–53.

Pauly M. V. *An Analysis of National Health Insurance Proposals*. Washington, D.C.: American Enterprise Institute, 1971.

———. "The Incidence of Health Insurance Costs: Is Everyone out of Step but Economists?" In *Proceedings of the Forty-First Annual Meeting of the Industrial Research Association*. New York, December 1989: 387–410.

———. "The Normative and Positive Economics of Minimum Health Benefits." In *Health Economics Worldwide*, edited by Zweifel, P. and H. E. Frech. Netherlands: Kluwer Academic Publishers, 1992: 63–78.

Pauly, M.V., et al. "A Plan for 'Responsible National Health Insurance.'" *Health Affairs* 10–1 (Spring 1991): 5–25.

President's Commission for the Study of Ethical Problems in Medicine and Biomedical and Behavioral Research. *Securing Access to Health Care*. Washington, D.C.: Government Printing Office, 1983.

Usher, D. "The Welfare Economics of the Socialization of Commodities." *Journal of Public Economics* 8 (1977): 151–69.

14

The Search for Adaptable Health Policy through Finance-based Reform

C. Eugene Steuerle

Government policy toward health care can never be separated from financing or tax issues, or from alternative uses and expenditures to which tax dollars might be devoted. In many policy discussions, health policy is treated as isolated from tax policy. Inevitably and irreducibly, however, they are the two sides of the same accounting ledger. Similarly, since presumably the total well-being of the individual is the concern, health policy must be treated as a subset of social or welfare policy.

This chapter examines health policy from this broader, public finance perspective. The first section presents data on health expenditures from the financing or source side, rather than from the uses or health expenditures side. The second section discusses how and why health policy expenditures have an impact on other social and budgetary policy. The third section indicates how the existing tax provisions toward the purchase of health insurance might be reformed to produce greater equity and efficiency, as well as leave a flexible instrument to which other reforms might be added or rejected on their own merits. The fourth section demonstrates surprisingly that play-or-pay schemes—requirements that insurance be purchased or that a tax be paid—have become a component of almost every proposed plan for reforming health policy. After showing that the common underlying public finance principle justifying play-or-pay is one of horizontal equity or equal treatment of equals, the section discusses some efficiency and administrative aspects of alternative ways to reach this goal. The final section summarizes the lessons learned by viewing health policy from these public finance vantage points. Although policy analysts and officials will disagree over many options for the future, this chapter proposes a common meeting ground and basic plan for action.

Sources of Financing for Health Expenditures

Health expenditures can be examined from the source or financing side, as well as the uses side. This requires that numbers be rearranged in a way slightly different from normal.

Private and Public Expenditures, Including Tax Expenditures. Figure 14–1 presents estimates of the sources of financing for health care for fiscal year 1992. Numbers provided by the Health Care Financing Administration must be modified to take into account the value of tax subsidies that operate like other expenditures but are often neglected. Here tax subsidies are treated roughly in the manner that would occur if they were put into the budget of the Department of Health and Human Services. Note, however, that when the governmental subsidies are treated as the source of payment, then the net amount contributed by purchasers is less by the amount of the subsidy. Tax reductions that apply to employer-provided health, for example, effectively reduce the net amount contributed by employers to employer-based plans. For technical reasons, conventional revenue-loss figures are used to estimate tax subsidies, even though this procedure understates their real value.[1]

These simple calculations strikingly show that federal, state, and local governments pay for more than one-half of total health expenditures in the United States—not the smaller fraction usually shown. When everything is counted, various levels of government in the United States will spend $390 billion to subsidize health care in fiscal year 1992.

---

1. The tax subsidies themselves are nontaxable. In effect a $10 nontaxable subsidy, whether floated through the expenditure or tax system, is worth more than a subsidy that is taxable. In the Tax Expenditure Budget of the United States, the difference is accounted for as that between the "revenue estimate" of the tax expenditure and its "outlay equivalent" cost.

The issue is complicated further by a fundamental accounting problem when something is subsidized. If the government pays 50 cents out of every dollar of expenditure, then the value of the expenditure in theory should equal only 50 cents to the purchaser; yet one dollar's worth of goods and services are used in the economy. A subsidy, therefore, acts like a negative excise tax that drives a wedge between total income and total product in the economy. Because this table derives sources of financing for expenditures, it follows conventional accounting for health expenditures and forces income and product to be equal when, in fact, many subsidies make them unequal. The problem applies not only to the nontaxation of the tax subsidies, but also to items like Medicare that are nontaxable and, hence, in theory, have a value in product that is different from the income received by suppliers of medical services. For an analysis of some similar problems, see Tolley and Steuerle (1979).

FIGURE 14–1
Estimated Sources of Financing for U.S. Health Care Expenditures, Fiscal Year 1992

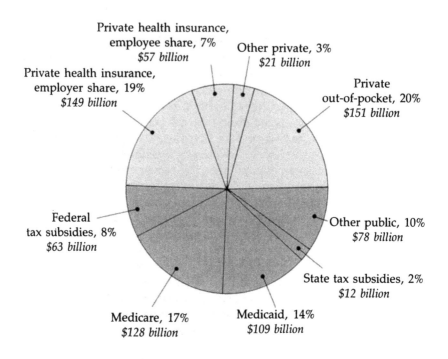

Private health insurance, employee share, 7% $57 billion

Other private, 3% $21 billion

Private health insurance, employer share, 19% $149 billion

Private out-of-pocket, 20% $151 billion

Federal tax subsidies, 8% $63 billion

Other public, 10% $78 billion

State tax subsidies, 2% $12 billion

Medicare, 17% $128 billion

Medicaid, 14% $109 billion

NOTE: Tax subsidies are subtracted out of applicable expenditure categories. All tax subsidies are in revenue-loss terms. Revenue effects derive from exclusions and deductions from the federal and state income tax and the employer and employee portions of the social security payroll tax. Tax subsidies for private health expenditures are subtracted out of their corresponding private categories and added to the government expenditure accounts, and thus they do not alter total net national health expenditures. Tax subsidies for public health expenditures such as Medicare are not subtracted from any other accounts, and thus they are treated as additions to total net national health expenditures. Calculations include $56 billion in subsidies for employer-provided health insurance.

SOURCE: Author's calculations, based on data from Levit and Cowan (1990), OMB (1991A), and the Joint Committee on Taxation.

Moreover, in real dollars and even as a percentage of GNP, federal, state, and local governments in the United States together contribute almost as much to health care as do governments in many countries with national health insurance programs for the entire population.

The sheer size of these numbers should warn us about exaggerating the effect of any particular reform, incremental or broad. On the one hand, additional increments of even tens of billions of dollars for any reform might change only moderately the allocations of funds among providers and payers and their way of doing business.[2] On the other hand, if the government cannot achieve a better allocation of funds and greater cost control with a $390 billion health budget, it is not clear that those problems would go away with a reform that required a $500 billion health budget. When a well-designed $500 billion package is compared with a poorly designed $390 billion package, it provides little information about which improvements to better design and which are due to the additional expenditures.[3]

Average Health Expenses per Household. Because individuals receive insurance, they are often unaware of the cost of the medical care they are receiving. By the time actual medical services are provided, the insurance policy usually makes the private cost of obtaining additional care either zero or quite low. This logic is often used to help explain how insurance boosts demand and leads to increases in health care costs.[4]

The logic, however, is usually not carried far enough. Although individuals may be ignorant of, and have little control over, the cost of medical care once they are insured, still they can be made conscious of the cost of insurance they are buying. As insurance costs increase, the amount of other goods and services people can purchase decreases. Conscious of the cost of insurance and the cost of other goods and services, consumers will make trade-offs between the two, although at a higher total cost of medical care than if there were no insurance at all.

In the United States, however, individuals are not only kept ignorant

---

2. Of course, an annual increment of at least $10 billion or more in real government expenditures is already scheduled to occur annually—but by budget conventions those scheduled increments are considered baseline, or current law, figures.

3. I recognize the argument that the government might be able to function more as a monopsonist if it controlled all of the health market. Even if one excludes the inefficiencies and inequities normally associated with a monopsony, however, a firm with a 50 percent market share is not without its levers over the market.

4. See, for instance, Phelps (1976), or more recently, Aaron (1991, 10–13). For a provocative discussion of how the medical profession's professional paradigm limits the ability of consumers to influence consumer choices, see also Havighurst (1990, 415–29).

of the cost of the medical care they receive; they are even deterred from knowing the cost of the medical insurance they purchase.

Table 14–1 shows how individuals pay for health care in the United States. The average expenditure per household is estimated at $8,000. Note that within categories, the averages reported in the table are per household in the United States, not per household that might incur the particular type of expense involved. Of the $8,000, only about one-third is paid directly by individuals, and even a large portion of that one-third is hidden. Premiums for federal supplemental medical insurance are taken directly out of social security checks and are set at such a low rate that there is almost no choice other than to buy the supplement. Personal payments toward employer-provided group health insurance also are typically set at low rates relative to total cost.

Even if individuals recognize the direct costs that come out of their paychecks and social security checks, they still have little idea of the other costs they are paying. An average of about $3,930 is paid per household through higher rates of federal income, federal social security, state income, state sales, and other taxes to support federal, state, and local health efforts. Employers on average contribute another $1,580 per household. Even though economic theory in general holds that these payments are actually paid by employees in the form of reduced cash wages, the employee is usually kept ignorant of these costs.

These figures demonstrate that individuals may fail to make cost-conscious decisions not only with respect to health services once they have insurance, but with respect to the cost of insurance itself. Recently there have been a number of initiatives by employers to introduce cost-sharing and offer options to employees. A number of firms have moved away from employer payment of the entire health insurance bill and toward a system whereby employees contribute some portion. The rise, if any, in percentage of payments coming from employees, however, has been rather modest.[5] Because employees pay either way—but the government penalizes direct employee contributions and knowledge of costs—any required employee contribution should be seen as a fairly expensive effort to raise the cost-consciousness of employees as buyers of health insurance.

---

5. The percentage of private health insurance financed by employee contributions declined steadily from 41 percent in 1965 to 18.9 percent in 1980, and then it began to increase, reaching 22.8 percent in 1989. See Levit and Cowan (1990). Surveys imply that more employers are requiring employee participation. See, for instance, Jensen, Morrisey, and Marcus (1987). On the other hand, many employers may face difficulty in trying to increase or even maintain the employee share during periods of rapidly rising costs.

TABLE 14-1
How Households Paid for Health Care, Fiscal Year 1992

	Average per Household $ [a]	% of GNP	% of Personal Income	% of Money Income
Paid indirectly				
Taxes: Federal Hospital Insurance Payroll Tax	860	1.4	1.6	2.1
Taxes: other federal, state, and local[b]	3,070	4.9	5.8	7.4
Reduced wages: paid by employers[c]	1,580	2.5	3.0	3.8
Other[d]	190	0.3	0.4	0.5
Paid directly				
Personal contributions: to private health insurance[e]	590	0.9	1.1	1.4
Out-of-pocket payments	1,580	2.5	3.0	3.8
Premiums—Federal Supplemental Medical Insurance	130	0.2	0.2	0.3
Total	8,000	12.9	15.1	19.4
Addendum				
Mean GNP per household	62,160	—	—	—
Mean personal income per household	53,130	—	—	—
Mean money income per household	41,320	—	—	—

NOTES: Estimated total health care spending in the United States in fiscal year 1992.
All tax subsidies are in revenue-loss terms. Included are revenue effects of exclusions and deductions from the federal and state income tax and both the employer and employee portions of the social security payroll tax. Tax subsidies for private health expenditures are subtracted out of their corresponding private categories and added to the government expenditure accounts, and thus they do not alter total net national health expenditures. Tax subsidies for public health expenditures such as Medicare are not subtracted from any other accounts, and thus they are treated as additions to total net national health expenditures.
a. Average household size in the United States was 2.63 persons in 1990. Amounts rounded to the nearest $10.
b. Includes taxes needed to finance direct government health spending out of general revenues, plus the amount general taxes must be raised in order to compensate for revenue lost due to special tax treatment of certain health-related income, about 26 percent of the total.
c. Employer contributions for health insurance, less government tax subsidies.
d. Nonpatient revenue for the health care industry, including charitable donations, interest income, hospital parking and gift shops, and so forth.
e. Includes both employee contributions to private group health insurance plans, plus individual policy premiums.
SOURCES: Author's calculations based on data from Levit and Cowan (1990), OMB (1991A), and the Joint Committee on Taxation.

The Growth in the Cost of Health Care. Health costs clearly have risen dramatically in recent years, and for all practical purposes they appear to be out of control. Nonetheless it is a mistake to argue that the rate of increase of health costs is by itself a justification for reform. The justification must always be that costs are too high per se and that inefficiencies and inequities are associated with these high costs. Even if costs were to stabilize, a reformed system should still be able to justify its superiority over the current system and other alternatives that were rejected.

As any student of natural or social science knows, moreover, health costs cannot continually absorb a larger and larger percentage of the nation's income. Mathematically it is impossible. Logically the cost associated with each additional, forgone, nonmedical good eventually rises, and the benefit of each additional medical service eventually falls, as health absorbs more of total output.

None of us really knows at what point the health cost curve would come down or stabilize independently from government action. We do not know which of the hypothetical curves in figure 14–2 we are on. It is important, however, to realize that many reforms being proposed are likely to be still in effect five decades or more after enactment. Any new health care system for the nation, therefore, must be designed to adapt toward an optimal level of spending, as determined in large part by future, unknown economic conditions, rather than toward a level of spending set by a late twentieth century view of how to control a nonoptimal growth rate.

Health Policy in the Broader Context of Budget, Tax, and Social Policy

Budget data make obvious the possibility that expenditures on health may be helping to deter government action on almost every other domestic front. This reinforces the notion that health policy choices are seldom matters merely of health policy, but of budget, social, and tax policy as well.

Health and Everything Else. One of the major factors driving concern over health policy is its effect on government budgets. While higher health costs may imply higher taxes sooner or later, it is just as likely that higher health expenditures imply lower spending on other social needs. Table 14–2 presents as an example changes in all major categories of spending between 1991 and 1996, as outlined in the Office of Management and Budget's Mid-Session Review of the Budget in mid-1991. Essentially everything in the budget pays for either increases in

FIGURE 14–2
Some Hypothetical Trajectories of U.S. Health Care Expenditures, as a Portion of GNP
(percent)

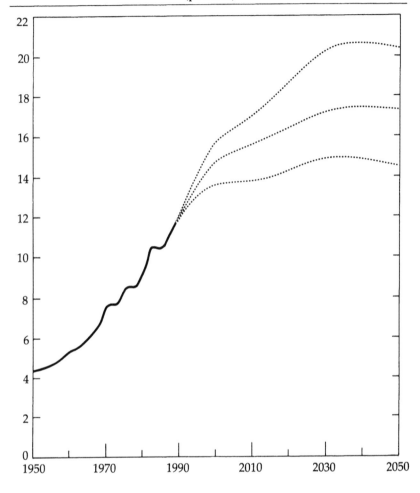

SOURCE: Historical data are from HIAA (1990). Future levels are author's extrapolations.

health outlays or deficit reductions. Within the human resource budget, for instance, health and Medicare would rise by almost 0.88 percent of GNP between 1991 and 1996, while every other category would decline. There are drops in every major educational function—primary and

TABLE 14–2
SELECTED FEDERAL GOVERNMENT OUTLAYS, AS A PORTION OF GNP,
FISCAL YEARS 1991–1996
(percent)

Outlays, by Budget Function	1991	1996	Change, 1991–1996
Medicare and other health	3.18	4.06	+0.88
Other human resources	9.22	8.43	−0.80
Elementary, secondary, and vocational education	0.21	0.18	−0.03
Higher education	0.20	0.08	−0.12
Other education, training, and employment	0.36	0.27	−0.08
Income security	3.10	2.88	−0.23
Social security	4.79	4.57	−0.22
Veterans' benefits	0.57	0.46	−0.11
Energy, natural resources, and environment	0.38	0.29	−0.10
Transportation, community, and regional development	0.70	0.54	−0.16
International affairs	0.32	0.24	−0.08
Agriculture	0.28	0.18	−0.10
Other: net residual	0.15	0.18	+0.03
Total outlays, excluding deposit insurance, net interest, and defense	14.25	13.91	−0.33

NOTE: Details may not add to totals, because of rounding.
SOURCE: Author's calculations based on data and assumptions from the Office of Management and Budget (1991A and 1991B).

secondary education, higher education, and other education, training, and employment. Expenditures for various forms of income security would also be reduced relative to GNP. Outside the human resource budget, expenditures on energy, natural resources, and the environment would fall by 1996, as would outlays for transportation and for community and regional development. International affairs would be run "on the cheap." Expenditure patterns in the 1980s show a similar trade-off between growth in health spending and decline in almost all other types of spending.

A similar story can be told at the state and local levels. For example, Drew Altman, the former commissioner of Human Services in New Jersey, states, "In New Jersey, in any given year, the increase in Medicaid necessary just to maintain current services consumed about one-half of all new funds available for our department. This left the homeless, the mentally ill, the elderly, the disabled, veterans, welfare recipients and other needy groups to fight for the leftovers" (Wessel 1991).

These data provide empirical support for the theoretical proposition that expenditures on health displace other government efforts and functions. One connection among health, tax, and other social policy is the following: increased government spending on health care, or any item, raises tax rates. At higher rates, the inefficiency associated with maintaining any other category of spending rises, and correspondingly the efficiency gains from reducing that category also increase. That is, the higher the initial rate, the more distorting are equal rises in the tax rate. Thus raising tax rates 40–41 percent to support education is much more distorting than raising those rates 30–31 percent to support the same level of educational spending.

Raising tax rates by ten percentage points or more just to pay for health care is not an exaggeration. See, again, table 14–1. One can approximate the tax rates faced by workers to support health care under current law and under various proposals. Roughly speaking, a typical worker already loses an additional eight to ten percentage points of earned income simply to support current government health programs.[6] When fully implemented, a typical, recent national health bill would raise tax rates by eleven percentage points or more for those participating in a government, rather than employer, plan.[7] This rise implies that workers could easily pay as much as one-fifth of any additional income, or their marginal tax rate would be higher by about twenty percentage points, simply to support government health programs.[8]

The point is not that the tax increases per se make the worker worse off. If taxes merely displaced other private payments for the same

---

6. For simplicity, I assume the worker consumes what he earns and that all expenditures to support current health programs eventually come out of taxes, even when there is temporary deficit financing.

7. The Health Insurance Coverage and Cost Containment Act of 1991 introduced by Dan Rostenkowski, Chairman of the House Ways and Means Committee, for instance, would impose initial tax rates of 9 percent of payroll subject to Medicare and then raise those rates to about 11 percent over the next few years to support increased outlays. Alternatively, an employer health plan must be provided. In addition, there would be a 10 percent surcharge on the current Medicare rate of 2.3 percent, thus implying a surcharge rate of 0.23 percent. A portion of these taxes might be used to lower other government health costs, but such an exchange is not clear. See Ways and Means Committee (1991A, 1283–85).

8. As seen in table 14–1, the percentage of money income paid for health is much higher than the percentage of GNP or even of personal income. GNP figures have not yet netted out such items as depreciation, while personal income includes many nontaxed sources of income such as fringe benefits.

343

amount of insurance, a worker would not be worse off in terms of total income or total consumption. By raising marginal tax rates, however, health reform can significantly raise the costs—in terms of distortions and inefficiencies—that must be borne to maintain other social and government programs. Again, health policy cannot be treated as isolated from tax policy or from other social policy.

The trade-off among social policies may look even worse if we ask to what degree real benefits increase because of government health programs. In 1992, for instance, direct federal, state, and local expenditures on health, excluding the tax expenditures included in figure 14–1, will equal approximately \$315 billion. Had medical prices since 1965 risen only as fast as the price index for other goods and services, however, the same amount of health care could have been purchased for \$204 billion. Without this excess medical inflation, therefore, governments could have purchased \$111 billion more in goods and services, health or otherwise, without raising taxes.

Another way of stating this phenomenon is that many government health expenditures increase the amount received by suppliers of health services, but not the care provided to individuals. To the extent that the design of the government programs is partly responsible for the increase in medical prices, the efficiency of the transfer is further called into question.[9]

Government health care programs are in-kind programs, similar to housing. Traditionally the public finance literature has frowned upon the provision of in-kind benefits because they reduce consumer choice and raise prices of the goods being subsidized. Even without any induced price increase, recipients would almost always prefer cash to an in-kind benefit. Not only might they choose to spend the cash on some preferable item; they might also choose different providers of the same item. Thus public housing is inefficient not simply because it displaces food, clothing, and other goods, but because other forms or locations of housing might be preferable to the one determined by the government. This line of logic is also used to support the conclusion that, if in-kind benefits are to be provided, vouchers may be superior to the provision of goods and services in a manner that more narrowly restricts choices

---

9. The calculation is not precise. Some government expenditures are for items that are not really part of the total deflator. Finally, health prices are not well measured. For a discussion of this latter issue, see Aaron (1991, 41–42). These qualifications, however, do not eliminate the basic argument that the value of medical goods and services provided by the government in 1992 is seriously eroded by medical price inflation.

and decisions by participants.[10]

Open-ended Government Programs. Many reasons are offered for the government's inability to contain the health care part of the budget. Insurance lowers the price of health care and drives up demand beyond the point at which benefits are equal to costs. Government subsidies have also increased demand and price. New technology is expensive, and society has been unwilling to admit that it must ration that new technology. All this is true. None of it, however, is quite adequate to explain the government's inability to get this part of the budget under control, nor to designate exactly where and how the next health dollar should be spent.

Almost any time a government expenditure is out of control, that expenditure has been enacted in a way that is open-ended. Traditionally the term "open-ended" has been applied to programs such as government loans, financial credits, or guarantees, where no limit has been placed on the number of transactions that can be made to fall into the subsidized or guaranteed category. More broadly, however, the term can be applied to any program where the costs are determined outside the budget by the level of activity of private citizens. In truth, no program is perfectly open-ended with respect to all its features. Under deposit insurance, for instance, a person may hold an endless number of guaranteed accounts, but personal saving creates some constraint on how much is guaranteed.

Government health care policy traditionally has been open-ended. Excluding some small copayments by beneficiaries, most hospital expenses have been covered by Medicare. Gradually, more regulations have come to be adopted in an attempt to limit charges, but the container has hardly been made airtight. Hospital payments became displaced by government payments for outpatient care. One type of procedure was limited, only to be replaced by another.

More generally, the whole definition of health has been left rather vaguely defined and, as a result, open-ended. From one perspective, there is value to a vagueness of definition. Why should psychological care, dental care, or other types of care not be insured? Why should new technologies not be subsidized along with the old? The difficulty is that with an open-ended subsidy, the definition itself becomes biased toward inclusion, rather than exclusion, and the recipients of the subsidy, including suppliers of medical services, are in charge of the definition.

---

10. Suppose, for instance, that cash benefits are opposed because of a fear they will be misused by recipients. There are many ways of restricting assistance without specifying exactly where, when, and how specific consumption should take place.

Vouchers or Credits as Replacements for the More Inefficient and Unfair Tax Exclusion for Employer-provided Insurance

The principal tax subsidy for health is one of the government's open-ended health programs. Employees are granted an exclusion from federal income taxes, state income taxes, and federal social security taxes for any costs of health insurance paid on their behalf by an employer. Almost any insured procedure, no matter what its cost or reasonableness, can qualify for this subsidy. Again the definition of health is left vague enough for much to fall under its umbrella, for doctors to determine what is ordinary or necessary, for new technology to be applied immediately, and for multiple health care providers to be present for any particular procedure, so as to give the patient further protection against anything going wrong.

The subsidy violates almost every principle of both tax and health policy: it raises costs, it encourages excess consumption of health care and excess purchase of health insurance, it grants greater benefits to higher-income individuals than to lower-income individuals, and it discriminates greatly in the amount of benefits provided to persons equally in need of assistance.[11] It even causes distortions in the way labor markets are organized (Kosters and Steuerle 1981, 86–92).

If employees receive $100 more in employer-provided health insurance rather than cash wages, typically they will generate additional tax saving of approximately $35 in income tax, social security tax, and state income tax. Employees therefore will purchase $100 worth of insurance even when it has a value to them of only $65. Natural consequences are both cost inflation and inefficiency in the purchase of health insurance. The cost escalation is compounded to the extent that the insurance itself leads to a lack of cost-consciousness when actual medical expenses are incurred.

The tax benefits of employer-provided insurance also significantly favor higher-income individuals. These individuals are favored partly because they are more likely to receive health benefits from an employer. Figure 14–3 shows the percentage of the U.S. population at various income levels who are covered by employer-provided insurance. An individual at 250 percent or more of poverty is more than four times as likely to have this health insurance coverage as one at 50–99 percent of the income level necessary to move out of poverty.

Higher-income individuals are also more likely to have a generous plan than lower-income individuals, even if covered by an employer. In addition the benefits of the tax exclusion are greater at higher rates of

---

11. Earlier discussions of some of these problems can be found in Enthoven (1979) and Steuerle and Hoffman (1979, 101–15).

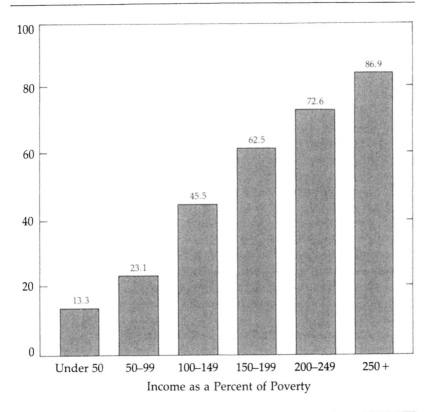

NOTE: Calculations exclude the institutionalized and the Medicare-eligible.
SOURCE: Author's calculations, based on Congressional Research Service analysis of data from the March 1990 Current Population Survey. See Ways and Means Committee *Green Book* (1991B, 309).

tax, although differences are not nearly so great as before passage of the Tax Reform Act of 1986.

Taken together, these last two factors imply a rise with income in the average value per recipient household of federal tax subsidies for employer health insurance. Although available data are limited, the rough estimates in figure 14–4 demonstrate that the average value for households in the fifth quintile of income—the richest 20 percent of households—is about $1,560, versus about $525 for households in the second quintile—the second poorest 20 percent of households.[12]

Even at the same income levels, there is little justification for providing substantially different tax benefits to individuals based solely on whether they work and the type of health insurance their employer offers.

Credits or Vouchers. A logical step toward greater equity and efficiency would be to cut back on the value of the employer exclusion and make a credit available to all taxpayers, or more specifically all taxpayers without access to Medicare or any remaining subsidy for employer-provided insurance. Far greater equity would be established among all taxpayers, whether or not employed, whether or not beneficiaries of employer-provided plans, and whatever the size of their plans. A credit would clearly be more progressive than an exclusion that mainly benefited higher-income classes.

Moreover, in keeping with the argument for economic efficiency, a credit rate of 100 percent of the first dollars of health expenditure is likely to be superior to an exclusion that applies to all expenditures, including the last and least valuable ones made. In effect a credit—combined with a cap or elimination of the existing exclusion—can be designed easily to avoid subsidizing the last dollars of expenditure on health insurance. This credit would help remove some of the cost-increasing features of existing law.

Relative to alternative health policies, a credit also has much to commend it. Perhaps one of its principal advantages is that it is much more likely to be finance-controlled, by design. That is, legislators would decide over time the amount to be devoted to the subsidy, according to finances available and other needs of society.

Assume, for example, that under a credit approach, the rate of credit would be 100 percent of certain health expenditures up to some fixed amount.[13] In this case, presumably almost all eligible citizens would buy at least the minimal policy that the credit would cover.[14] The total

---

12. This table is derived from census data that includes, in the definition of income, the market value of employer-provided health insurance and excludes the effects of taxes and transfers. Households falling into various quintiles are affected by this definition.

13. The suggestion that a rate of 100 percent be used is contained in Steuerle (1990A, 22–28), and in Steuerle (1990B, 38–40).

14. Certain beneficiaries of other government programs, such as Medicare or a remaining exclusion for employer-provided benefits, might not be eligible for the credit.

FIGURE 14–4

ESTIMATED AVERAGE VALUE PER RECIPIENT HOUSEHOLD OF FEDERAL
TAX SUBSIDIES FOR EMPLOYER HEALTH INSURANCE, FISCAL YEAR 1992
(dollars)

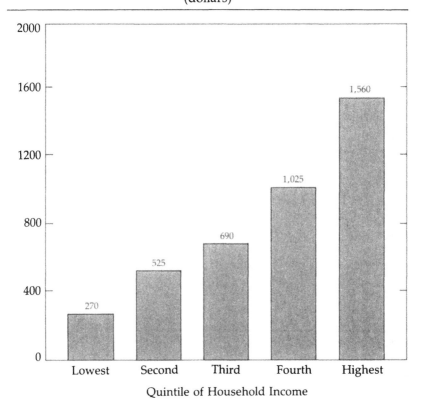

NOTE: Calculations are author's estimates for revenue loss, including both FICA and income tax. Marginal tax rate assumptions for each quintile are based on unpublished estimates from the Congressional Budget Office. The average value of employer-provided health insurance per recipient household by income quintile is derived from a U.S. Bureau of the Census study (1991A), which developed estimates for 1989 based on data from both the March 1990 Current Population Survey and the 1977 National Medical Care Expenditures Survey. Note that the definition of income used here to divide households into quintiles excludes the effects of taxes and government transfers, and includes the estimated market value of employer-provided health insurance.

SOURCE: Author's calculations, based on data from the U.S. Bureau of the Census (1990B) and the Congressional Budget Office.

budgetary cost of the credit for each succeeding year would be determined primarily by the size of the maximum credit amount. If fixed in nominal terms, or even indexed for general price inflation, the cost of the credit would actually decline over time relative to GNP—except as future legislators each year added to its maximum amount.[15]

With this type of health subsidy, current legislators would not need to predetermine the needs of society for decades to come, but could allow future legislators and voters to determine how much to spend on a particular program such as health. This would be determined not simply by the health needs of the population but by other needs, such as education and research.

All health needs would not be treated as equal, either. At one point, preventive care may be favored over expansion of the credit; at another, it might be research on a newly recognized problem, such as AIDS; at another, long-term care for the disabled; at still another, hospice care, meals-on-wheels, or assistance for chronic rather than acute care. The credit may be increased to allow for expansion in services covered under insurance; many new demands, however, could be subsidized or funded better through other programs. It is impossible to determine in advance which needs are most important and which procedures can be expanded most efficiently through additional subsidy.

An added attraction of a credit or voucher approach—especially one that would apply at a rate of 100 percent—is that it would provide a mechanism to start dealing with the so-called notch problem in Medicaid. For most low-income individuals, Medicaid either is available or is not. If one receives Aid to Families with Dependent Children (AFDC), Medicaid insurance is provided. If additional income of one dollar moves a person just beyond eligibility for AFDC, Medicaid benefits are not available.

With a credit or voucher, health insurance benefits can be designed never to be completely lost when Medicaid eligibility ends. If the size of the voucher is small relative to the value of the Medicaid, either states or the federal government could also supplement the basic federal voucher for moderate income households without making medical assistance an all-or-nothing proposition.

In summary, a credit or voucher for health insurance would recognize different forms of health care as competing both with each other and with other important needs of society. A credit-based scheme

---

15. By the same token, a credit need not be finance-constrained. A credit could be given for a given percentage of any cost incurred, in which case the cost of the credit would rise over time without limit and regardless of available funding and other social needs.

tries to avoid imposing on policy makers the types of straitjackets that have so constrained budget making in recent years. This flexibility and adaptability is one of its greatest strengths relative to both current law and most national health insurance proposals.

Play-or-Pay

In the broadest sense, play-or-pay proposals are also finance-based schemes requiring that either insurance be purchased (play) or a tax be assessed (pay). At their core, play-or-pay plans are justified by the notion that it is unfair and often inefficient for some to impose costs on others who are no more capable of bearing those costs.

Under the current health care system, many individuals do not pay for their own insurance. Later when they become ill they may fall back on subsidized parts of the system, such as charitable care or welfare. Even those not initially eligible for such assistance may become eligible if health conditions become severe enough and income falls adequately. In effect many of those labeled as uninsured have a backup insurance system.

Who pays for this insurance? Where public assistance is involved, the taxpayer pays. Hospitals have found it difficult to turn away patients, however, even when the government does not provide support. In these cases, other paying patients usually cover the cost of the uninsured. These costs show up indirectly in higher hospital charges and higher premiums for health insurance. Certain inefficiencies are also introduced, as these additional costs come to be treated like a hot potato that different insurers and providers try to pass on to others. These considerations have led some employers with generous health plans to support play-or-pay requirements as a means of reducing their own costs of subsidizing others.

Note, by the way, that the equity principle underlying play-or-pay must be distinguished from the goal of establishing greater progressivity. Although advocates of health reform often talk about increasing the supply of health care or lowering its cost for low-income individuals, this claim mixes two independent goals. The first is helping low-income individuals to have sufficient available income for the purchase of health insurance—and possibly other goods. The second is requiring individuals to purchase health insurance or, more specifically, health insurance with particular characteristics. Each goal—greater progressivity and required health insurance coverage—must be justifiable in its own right. If greater income is desired for low-income individuals, then why require income to be spent on health insurance? Perhaps education or job training would make a better investment, or food and clothing would be preferred forms of consumption. Similarly, if requiring everyone to buy health insurance makes sense, then its merits cannot depend mainly on the amount of redistribution achieved along the way.

The ability of some to ride free on others' payments of taxes and insurance is a problem that applies at all income levels. Even at higher-income levels, many people are not covered by insurance.[16] At the opposite end, many individuals with low wage rates purchase health insurance. Economists would assert that employees receiving $10,000 in cash wages and $5,000 in a health insurance policy from an employer essentially earn $15,000 of income, $5,000 of which goes to purchase health insurance.[17] If other employees earning $15,000 a year do not purchase health insurance, they may ride free on the contributions of those who were no better off in the first place. In public-finance terms, this is a problem of unequal treatment of equals, or horizontal inequity.

Although not precisely the same, the requirement that individuals purchase automobile insurance is based on similar considerations of equity. Injured parties should not be made to bear the costs imposed by uninsured motorists who are equally capable of buying insurance.

Employer versus Individual Play-or-Pay. The term "play-or-pay" has been applied almost exclusively to mandates on employers such as those contained in plans offered by the Pepper Commission (Pepper Commission 1990), the National Leadership Commission on Health Care (National Leadership Commission on Health Care 1989), the Chairman of the Ways and Means Committee (Ways and Means Committee 1991), Alain Enthoven and Richard Kronick (Enthoven and Kronick 1989), Karen Davis (Davis 1989), Henry Aaron of the Brookings Institution (Aaron 1991), and the Urban Institute's John Holahan, Marilyn Moon, Pete Welch, and Stephen Zuckerman (Holahan, Moon, Welch, and Zuckerman 1991).

This is confusing. In fact, a wide variety of proposals without employer mandates also follow a play-or-pay logic. For instance, Mark Pauly, Patricia Danzon, Paul Feldstein, and John Hoff (Pauly, Danzon, Feldstein, and Hoff 1991) would require increased individual income taxation of individuals who do not buy health insurance. This is nothing more than play-or-pay at the individual level. Uwe Reinhardt has proposed that non-poor Americans without health insurance essentially play by buying a mandated insurance package or pay an additional individual tax (Reinhardt 1989). The Heritage Foundation recently proposed not only that a credit be made available for purchasers of health insurance—a part of their plan that is often highlighted—but also that

16. Katherine Swartz, for instance, found that 22.9 percent of the uninsured have family incomes of three times the poverty level or more. See Swartz (1989, 10).
17. For this simple example, tax considerations are ignored.

all individuals pay a penalty if they do not purchase health insurance (Butler 1990). The latter part of their proposal, again, is a play-or-pay scheme at the individual level.

Jason Juffras and I have proposed that any new child credit made available to middle- and upper-income households be conditioned upon the purchase of health insurance for those children. In the absence of a child credit, we have also suggested that personal and dependent exemptions be denied to middle- and upper-income taxpayers who do not provide health insurance to their households.[18] These, too, are modest play-or-pay schemes. Four contributors to this volume alone—Henry Aaron, Stuart Butler, Mark Pauly, and I—are among those associated in different ways with play-or-pay.

How can characters thought to be so disparate (some might say, desperate) be found to support a similar logic for health reform? At the core, each falls back implicitly or explicitly on principles of public finance. Assuming it can be made to work, a penalty for not purchasing health insurance is a means of trying to create greater horizontal equity and eliminating inefficient cross-subsidization.

In design and implementation, play-or-pay proposals differ significantly from each other. Since the equity argument is undoubtedly an individual one, however, mandates on employers turn out to be rather blunt instruments for achieving greater fairness. To begin with, if there is a common logic behind all play-or-pay schemes, then that logic clearly is not confined to a subset of the population who happens to work. In many proposals the requirements are limited even further to full-time employees—thus providing a significant incentive for employers to convert employees to part-time.

The employer requirement either to buy health insurance or to pay a tax also raises the effective amount of minimum wage that an employer must pay. Almost all economic analyses show that increases in the minimum wage decrease employment among low-income individuals. The adverse consequences are also most likely to show up in smaller firms—those that currently provide fewer health benefits than others.[19]

---

18. Unlike many of the other individual proposals, our penalty tax does not make a person eligible for a public plan. It is simply a penalty for the probability that the individual may fall back on public assistance or charitable care. See Steuerle and Juffras (1991).

19. In an especially illuminating study, Sheila Zedlewski details the effects of employer expansion on insurance costs for firms of various sizes. A broad mandate would raise health insurance costs for all employers, for example, by 34 percent, but by 81 percent for firms with fewer than twenty-five employees. See Zedlewski (1991, 4).

Note also that employer requirements may have undesirable consequences on groups that legitimately want to work for cash wages. Spouses of employees with health plans, for instance, may prefer to receive cash rather than another health insurance policy. Teenagers in families are often in the same situation. Elderly individuals who want to work may be unable to obtain jobs if their health costs must be covered by an employer, and firms with many senior workers may simply go out of business (Steuerle 1990B).

In most employer play-or-pay systems, the pay part pushes individuals into a public plan. Unfortunately, undesirable redistributions occur as employers and individuals then sort themselves into two groups: those for whom it is cheaper to pay than play, and those for whom it is cheaper to play than pay. The tax rate may not be stable as selection between these two groups takes place. Regardless, there seems little justification for employees in low-risk occupations, for instance, to subsidize the health insurance premiums of high-risk employees who might also receive higher cash wages. Nor does it seem justified for firms with older workers to move into the public pay part of the system, while firms with younger workers find it cheaper to stay within the private system.

Suppose that the rate of tax in the public plan is based on total compensation or, as in the bill put forward by Chairman Dan Rostenkowski, on the Medicare wage base. Then high-income employees in the public plan are forced to subsidize low-income employees, while high-income employees in mandated private plans are not required to help bear that burden. Similarly, low-income employees in the public plan would receive subsidies from the government, while low-income employees in private plans would be forced to pay for most of their insurance through lower wages.[20] In effect, on both the benefit and tax sides of the equation, employer play-or-pay schemes usually violate the very principles of fairness or equity, as well as efficiency, on which they are first developed.

In truth, if play-or-pay makes sense, it does so at the individual level—where the burden is really borne. Requiring individuals either to buy insurance or to pay a tax, however, may be more difficult to achieve politically, because it does not hide behind the illusion that the employer is somehow covering the costs.

---

20. In a private plan, the cost to the employer of providing insurance to any employee equals the cost of the insurance policy. For employers using the public plan, the cost would be proportional to wages. Economic theory holds that employers will reduce cash wages by approximately the cost of other benefits that they provide.

Applying play-or-pay at the individual level, moreover, is not without its own technical difficulties. If an additional tax or penalty is to be paid by those who do not have health insurance, then some withholding system must be set up to ensure that those taxes are collected during the year. The IRS is simply incapable of going to millions of households, many of modest means, and collecting significant penalties or underwithheld taxes at the end of the year. Nor do many households have savings adequate to pay such a tax if there has not been withholding throughout the year. The regular income tax relies upon fairly flat rates of tax at moderate income levels, as well as upon overwithholding, to ensure that adequate tax is collected during each week and month of the year. Play-or-pay at the individual level must confront similar administrative issues.

It is therefore either impossible or enormously expensive to set up a separate tax structure to implement health policy goals. Each social policy in this country does not warrant its own tax system. Elaborate adjustment of the tax that would be paid by income level, for instance, probably is not feasible. Most people know only each April what their total income was for the past year. The tax system is confusing enough as it is, and people cannot guess their final annual income during each pay period of the year. Nor can they or their employers constantly adjust the insurance policy and withholding rate that must apply.

What are some play-or-pay taxes that could be administered at the individual level? Two are suggested here. A personal or dependent exemption might be denied for persons who are uninsured. An alternative procedure would be to apply a flat surtax rate to those without insurance. Both essentially would exempt lower-income individuals from the penalty.

Many schemes propose that individuals who pay must be made to join some public plan. Most of these proposals have not yet been developed in a way that could be made administrable. Individuals jump into and out of coverage quite frequently. According to the U.S. Bureau of the Census, approximately 31 percent of the nonelderly population went without health insurance for at least one month of the twenty-eight-month period between 1986 and 1988 (U.S. Bureau of the Census 1990a). The accounting for moving back and forth between private and public plans could be quite extensive and complicated. Some similar problems arise with the pay side of employer mandates, as well.

The tax system, moreover, is based upon an annual accounting period, whereas health insurance payments are made monthly or more frequently. If employers were required to report on whether individuals were covered at given times, those reports could take weeks to reach health officials who were to determine eligibility for the public plan. We could list many administrative issues that have been given little attention.

A simpler approach, at least to start, would be to let assistance rules determine who could use a public plan and let the penalty crudely represent a premium for the probability of falling back on public assistance—rather than have a penalty that provides unqualified access to a public plan. For middle- and higher-income individuals, the penalty would provide significant incentive to maintain health insurance policies. Increased coverage would reduce some public costs, and the penalties would also add moderately to revenues. Both these sources of revenues could be used to expand coverage at lower-income levels or, in the presence of a voucher or credit, to increase the size of the voucher or credit.

A note of caution is also in order. No significant change in tax or health policy can be achieved without some change in administrative burdens. Play-or-pay mandates require enforcement and reporting mechanisms. With individual play-or-pay, for instance, health insurance companies almost inevitably would be required to file information reports with the IRS and with the individual.

Conclusion

The public contribution to the nation's health care is even higher than commonly suggested. When tax expenditures are included, federal, state, and local governments will have spent close to $390 billion in this fiscal year for health. This amounts to about one-half of the nation's health care budget, and it is as much as is spent by many governments with national health insurance programs.

Individuals have little idea of just how much they are contributing for their own and others' health care. The average public and private expense per household is $8,000. Most of these costs are hidden from the individual and are paid through lower cash wages and higher tax rates. This leads to a lack of cost consciousness with respect to insurance itself and less pressure to keep underlying expenses of that insurance under control.

Expansions of public health care subsidies are forcing significant declines in spending on other social programs. One reason for the rate of expansion is the open-ended nature of most existing health programs. In addition, they are in-kind programs, and the value of the benefits provided is often less than the cost.

The major tax program applying to health—the exclusion provided for health insurance only if furnished by an employer—is not only open-ended, but is particularly unfair and inefficient. It directly leads to cost inflation and, additionally, is designed to be available if employers help to keep employees ignorant of the health costs they actually pay.

When the principles of public finance are applied to health policy, they suggest that it could be improved significantly by three means: by restoring greater equity and efficiency in existing programs; by allowing consumers to be more conscious of the costs they are bearing; and by eliminating the open-ended nature of most health programs, including the tax break for employer-provided insurance.

Conversion of the existing employer exclusion to a voucher or credit would create greater equity, would promote efficiency, and would lead to greater cost-consciousness. A voucher or credit has additional inviting features. It helps to reduce problems associated with the sudden elimination of eligibility for Medicaid when one more dollar is earned. Because it is not an open-ended mechanism for subsidizing health care, it grants future policy makers greater freedom on how to allocate money both within the health budget and between health and other social needs.

In addition, the principles of horizontal equity and efficiency establish a case for some play-or-pay mechanism. Employer mandates, however, turn out to be inefficient, unfair, and often regressive in their impact. Individual mandates avoid many of these problems, but they must be made as simple as possible in order to be administrable and to allow within-year withholding to be accurate.

While the case for a voucher over the existing tax exclusion and the case for some play-or-pay mechanism are separate, a combination of the two might provide a significant incentive for most households to purchase insurance. They would also lead to a substantial decline in the number of the uninsured. Moreover, they could easily be designed to provide even greater incentive for the coverage of children, if that were the preferred policy goal.[21]

Suppose that because of budget constraints these changes were made in an approximately deficit-neutral, expenditure-neutral, revenue-neutral manner. A modest voucher of $350 per person and a penalty of $387 per person (that is, the loss of a $2,150 exemption to someone in the 15 percent federal income tax bracket and a 3 percent state income tax bracket) could together provide a significant incentive for purchasing health insurance.[22] For a three-person household, the differential between purchasing and not purchasing insurance would then equal more

21. Since the cost of insurance for children is much less than for adults, an equal per-capita voucher and an equal per-capita penalty for not obtaining insurance would cover a much greater portion of the insurance costs of children than of adults.

22. The personal exemption actually equals $2,150 for 1991 and increases each year with inflation. If denial of this exemption is used rather than a surtax, there would be an additional penalty in states that piggybacked their income tax onto the federal system.

than $2,200 per year. Even more modest vouchers, credits, or penalties might provide a spur for many not to neglect their health insurance coverage.

These two changes could be designed not only to support but to enhance the basic structure of employer-provided insurance far more than most national health insurance plans do. First, employers are efficient purchasers of insurance, and they would maintain a strong incentive to act as administrative agents, bargainers, and withholding agents for employees. Second, if a voucher were made available, employers could be mandated to offer plans on which the vouchers could be spent.[23] Employers would then both withhold premiums from employees and adjust for advanced payment of the value of the voucher. Third, even as modest a penalty as the denial of a personal exemption would require adjustments in withholding by employers. This in turn requires a regular collection of data on whether employees and the members of their household maintain health insurance.

In effect, assessing the pay requirement of an individual-level play-or-pay scheme cannot be implemented without involving employers in some administrative responsibility for collecting the tax payments. Once again this would be an indirect way of mandating employer involvement in the health care of workers, but without most of the undesirable side effects of broad mandates that require employers to pay for the insurance itself.

Vouchers and individual play-or-pay requirements, therefore, could be designed in a way that would strengthen the role of the employer as an efficient intermediary for individuals. Some advocates of vouchers or individual play-or-pay schemes mistakenly skip over the important role of employer intermediaries in their advocacy of individual-choice models. They convey the misleading impression that the benefits of the existing employer-based structure would be abandoned, when in fact that structure could easily be reinforced and strengthened. In some cases, moreover, they complicate proposals for individually based vouchers or mandates in ways that may be too restrictive to be administered by employers.[24]

---

23. A similar employer requirement is contained in Meyer, Silow-Carroll, and Sardegna (1991).

24. For instance, Heritage would base the size of the credit upon anticipated health expenses compared with income (Butler 1990, 15), as would Herzlinger (1991, 78). Pauly, Danzon, Feldstein, and Hoff (1991, 10) would vary the maximum out-of-pocket expense for households according to their income. These types of variations could make it much more difficult for an employer to bargain over the price of plans, to know how much to adjust withholding, and to know how much credit would be available at the end of the year.

At the same time, advocates of national health insurance with play-or-pay requirements on employers sometimes hint that their schemes would rely on the basic employer framework already in existence, and that voucher schemes would abandon that framework. In actual fact the opposite is likely to occur. Employer play-or-pay schemes could easily lead to significant employer abandonment of private plans in favor of participation in a public plan. These employers simultaneously would give up some or all of the administrative functions associated with health insurance and would cease to worry about this aspect of the well-being of employees. Besides health insurance, such other effective interventions as physicals and inoculations might be forgone once those services were obtainable, even if less often used, under the public plan. Thus, despite the labels, a well-designed plan based on individual credits or mandates is more likely to maintain and reinforce the basic structure of employer-administered health insurance than are most employer-based mandates that encourage abandonment of private plans.

Would individual credits and mandates solve all problems in the medical marketplace? Hardly. They neither preclude nor prejudge debates on a wide variety of other issues, such as community rating for insurance policies, required acceptance of individuals with existing health conditions, establishment of subsidized reinsurance funds, malpractice reform, controlled evaluation of medical procedures, and so forth. Each of these issues would be debated on its own merit and is beyond the scope of this chapter. Finance-based schemes such as vouchers or credits and individual play-or-pay requirements, however, do not foreclose action on any of these fronts.

Even in the presence of widespread disagreement over how far the public health care system can be stretched, adherence to public finance principles still should lead to some similar conclusions among researchers and analysts of very different stripes. The creation of a mechanism more equitable and efficient than the existing employer exclusion should be recognized as a worthwhile objective in and of itself. In addition, the widespread use of play-or-pay schemes in health reform proposals implies at least an acceptance of the notion that individuals without insurance should not automatically be able to spread their costs onto others. A common meeting ground is suggested.

References

Aaron, Henry J. *Serious and Unstable Condition: Financing America's Health Care.* Washington, D.C.: The Brookings Institution, 1991.
Butler, Stuart M., ed. *Is Tax Reform the Key to Health Care Reform?*

Washington, D.C.: The Heritage Foundation, 1990.

Davis, Karen. "National Health Insurance: A Proposal," *American Economic Review* 79 (July 1989): 349–52.

Enthoven, Alain. "Recommended Low-Cost Changes to Existing Laws to Enhance Competition among Health Care Financing and Delivery Plans" (unpublished note, 1979).

Enthoven, Alain, and Richard Kronick. "A Consumer Choice Health Plan for the 1990s," *New England Journal of Medicine* 320 (January 5, 1989): 29–37 and (January 12, 1989): 94-101.

Havighurst, Clark C. "The Professional Paradigm of Medical Care: Obstacle to Decentralization." *Jurimetrics Journal* (Summer 1990).

Herzlinger, Regina E. "Healthy Competition." *The Atlantic Monthly* (August 1991): 69–80.

HIAA (Health Insurance Association of America). *Source Book of Health Insurance Data.* Washington, D.C.: HIAA, 1990.

Holahan, John, Marilyn Moon, W. Pete Welch, and Stephen Zuckerman. *Balancing Access, Costs, and Politics: The American Context for Health System Reform.* Washington, D.C.: The Urban Institute Press, 1991: 4–25.

Jensen, Gail A., Michael A. Morrisey, and John W. Marcus. "Cost Sharing and the Changing Pattern of Employer-sponsored Health Benefits." *The Milbank Quarterly.* 65 (1987): 521–50.

Kosters, Marvin H., and Eugene Steuerle. "The Effect of Fringe Benefit Tax Policies on Labor and Consumer Markets." *Proceedings of the National Tax Association* (1981).

Levit, Katherine R., and Cathy A. Cowan. "The Burden of Health Care Costs: Business, Households, and Governments." *Health Care Financing Review* 12 (Winter 1990): 127–37.

Meyer, Jack A., Sharon Silow-Carroll, and Carl J. Sardegna. "Universal Access to Health Care: A Comprehensive Tax-Based Approach." *Archives of Internal Medicine* 151 (May 1991): 917–22.

National Leadership Commission on Health Care. *For the Health of a Nation: A Shared Responsibility.* Ann Arbor, Mich.: Health Administration Press, 1989.

OMB (Office of Management and Budget). *Budget of the United States Government FY 1992.* Washington, D.C.: U.S. Government Printing Office, 1991a.

———. *Mid-Session Review of the Budget.* Washington, D.C.: U.S. Government Printing Office, 1991b.

Pauly, Mark V., Patricia Danzon, Paul Feldstein, and John Hoff. "A Plan for Responsible Health Insurance." *Health Affairs* (Spring 1991): 4–25.

The Pepper Commission (U.S. Bipartisan Commission on Comprehensive Health Care). *A Call for Action.* Washington, D.C.: U.S. Government Printing Office (1990).

Phelps, Charles E. "The Demand for Reimbursement Insurance." In Richard N. Rosett, ed., *The Role of Health Insurance in the Health Services*

Sector. New York: National Bureau of Economic Research, 1976.

Reinhardt, Uwe. "Toward a Fail-Safe Health Insurance System." *The Wall Street Journal* (January 11, 1989): A16.

Steuerle, C. Eugene. "Comments on the Proposal." In Stuart M. Butler, ed. *Is Tax Reform the Key to Health Care Reform?* Washington, D.C.: The Heritage Foundation, 1990a.

———. "Mandating Employer Provision of Health Insurance." Washington, D.C.: American Association of Retired Persons, May 1990b.

Steuerle, Eugene, and Ronald Hoffman. "Tax Expenditures for Health Care." *National Tax Journal* 32 (June 1979): 101–15.

Steuerle, C. Eugene, and Jason Juffras. "A $1,000 Tax Credit for Every Child: A Base of Reform for the Nation's Tax, Welfare, and Health Systems." Policy paper. Washington, D.C.: The Urban Institute, 1991.

Swartz, Katherine. *The Medically Uninsured: Special Focus on Workers*. Washington, D.C.: The Urban Institute Press, 1989.

Tolley, George S., and C. Eugene Steuerle. "The Effect of Excises on the Taxation and Measurement of Income." In *Compendium of Tax Research, 1978*. Washington, D.C.: U.S. Department of Treasury, 1979.

U.S. Bureau of the Census. *Health Insurance Coverage: 1986-88*. Series P–70, Current Population Reports. Washington, D.C.: U.S. Government Printing Office (1990a): 5.

———. *Measuring the Effect of Benefits and Taxes on Income and Poverty: 1989*. Series P–60, Current Population Reports. Washington, D.C.: U.S. Government Printing Office (1990b).

Ways and Means Committee. "The Health Insurance Coverage and Cost Containment Act of 1991." Reprinted in *Tax Analysts Highlights and Documents* (August 5, 1991a).

———. *1991 Green Book: Background Material and Data on Programs within the Jurisdiction of the Committee on Ways and Means*. Washington, D.C.: U.S. Government Printing Office, 1991b.

Wessel, David. "Medicaid Is Beginning to Look More Like Part of the Problem with the Health Care System." *Wall Street Journal*, August 8, 1991b.

Zedlewski, Sheila R. *Expanding the Employer-Provided Health Insurance System*, Report 91–3. Washington, D.C.: The Urban Institute, 1991.

15

Elimination of Employer-based Health Insurance

Warren Greenberg

Many have recognized the need to improve efficiency in the health care marketplace. Indeed, until the late 1970s, the U.S. health care system was remarkably inefficient and regulatory. It was driven by cost-based reimbursement, state regulatory controls on hospital costs and prices, federal and state health planning and certificate-of-need laws, severe limitations on hospital privileges for nonphysician providers, and a complete absence of information about the quality of care and price of providers.

During the past decade and a half, major gains in efficiency in the delivery and financing of health care services have come about.

In 1976, 175 HMOs had 6.016 million individuals enrolled. In 1990 569 HMOs had 36.5 million enrolled (Lane 1991; *HMO Fact Sheet* 1991). In 1976, there were no preferred provider organizations (PPOs); in 1990 there were approximately 800 PPOs with about 55 million persons eligible to enroll (Pickens 1990). In 1981, 23.9 percent of employees of medium and large firms had a choice of health plans, while in 1985, the most recent year for which data are available, 34.5 percent had a choice of health plan (Jensen et al. 1987, 530).

Before 1975 the professions, including health care, were exempt from antitrust prosecution by the Justice Department and the Federal Trade Commission. After the *Goldfarb v. Virginia State Bar* decision in 1975, which lifted immunity from antitrust legislation for professionals, federal antitrust litigation in the health care industry grew faster than in any other industry on the agenda of the Federal Trade Commission. Physicians could no longer boycott cost-containment efforts of third-party insurers, anticompetitive hospital mergers could no longer take place, and physicians could no longer interfere with HMO growth.

I would like to thank Avi Dor, Wynand van de Ven, and Deborah Kamin for their helpful comments.

The number of state regulatory programs has also declined. Currently, only the state of Maryland has an all-payer system, compared with nine states with prospective reimbursement systems in 1975 (Merritt 1991; Fanara and Greenberg 1985). No longer are there federal certificate-of-need regulations; in addition, state health-planning legislation has largely been abolished.

Consumer information on the quality and price of providers is still scarce. Yet the Health Care Financing Administration (HCFA) has published total Medicare patient mortality rates as well as those for sixteen diagnostic categories for nearly every nonmilitary hospital in the country since 1986. In the private sector, a large number of PPOs have begun to include only the hospitals in their organization that they believe to be of high quality. The Travelers Companies, for example, have preferred provider relationships with twelve transplant programs chosen on quality-of-care standards (*Health Care Competition Week* 1991).

Imperfections in the Health Care Marketplace

Nevertheless, there are still a number of imperfections in the health care marketplace. The diagnostic related groups (DRGs), for example, established in 1983 for the Medicare program, are directed only at the in-hospital segment of the health care sector. Under DRGs, unlike in other industries, the government (the buyer), rather than the provider of care, establishes the price for approximately 475 diagnoses. Hospitals with different levels of demand, quality of care, or marginal costs receive the same payments, although there are some broad differentials for urban-rural, teaching-nonteaching, and the like.

The resource-based relative value scale now sets the payments for physicians' fees. Physicians within specialty groups are paid the same amount for services delivered regardless of the demand or quality of physicians. Similar to the DRG payment, the government (as buyer) sets the amount to be paid for each service delivered.

Another imperfection in the medical marketplace is the barrier to entry to key resources. Physicians, for example, have attempted to bar staff privileges at hospitals to allied health professionals. In 1990, physician groups were found to have violated the Sherman Act by denying hospital staff privileges to chiropractors (*Wilk v. American Medical Association*, 1990).

Moreover, because employer-paid health insurance premiums are still not subject to an individual's federal, state, and local income taxes, people have an incentive to purchase more insurance than they would if health insurance were subject to taxes.

Clearly, an efficient marketplace in health care has not yet been achieved. It will continue to be an important concern for academic researchers and public policy makers.

In contrast to an emphasis on efficiency, less attention has been focused on improving equity in the financing and distribution of health care services, perhaps because economists have found it difficult to measure and evaluate equity scientifically. Moreover, inequities in health care may stem from differences in health status as well as from differences in income. Yet it appears that some semblance of equity appears to be a goal among Western nations. Even the United States has periodically discussed national health insurance with a minimum amount of coverage for all. Community rating, which groups all individuals in a single employer group, regardless of health status, into a single payment catchment was a dominant form of health insurance in the United States until the 1970s. Medicare and Medicaid made at least a nod toward equity when they were adopted in 1965.

This chapter emphasizes equity as well as efficiency in health care. A nation with 35 million people uninsured and 30 million people underinsured, while others in the population may have unlimited access to the latest advances in medical technology, can use improvement in distributing services more equally. A more equal distribution of health care services may improve the human capital of the population and reduce some costs if preventive care is used.

Can the United States improve efficiency in its health care system and at the same time achieve some much needed gains in equity? In this chapter I examine the current Dutch health care system, which appears to be highly regulatory, inefficient, and inequitable. Second, I explore the Dutch government's proposals and rationale behind a new, market-oriented health care system, due to be implemented by 1995, which would be less regulatory but more efficient and equitable. Third, I suggest how elimination of employer-based health insurance, and other tenets of the proposed Dutch health care system, may provide more efficiency as well as improve equity in the U.S. health care system. Adopting the Dutch proposals may also increase the productivity of the U.S. work force.

The Current Dutch System

Until the late 1980s, the Dutch health care system suffered from a lack of both efficiency and equity, suggesting that a highly regulated system is not necessarily equitable. In other countries in which health care is heavily regulated, such as Canada, Great Britain, and Israel, there are inequities in the distribution of such services as well.

Two insurance components in the current Dutch health care system make for a built-in two-tiered system. Those earning less than $25,000 a year (approximately 60 percent of the population) and the unemployed must enroll in a sickness fund in their geographic region. There is, therefore, no competition among sickness funds. (Price competition among sickness funds would be nonexistent in any event since all sickness funds are required to charge the same premium.)

Sickness funds have standard benefit packages of physician, hospital, and some dental services. Payments for hospitals and physicians are negotiated with the sickness funds and are the same for each physician type and hospital. In each sickness fund, medical specialties practice on a fee-for-service basis, while general practitioners are paid on a capitation basis. Selective contracting is not allowed. Physicians or physician groups are exempt from antitrust prosecution. Sickness funds have no incentives to be efficient since they are reimbursed by the government according to the health expenditures of their members. If sickness funds are able to reduce costs through efficiency, reimbursement is reduced in the same year. In general, half the premium of the sickness funds is paid by the employer and half by the employee.

Individuals with wages of more than $25,000 a year and those who are self-employed have the opportunity to enroll with one of seventy commercial insurers. (Those with incomes less than $25,000 a year are eligible to enroll with a commercial insurer but rarely do, since they would have to pay an additional premium.) Uniform payments for physicians and hospitals are negotiated with all the commercial insurers. Although one may have a choice among commercial insurers, they have generally not competed on a cost-containment basis. The uniform fees of physicians and the potential boycott (due to the absence of antitrust legislation against providers) by providers against the insurers if cost-containment activities were to be put into place have inhibited cost containment. Commercial insurers may, however, compete on price as well as on a risk selection basis by attempting to attract the healthiest individuals. Therefore, higher-income, healthy individuals who are enrolled with a commercial insurer may pay less for their health insurance coverage than lower-income individuals enrolled in a sickness fund. In addition, some commercial insurers may provide better service since they must compete against one another for business. As in the sickness funds, premiums are generally paid by the employer and the employee.

Although the commercial carriers may elect not to enroll high-risk individuals, less than 1 percent of the Dutch population does not have health insurance. Individuals eligible for insurance in a sickness fund are automatically enrolled without regard to health status. In addition, individuals may continue with commercial coverage, regardless of health status, if they leave their employer group.

In addition to the absence of choice of sickness fund for the majority of the population, the Dutch government has attempted to restrict the supply of providers. Family physicians cannot open new practices in areas where an ample supply exists. The number of medical specialists is restricted. Hospitals must receive governmental approval to increase the number of their beds or to invest in new, expensive technology. The government must also approve expansion and location of nursing homes.

For catastrophic illnesses, the compulsory Exceptional Medical Expenses (Compensation) Act covers nursing home stays, special institutional care, and prolonged hospital stays. It is financed by income-related premiums paid by employees (van de Ven 1990, 1991).

The Proposed Dutch System

The current Dutch Left-center government and the former Right-center government have both approved a new health care system. Dissatisfaction with the present arrangement stems from a lack of choice among sick funds and the inequities of cream-skimming behavior by the commercial insurers. Health care costs also continue to climb. They were approximately 8.5 percent of the gross national product in 1990, up from 6.0 percent in 1970 and 3.3 percent in 1953. The lack of incentives for cost containment by the sickness funds and the prohibitions against limited provider plans were identified as contributors to this rise in costs. Finally, both the providers and the Dutch government believed that regulation had become unworkable. Calculation of the optimum number of providers in an area, for example, was an unachievable task for government and at the same time created barriers to entry for many providers.

Influenced by the academic work of Alain Enthoven of Stanford University (1978), in 1987 a health care commission created by the government and headed by W. Dekker, former president of the Phillips Corp., proposed a new system that increases efficiency while it stresses equity. The proposals are targeted at an individual—not an employer-based health insurance system.

Under the proposed system, each individual must pay an income-adjusted premium into a central government fund. Plans would be reimbursed by this fund based on a case-mix adjusted formula, which could include the degree of cost containment the population desires. If calculated properly, the case-mix adjusted formula would curtail any incentives for avoiding high-risk individuals since plans would be reimbursed for poor risks. The case-mix adjusted formula would also act as an upper limit on the amount of total health care expenditures a nation would tolerate. Limits are important since many procedures are performed, because of insurance, in which incremental costs exceed the incremental benefits. Without a limit, health care costs will continue to grow rapidly. Thus far, the Dutch government has not provided ground rules on what the limit should be.

Plans would be expected to contain costs by selective contracting, by utilization review, and by more efficient use of resources. Since each health care plan encompasses a broad health care package, providers would not have incentives to shift utilization to an unregulated segment to make higher incomes.

Individuals could then choose the health-insuring organization of their choice. Health-insuring organizations might be managed-care plans such as health maintenance organizations, preferred provider organizations, or traditional fee-for-service plans. All insuring organizations would be free to negotiate any kind of payment arrangement with providers. In addition to the income-adjusted premium, individuals could pay up to an additional 15 percent of the premium to enroll in the plan of their choice. Individuals could also choose plans based on the quality of providers, the conveniences, and the services. Plans must, however, have substantially similar benefit packages to prevent the plans from modifying the packages (with, for example, extremely high deductibles) to discourage high-risk individuals from joining.

Plans are encouraged to advertise price, quality, and any amenities. Government would ensure the financial solvency and truthfulness in advertising of each plan. Government would also be expected to help consumers evaluate the plans. In addition, private employers could help assess them and, in fact, could help pay the employee's premium. Specialized consulting firms might provide additional information about these plans in the same way that counseling firms offer information to high-school students on prospective colleges. Health care plans would be prohibited from colluding on price or on any other dimensions of performance, and neither providers nor plans would be exempt from antitrust action.

Under the proposed Dutch health care system, competition among health plans would increase efficiency to meet the needs of prospective buyers. The case-mix adjusted formula, an open enrollment period every two years, and the similar benefit package for each plan would enhance equity in access. Each person would be eligible to purchase a health care plan regardless of his or her income or health status. The unemployed, for example, would be required to pay only a nominal premium to the insuring organization of their choice to prevent individuals from free riding on the health care payments made by others. Cost containment could be achieved by a budget cap on each of the plans. Thus, the

Netherlands would move from a highly regulated, inequitable system of health care delivery to a more competitive and equitable system (van de Ven 1990).

Advantages of the Proposed Dutch System in the United States

The U.S. health care system could be made more efficient and equitable as well as more productive by eliminating employer-based health insurance and gradually moving toward the proposed Dutch system.

Gains in Efficiency. With the elimination of employer-based health insurance all individuals, regardless of employment status, would have a choice of health care plans during an open enrollment period. They could choose a plan based on what they perceive as the best quality-cost trade-off for them. In 1985, only 34.5 percent of employees of medium and large firms had a choice of health care plans (Jensen et al. 1987, 530). Before experience with the system, it is not clear how many plans or what types of plans might be offered under an individual-based system; the number and type would be a function of demand and any economies of scale in administering and controlling costs.

The current inefficiencies from nontaxable health care premiums paid by employers would be removed. Premiums now paid for health insurance by employers are exempt from an employee's federal, state, and local income taxes. This exemption creates incentives for employees to carry greater amounts of insurance and disproportionately benefits those in the higher tax brackets. Under the Dutch proposal all individuals would purchase health insurance with after-tax dollars; the incentive to purchase the more expensive plans would be reduced.

The transactions costs of firms with a high turnover of employees would be substantially diminished. Firms would not continually have to register new employees for health care benefits in such high-turnover industries as real estate, automotive repairs, and building construction, which currently employ approximately 27 million individuals (Schorr 1990).

Gains in Productivity. It has been estimated that 15 percent of the adult work force retain their current jobs or have changed jobs because of health care benefits (International Communications Research 1990). Such benefits might be difficult to obtain from an employer because, for example, one might have a preexisting condition or work for an employer who does not provide health insurance. Moreover, some individuals would like to return to school, to work part time, or to leave their job entirely; yet they continue with unproductive jobs because they would be unable to get health insurance or would have sharply reduced benefits without a full-time job. As yet, we have no estimates of the loss of productivity to society for those who cannot change jobs or who have switched jobs because of health benefits. There were, however, some 115 million employed civilians in the U.S. work force in 1988 with an average income of $16,000 a year (*Statistical Abstract of the United States* 1990, table 624, p. 378 and table 660, p. 400). Assume that forced retention or job change would have resulted in a productivity loss of just 5 percent of income or $800 per worker. Fifteen percent of 115 million workers (or 17 million) multiplied by $800 is equal to a $13.6 billion productivity loss. Additional research will be needed to estimate this loss more accurately.

Gains in productivity may also result if those who are currently uninsured acquire health care coverage. Studies have shown, for example, that women with diabetes mellitus who receive prenatal care incur less risk for themselves as well as for their children. Thus preventive care can increase the human capital of the work force as well as its subsequent productivity. In addition, such prenatal care appears to reduce expenditures on health care in later years (Hinman and Koplan 1984; Elixhauser et al. [forthcoming].

Gains in Equity. The proposed Dutch system ensures that everyone has insurance for basic health services. Individuals who formerly could not secure such coverage because of financial barriers or poor health would be able to purchase insurance. Those who have been unemployed or have recently lost their jobs because of a company's bankruptcy would be able to secure insurance (*New York Times*, July 2, 1991).

No longer would insuring organizations have incentives to compete by avoiding entire groups of high-risk employees such as groups of gay activists or those who work with asbestos. No longer would individuals employed with one firm pay higher premiums for the same benefits package than individuals employed in another firm simply because of the case-mix of employees (Swartz 1990). No longer would individuals employed in the same firm pay increasingly differentiated rates based on risk status. Individuals, however, would also be able to purchase supplemental coverage for such discretionary procedures as cosmetic surgery and amenities such as private hospital rooms.

In addition to improved equity of access to health services, health care premiums would be paid on an income-adjusted basis to improve equity in payment. This approach may be compared with the current employer-based system where nontaxable health care premiums paid by employers benefit the wealthiest individuals.

Potential Problems in the Elimination of Employer-based Health Insurance. Elimination of employer-based health insurance might involve less governmental bureaucracy and intrusion than any other health care proposals of which I am aware. Nevertheless, implementation poses a number of potential problems.

First, the capitation formula is difficult to compute. A valid prediction of utilization of health services may be based on such variables as previous utilization, functional health status, previous medical expenditures, disability, diagnostic information, and indicators of chronic medical conditions. Thus far, researchers have been able to account for about two-thirds of the maximum explainable variance of about 15 percent in individual health expenditures with case-mix measures (Newhouse et al. 1989; van de Ven and van Vliet 1990). Case-mix measures, however, need not be perfect because insuring organizations will also probably be unable to forecast the case-mix of their population and their future expenses with precision. Clearly, more research on case-mix measurement is needed.

Second, an "optimal" budget cap will be difficult to compute. Should the budget cap, for example, be set so that the marginal benefits of medical procedures to individuals as an aggregate are equal to the marginal costs to society or equal to the marginal costs to individuals as an aggregate? If the former criterion is selected, far fewer procedures will be performed since society's costs for a heart-lung transplant, for example, will be considerable, while the marginal costs to the individual (if he or she is insured) will be nominal. Calculating the marginal benefits and marginal costs will be a difficult task in any event. Budget caps may also be based on simpler criteria such as a review of health care expenditures in previous years.

If a budget cap is computed, it is not clear how insuring organizations will limit care. With a budget cap, however, they would have the flexibility to move individuals to the lowest-cost setting and deliver care in the most efficient manner. Insuring organizations, depending on the liability laws, may provide lesser amounts of care to individuals in the terminal stages of illness with little chance of recovery.

Third, a continual trade-off between efficiency and equity would exist at the maximum level to which insuring organizations may price their standardized benefit package. The ability to charge a higher price than 15 percent of the benefit package currently contemplated will allow for greater choice, price flexibility, and efficiency. It may, however, reserve the better-quality insuring organizations for only those who can afford it.

Fourth, the collection of increased payroll or income taxes may affect the hours worked and the labor supply (work effort) of individuals. Individual work effort may decline with an increase in such taxes. Employers, however, may no longer pay for health benefits, which could lower prices. The demand for additional workers might thereby increase unless higher wages are substituted for health benefits.

Fifth, the provision of insurance for those now underinsured and uninsured will raise health care expenditures. As yet no estimates are in on what the proposed Dutch system would cost, but increased preventive services and higher productivity could help offset the greater expected costs of coverage for more people.

The Low-Risk Equilibrium of the U.S. System

Given the current competition among insuring organizations, (1) it is not difficult to imagine an equilibrium that will make employers more hesitant to employ high-risk individuals; (2) if high-risk individuals are employed, they will pay increasingly higher rates for health insurance' and (3) insuring organizations will set higher and higher prices for high-risk employee groups. This possibility is not far removed from the Rothschild-Stiglitz equilibrium of insurance markets set out fifteen years ago (Rothschild and Stiglitz 1976). Moreover, smaller firms will become more reluctant to offer health insurance since the potential cost of a few high-risk individuals could not be spread out over many employees. If smaller firms do not offer health insurance, they will enjoy a cost advantage of about $3,200 per employee over the larger firms (*New York Times* January 29, 1991).

Larger firms, in turn, will also be reluctant to offer health insurance. As the costs of health care continue to rise, fewer firms will offer health insurance in the future. An equilibrium may exist where a handful of firms provide insurance to the healthiest individuals. It is not surprising that as the number of employees decreases in a firm, the percentage of firms in that size category that offer health insurance decreases (Helms 1991). If all firms are mandated to provide health insurance, employers will have the same incentive to avoid hiring high-risk workers, firms will pay higher rates for high-risk employees, and insuring organizations will set increasingly higher prices for high-risk employer groups.

The result may be not only a lack of health insurance for high-risk individuals but also increased unemployment. Such individuals may have a risk pool available to them, but it is not clear what the benefit package of the risk pool would be, what the terms of financing would be, and what form competition would take among insuring organizations, if any. Moreover, the unemployed or those employed in firms exempt from mandated coverage will not benefit from such coverage. (The Consolidated Omnibus Budget Reconciliation Act of 1985, however, allows workers to continue with their employer's health insurance coverage for eighteen months after termination if workers are willing to pay the premium for individuals.)

Toward Efficiency and Equity

Elimination of employer-based health insurance would bring about a substantial change in the financing and distribution of health care services in the United States. Some incremental steps, however, could be taken to alter our current system gradually.

First, the standardized benefit package requirement may be abandoned if it does not allow enough flexibility in benefit design. Insuring organizations may, therefore, compete by altering their benefit packages, but the case-mix adjusted reimbursement should prevent avoidance of high risks. With more high risks, insuring organizations would receive greater reimbursement. (The standardized benefit package would discourage discrimination if the case-mix adjusted formula had flaws or was not calculated correctly.)

Second, a budget cap need not be implemented. The United States may not desire, for example, a cap that might reduce funds for technological advancement or deny needed care to the terminally ill. If a budget cap is not instituted, however, health care costs will continue to grow.

Third, in the short run, employers might continue to offer health benefit packages. At the same time, the government could begin reimbursing competing, non-employer-based health insurance organizations on a case-mix adjusted basis with premiums paid by individuals to the government. The demand for non-employer-based insurance would grow as high-risk individuals found it increasingly difficult to get health insurance coverage from employers; an equilibrium would prevail where only healthy twenty-two-year-olds could get employer-based health insurance from large firms. Finally, employer-based health insurance would disappear. Employers, however, could still choose to pay the premiums for the employees' health insurance even under an individual-based system.

The Political Economy of Eliminating Employer-based Health Insurance

Political lobbying groups generally act in their own interest. Groups such as the American Medical Association and the American Hospital Association might therefore support the elimination of employer-based insurance, since universal coverage would generate greater demand for their services. The Health Insurance Association of America, Blue Cross–Blue Shield, and other health-insuring organizations would support the elimination of employer-based coverage because more individuals would then be covered under their policies. Large business firms might support it because the costs of health insurance would no longer add to the prices of their goods and services and consequently they would be more competitive with foreign firms, assuming that potential increases in wages would not equal the cost of health benefits. Small businesses would support it because a proposed mandated health benefits policy would no longer be a threat to their cost structure. Individual employees might support it because the uncertainty of being without health insurance would be removed. Those currently without health insurance and those underinsured would support it because they could then secure insurance.

Conclusions

This chapter has suggested that the elimination of employer-based health insurance, modeled after the proposed Dutch health care system, would improve efficiency, equity, and productivity in the United States. While the proposed Dutch system relies heavily on competition among insuring organizations and among providers to ensure efficiency and quality, it uses a case-mix adjusted budget cap to improve access and equity as well as to curb rising costs. The government would also play a necessary role in disseminating reliable information on insuring organizations and in prosecuting anticompetitive behavior of providers or insuring organizations.

Elimination of employer-based health insurance might be a gradual process in the United States. Case-mix reimbursement of competing insuring organizations by the government would be a good beginning step.

The Dutch government is now making changes in its highly regulatory health care system. A greater reliance on market forces along with government case-mix reimbursement could help achieve a more efficient and equitable system. If the United States is to bring greater efficiency and equity into its system, the Dutch proposal might be the road map to follow.

References

Elixhauser, Anne, et al. "Financial Implications of Implementing Standards of Care for Diabetes and Pregnancy." *Diabetes Care* (forthcoming).

Enthoven, Alain. "Consumer Choice Health Plan." *New England Journal of Medicine* 298, nos. 12, 13 (1978): 650–58, 709–20.

———. "Multiple Choice Health Insurance: The Lessons and Challenge to Employers." *Inquiry* 27 (1990): 368–75.

Fanara, Philip, Jr., and Warren Greenberg. "Factors Affecting the

Adoption of Prospective Reimbursement Programs by State Governments." In *Incentives v. Controls in Health Policy*, edited by Jack A. Meyer (Washington, D.C.: American Enterprise Institute, 1985).

"Health Care a Growing Burden." *New York Times*, January 29, 1991.

Health Care Competition Week. "Travelers, Blues Announce Organ Transplant Networks." June 24, 1991: 1.

Helms, W. David. "Expanding Health Insurance Coverage." Paper presented at the meeting of the Association for Social Sciences in Health, Bethesda, Md., April 1991.

Hinman, Alan R., and Jeffrey P. Koplan. "Pertussis and Pertussis Vaccine: Re-analysis of Benefits, Risks, and Costs." *JAMA* 251 (1984): 3109–13.

HMO Fact Sheet, Group Health Association of America, August 1991: 1.

Jensen, Gail A., et al. "Cost Sharing and the Changing Pattern of Employer-sponsored Health Benefits." *Milbank Quarterly* 65, (1987): 521–50.

Lane, Nina, of Group Health Association of America, Washington, D.C. Personal communication with author. August 14, 1991.

Merritt, Richard, director. Intergovernmental Health Policy Project. George Washington University, Washington, D.C. Personal communication with author. August 5, 1991.

Newhouse, Joseph P., et al. "Adjusting Capitation Rates Using Objective Health Resources and Prior Utilization." *Health Care Financing Review* 10 (1989): 41–54.

Pickens, Edward, director of special projects. American Managed Care and Review Association. Personal communication with author. October 1990.

"Retirees' Plight in Bankruptcies." *New York Times*, July 2, 1991.

Rothschild, Michael, and Stiglitz, Joseph E. "Equilibrium in Competitive Markets: An Essay on the Economics of Imperfect Information." *Quarterly Journal of Economics* 90 (1976): 629–49.

Schorr, Alvin L. "Job Turnover—A Problem with Employer-Based Health Care." *New England Journal of Medicine* 323 (1990): 543–45.

Statistical Abstract of the United States, 110th ed. Washington, D.C.: U.S. Bureau of the Census (1990).

Swartz, Katherine. "Why Requiring Employers to Provide Health Insurance Is a Bad Idea." *Journal of Health Politics, Policy and Law* 15, (1990): 779–92.

van de Ven, Wynand P.M.M. "From Regulated Cartel to Regulated Competition in the Dutch Health Care System," *European Economic Review* 34 (1990): 632–45.

———. "The Dutch Health Care System." Paper presented at George Washington University, Washington, D.C., May 1991.

van de Ven, Wynand P.M.M. and van Vliet, René C. J.A. "How Can We Prevent Cream Skimming in a Competitive Health Insurance Market?" Paper presented at the Second World Congress on Health Economics, Zurich, Switzerland, September 1990.

Commentary on Part Four

Mark Pauly places considerable emphasis on the value of choice with respect to consumption in general and to health insurance in particular. It is impossible to exaggerate the value of consumer choice in directing most market outcomes. The failure of economies that have relied on central planning is glaring and tragic. *Plan* has become a four-letter word. Out of politeness, those of us who have advertised the value of market allocation must suppress the temptation to say aloud what a little voice inside us keeps repeating, "We told you so." But we may be excused for gloating a bit.

When it comes to health insurance, however, I find the emphasis on retaining and expanding choice as an important objective of financing reform to be grossly exaggerated and the argument supporting this emphasis weak and unpersuasive. I believe that given the range of objectives in reforming health care financing, maintaining consumer choice in the selection of health insurance plans is not worthy of serious attention.

I have two reasons for suggesting this starting point. First, emphasis on choice rests on the premise that the one making the choice is the one who will enjoy or suffer the consequences of that choice. That assumption is not justified in the case of health care. The Mark Pauly who might elect to forgo mental health benefits is not the Mark Pauly whose daughter is later raped and requires extensive psychotherapy. The Henry Aaron who accepts a plan with strict limits on physical therapy is not the Henry Aaron whose spouse later suffers spinal cord injury in an automobile collision. The Mark Pauly and Henry Aaron of here and now are far more similar to one another, however different our tastes in health insurance may be, than would be the two Henry Aarons or the two Mark Paulys whose personalities, lives, and wants are separated by the chasm of physical catastrophe. Nothing could prevent the healthy Henry Aaron and Mark Pauly from making choices that the less fortunate Henry Aaron and Mark Pauly would rue, unless society intervenes in these choices. To be sure, although some loss would result from the imposition of

375

society's judgments about the appropriate scope and reach of insurance for health care, such loss is trivial compared with the gains to be achieved from preventing people from making mistakes they may later regret.

At a minimum, the emphasis on the loss from suppressing insurance choice requires some demonstration that the loss matters: I assert that choice among insurance plans does not matter much. Mark Pauly presents absolutely no evidence that it does. On the contrary, he reports, "Recent research on the relationship between income and the use of medical care, given a uniform illness level and uniform out-of-pocket payment, keeps turning up the surprising result that there is very little variation (at least in quantity of services and total expenditure), although there is substantial variation with income in the health levels achieved."

Why should one be surprised? Most medical spending occurs during high-cost episodes when patients under plans of almost any sort are fully insured and physicians make decisions about care based on medical criteria. Since Mark Pauly presents no information to document or quantify the importance of choice among insurance plans and the lonely wisp of information in the quotation I read disputes it, I urge that we start with the assumption that choice in types of insurance really does not matter very much.

Choice, of course, is a many-dimensioned thing. Choice among providers and the attendant competition among providers are or could be surpassingly important. That form of choice should be preserved and strengthened. But until someone presents at least a few shreds of evidence on the importance of choice among insurance plans, a decent respect for science requires skepticism. I stress this point because a large part of the case against proposals to mandate core benefits rests on the alleged loss of choice. That case has not even begun to be made.

Second, I, along with virtually every other economist I know, share the view that Mark Pauly and Eugene Steuerle advance on the desirability of either capping the exclusion of employer-financed health insurance from personal income tax or replacing the exclusion altogether with a credit. Mark Pauly refers to such a policy as "the good politician's dream policy." He raises, but does not really answer, the question of why politicians good enough to get reelected with almost plebiscital certainty have shown such seamless resistance to this dream idea. Those of us skeptical of the idea that real economic opportunities go unexploited— "You don't find $500 bills lying on the street"—should wonder why, if capping the exclusion is such a dream policy, consummately successful politicians run and hide whenever this idea is put forward by one of us good-government economists. Maybe we are missing something they see.

Finally, I have two comments on Eugene Steuerle's emphasis on the "undesirable redistributions" that arise under play-or-pay plans. He is perturbed that adverse selection between public and private plans may occur. Since health status is inversely related to income and age, high-wage and younger workers will tend to reap windfall benefits. Others worry that premiums, which standard wage theory tells us will depress wages dollar for dollar, are a regressive head tax.

At the risk of imperiling my credentials as a liberal whose heart regularly bleeds about income inequality and who does not feel that the economic juices would dry up if tax rates were higher and more progressive than they now are in the United States, I urge that not every public policy has to be "distributionally correct." A system of taxes, direct expenditures, and transfers may be improved by the addition of even a regressive element if such an addition deals with a serious national problem. Our current methods of paying for health care constitute a serious national problem. They breed inequity and inefficiency and in my view lead to excessive outlays, Mark Pauly's agnosticism on this subject notwithstanding. Let's adopt the policy with the best chance of dealing quickly with these problems and address issues of income distribution with other instruments.

Stuart M. Butler

An interesting aspect of all the chapters is the consensus that the current system of employer-based insurance for most individuals in this country has failed to achieve equity, affordability, and cost control, and the conclusion that the current system cannot achieve these goals. This observation leads to some rather interesting points about efforts to deal with our problems in health care through a play-or-pay approach.

Gene Steuerle tried to argue, "We're all play-or-pay advocates now." I resist this argument, even though technically each approach under discussion does suggest either a penalty or an encouragement through financial incentives for people to play rather than pay. In the discussion of the politics of health care, however, arguing that all these approaches are in fact a version of play-or-pay adds to the confusion. In this one case Gene Steuerle is more an academic than a political player in his discussion of actual politics.

From a purely political point of view, there is no question that play-or-pay is very attractive to politicians. It allows them to hide the cost of promised new benefits and to shift those costs to a part of the economy that is to some extent invisible. As Gene Steuerle points out, many inequities and problems are associated with that kind of approach.

Inside Washington play-or-pay has political problems. The complexities associated with trying to make play-or-pay equitable lead to complications: dealing with small employers, preventing employers from dumping high-cost individuals into the public program, designing two parallel systems that essentially run together, and the like.

These aspects of play-or-pay create political problems. While on the surface it is an attractive approach, in practice, as we try to design legislation to implement it, we have more and more problems.

In addition, creating institutions to operate a dual but parallel system is politically destabilizing. Moreover, institutions created to look at such things as fee structures in the medical profession and the design of insurance will take on a life of their own and become players in the political equation itself. This will lead to a transformation of play-or-pay into some kind of all-payer system.

Thus we are in practice talking about a radical reform, since a play-or-pay system ultimately would move decisively away from an employment-based system.

All the authors have considered how to move to some kind of alternative to play or pay, bearing in mind the political realities of the way Washington works—or as Mark Pauly put it, to create a "positive political economy" to move us in a certain direction.

I agree with Henry Aaron that capping or reducing the employer exclusion to finance some alternative will not work, whether it is a direct payment system, a Dutch-style sickness group arrangement, or the kind of voucher or tax credit approach that many of us have looked for. In the past, we have run into very heavy political weather with proposals to cap the exclusion. It has been proposed on many occasions. David Stockman opposed it quite vigorously in the early 1980s. He generated hostility from both sides of industry and very little support.

The key to breaking the impasse on this kind of approach is to combine a limit on the tax exclusion with very distinct benefits in one package, designed to provide some horizontal equity. In this way the inequity problems that Gene Steuerle and others mentioned in the current system are addressed. A new constituency to support a cap is created, with a new set of winners to challenge those who support the existing system. The package should make potential winners out of former losers in various ways. I favor approaches that would cap the benefits at the place of work and give credit for out-of-pocket expenses and that offer the possibility of portability, so that a person could continue with a plan and still get tax relief if he changes jobs.

These methods of capping the existing benefits system, while being politically sensitive to the need to create new winners, are needed to bring about political change. So there is a big difference between some of the proposals now being offered by the presenters and others that involve merely a cap on the existing exclusion. There is quite a big difference between the new approaches and what we saw in the early 1980s.

One other important point is the role of employers in any kind of transformation to tax credits. Some alternative to employment-based systems seems to be the only real choice for radical reform. Yet, that does not rule out any activity for employers. In some instances, of course, employers are a natural group for insurance purposes, because they offer economies of scale. Furthermore, as Gene Steuerle points out, even in an individualized system, employers can have very important functions managing the system, to make sure, for example, that people comply. Employers can be good at ensuring that individuals do, in fact, seek and obtain insurance in their own right, by providing proof to the government that their employees are obeying the law.

Employers can also be very helpful in making a simple payroll deduction of premium payments and sending those premium payments to the insurance company of the employee's choice—in other words, the bookkeeping function.

Alternatives based on individual credits would force employers to pay an extremely important and continuing role, but a very different one from that envisioned under the current system or any kind of play-or-pay system.

In ending, I concur with Mark Pauly's statement that we are gambling in an area of public policy and transformation of public policy, where we are trying to conjure a system that keeps various balls of cost control, efficiency, equity, public finance, and the like in the air.

Deborah Steelman

My single disappointment with all three chapters in this section is the exclusive focus on finance. In health care reform we must address delivery systems, lifestyle changes, and the public health role.

Moreover, all these proposals will require impractical levels of government regulation, and I am particularly worried about government's defining a single-benefit package. Such a definition would be a hindrance to innovation and adaptability.

Personal behavior responds not only to financing but also to factors in the culture and the society. My office building, for example, is a nonsmoking building. Two secretaries work for me in my small business, both of whom were smokers before they came to work in this building—they are now nonsmokers.

Some populations are very unlikely to be served through an insurance mechanism. These include the burgeoning non–English-speaking segment, for example, those who live in underserved areas, and those who are simply not capable because of alcohol abuse, drug abuse, or other circumstances to gain access to health care through the insurance mechanism.

A frightening statistic on this point concerns the four-year-olds who have been enrolled in the California Medicaid program since birth. Only a little over 30 percent of these AFDC children have seen a doctor or received a physical examination since birth; only 8 percent have had eye exams, and only 4 percent have received ear exams. Medicaid is failing a growing segment of the population. We must focus on these people to enable them to become an active part of our economy.

I believe that public policies for reform have to come about through politics. There is no public policy in a democracy without politics, and no true structural reform can occur without putting the current government programs on the table—Medicare, Medicaid, and the tax code.

We often discuss only the utopia that we want fifteen years from now. Yet, too often we neglect to apply real energy to taking the first step toward reform. And the first step is the most difficult politically.

The proposals in these chapters threaten such large change that many insured and satisfied people today prefer the status quo. When we attempt to destabilize a system that a vast majority of people are comfortable with, even if anxious over, the conservative tendencies of the most vested influences come to the fore. The first step must be to shake political alliances, rather than to destabilize the health care finance system itself. The conservative tendencies of Americans are very well known. While we may talk broad reform, many certainly do not want it applied to their lives today.

How then can we start to build the political alliances to achieve some of the policy reforms that have been described in these chapters? I believe we have to increase choices in every respect.

Medicare should have benefit packages among which Medicare recipients can choose. That population is clearly the most politically powerful, and until the concept of choice is embraced by that population, it will not be accepted by many federal politicians.

In Medicaid, we have to make choices possible for consumers, the states, and the communities. The federal government has to be much more willing to experiment, not only with the sort of additional benefits states can give but also in the delivery systems and how they meet the needs of the population that Medicaid is designed to serve.

In addition, I would recommend changes in the tax code. Today's tax code forces no choices. If we make changes in the tax code along the lines that have been proposed, the concept of choice as opposed to state-defined single-benefit packages must remain a priority.

Limiting choices will stabilize the current system and heighten the tolerance for the status quo, thus perpetuating the reliance on government and employers' responsibility, reducing the recognition of the need for greater personal responsibility, and continuing the economic threat posed by health care costs outlined so well in this volume.

The Role of Choice in
Health Policy Reform

Discussion of Part Four

ROGER FELDMAN, University of Minnesota: I am amazed that Henry Aaron is not willing to recognize the legitimacy of preferences for different health insurance arrangements. When people are asked what they want in a health insurance policy, some say low cost, others say freedom of choice, and yet others say no bother with paperwork.

At my university, with about 17,000 employees, when the freedom-of-choice policy was recently revoked, the protest was so great that we may withdraw from the larger group. Even though we probably would have a poorer risk selection, we may try to design our own policies.

While my example is anecdotal evidence, an increasing body of studies uses analytic methods to examine employee choice of health insurance arrangements. Maybe these studies do not meet Henry Aaron's standards for scientific acceptability, but at least they have been peer reviewed. They show that people can obtain a considerable amount of consumer surplus from being in their current health plan rather than in some of the alternatives offered to them.

Although I am certainly not in complete agreement with Mark Pauly and his colleagues in their proposal in *Responsible National Health Insurance* (AEI, 1992) one of its strongest points is that it recognizes diversity of preferences. I also felt very appreciative of Deborah Steelman's suggestion that offering more choices in Medicare might unblock some of the opposition to reforming that system.

CLARK C. HAVIGHURST, Duke University: I am right in the middle on this choice question. I would say to Henry Aaron that the glass is half full, that choice does have some benefits. Some very significant innovation in health insurance occurred in the 1980s. We had no choice to speak of before the 1980s, and we finally got some. The changes in health insurance in the 1980s were dramatic and important. I think it is a mistake to say that innovation stimulated by choice is not beneficial.

Earlier I talked about how we do not get enough choice from the health care financing system. So I would say to Mark Pauly and Roger Feldman that this choice glass is only half full. We need to work harder at trying to get more choice.

In response to Deborah Steelman's notion that we can have reform only through politics, I think some very useful reform can come through markets. We do need some cooperation from the courts, but I do not know that we have to have legislation. One could argue that legislation would help, but I would put more emphasis on contracts as well as vehicles of change. Earlier I challenged the health insurers to say how they would expand our choices. They refused to rise to that bait, but maybe in time markets will push them to give us more choice.

I am not prepared to go along with Henry Aaron, even though I agree that we are not getting all the choice that the market could deliver and that choice is currently not nearly as valuable to the consumer as it ought to be.

PATRICIA M. DANZON, Wharton School, University of Pennsylvania: I would like to respond to Henry Aaron's point about the schizophrenic Mark Pauly and the schizophrenic Henry Aaron, partly in defense of the Pauly-Danzon-Feldstein-Hoff health plan. Our plan does recognize the need for specifying some minimums, and we do stress minimum medical services that would be covered. We also specify a maximum out-of-pocket payment that individuals could take on and set a maximum stop-loss in the insurance part, which could vary by income. We specified those minimum benefits and the maximum stop-loss out of concern for free-ridership and myopia, which are the reasons for mandating in the first place.

Given the minimum benefits and a maximum stop-loss for out-of-pocket payments on those minimum benefits, the possibility of facing the sort of catastrophic loss described by Henry Aaron is protected against. Someone may have some regret, but he would not face anything like catastrophic schizophrenia under our plan.

In reference to Stuart Butler's suggestion that we trade some tax subsidies for out-of-pocket payments as a sort of quid pro quo for giving up some tax subsidies on the premium side, it is better to put all the tax subsidies on the premiums but leave out-of-pocket payments to perform the deterrence function that they are supposed to perform to control moral hazard.

DAVID DRANOVE, Kellogg Graduate School of Management, Northwestern University: It was very interesting to note the difference between the examples given by Roger Feldman and those given by Henry Aaron.

These reflected the types of diversity in the health insurance choices that individuals might make. Roger Feldman mentioned things like free choice of provider and the incentives that providers may face. Henry Aaron referred to specific service coverage—mental health care, optical care, and the like.

I have another example of why I think Henry Aaron's point is valid one: someone like me who wears contact lenses and eyeglasses may choose a health insurance plan with optical care; what I am really doing is seeking out a tax-subsidized purchase of a service that I expect to consume. That free choice allows us to take advantage of the current tax code is not, I think, a benefit of encouraging expanded choice.

GREG SCANLON, Health Benefits Letter: Mr. Greenberg, is the Federal Employee Health Benefits Program (FEHBP) a demonstration project of the Dutch system in this country, and if so, are there lessons to be learned from that?

WARREN GREENBERG, George Washington University: I like the idea of choice in the FEHBP. As I understand it, there are a large number of choices of plans, and I think that is a good thing. Some problem with risk selection exists among the plans, so I think we need to undertake more research on adjusting plans for case-mixes. It is an extremely difficult task.

To comment again on Henry Aaron's views on the role of choice, I gave an earlier example about the choice of universities. I would not be happy about having only one university in this country. I think we benefit by being able to choose among various universities or among various think-tanks. The burden is on Henry Aaron to show why we need one payer rather than multiple payers in the health industry. Why are we picking out this particular industry to limit choice?

H. E. FRECH III, University of California, Santa Barbara: Regarding choice in health care, Henry Aaron has staked out a really radical position here, and it deserves more discussion than it has gotten.

What he is most concerned about is that a person will decide not to cover catastrophic problems and later regret not getting the coverage. These regrets are a normal result of choice under uncertainty. When people buy fire insurance for their house and the house does not burn down, they may regret that they bought too much insurance. If, however, they bought little or no fire insurance and the house burns down, they may regret that also. Their response does not indicate market failure or necessarily any social problem because the rest of us feel that they should have it.

In the past, people often chose insurance with poor catastrophic coverage, partly because of the bad example of the Blues, who started health insurance in this country. But that problem is rapidly declining with the growth of coverage. People are more likely now to get catastrophic insurance.

Henry Aaron is trying to make a distinction between choice of insurance benefits and choice of providers. In a world with more and more types of managed-care schemes with different types of providers, the issue of choice cannot be separated in that way. If we want to preserve good, rational choices of provider, those choices have to be made beforehand through a choice of types of insurance benefits.

Moreover, if we have group insurance or sponsored insurance like that proposed by Alain Enthoven and Richard Kronick in *Consumer Choice Health Plan*, the important choices will be made by the sponsor, not the individuals. At that level it is especially unlikely that coverage of major catastrophic events will be omitted.

STEPHEN ZUCKERMAN, Urban Institute: I think the choices that we are discussing may not be as meaningful as people are led to believe. What happened over the 1980s was a lot of emphasis on choice of plan. There was segmentation in the provider market where HMOs and PPOs offered panels of physicians to different individuals. This trend is forcing changes in the choice of provider.

There is much agreement about catastrophic coverage in the various health reform proposals. The Pauly-Danzon-Feldstein-Hoff plan, for example, suggests a minimum benefit package with maximum stop-loss provisions. How such catastrophic coverage gets provided will be fairly similar in most proposals.

The education analogy, however, is not a good analogy here because people can make different choices about what they want out of education. There are fairly well-established clinical standards governing what the outcome is in health care, especially in the case of serious illnesses. We can detect whether people have, in fact, bought effective treatments.

When people talk about restricting choice, then, they are not really talking about restricting choice on less-serious benefits—the David Dranove example. Should we subsidize the purchase of contact lenses or health club memberships? I think not.

ROBERT HUNGATE, Hewlett-Packard: I would like to point out that Henry Aaron has added a very important element to the discussion of choice by focusing on the provider choice, which is another opportunity to make the market work better in the health care management system. Focusing purely on the choice of insurance plan ignores the health services part of the management of the activity.

JACK A. MEYER, New Directions for Policy: I think choice is very important. I will stand up for it, but I think it is a much more burning issue among economists than among the public at large, who seem to be primarily concerned with the issues that Warren Greenberg raised about the fairness of our system and rising costs.

At a recent conference the moderator began by saying we face a tough choice in health care today, whether to go with a national health plan or some sort of all-payer rate-setting and mandated-benefits approach. I was caught by surprise and tried to point out another option; I seemed to be the only one there concerned about the market alternative.

I see a wide disparity between the spectrum of opinion in our intellectual debates and the spectrum of opinion in the political arena. Those of us who have been advocating market-based approaches over the years lack an operational plan. In fact, the word *plan* came in for some tough sledding a while ago. But while planning may have fallen into disrepute in some quarters, in fact to sell something and get it done, we have to package it and tell people what we want to do in some detail. Many proposals coming out now have done that.

What the choice-market-incentive school of thought lacks is some way to translate theory into action. Therefore, what we have is two kinds of plans and a school of thought, and the school of thought is not really in the arena right now in my view.

We need to do some hard thinking about what needs to be done to translate some interesting theories and ideas into an approach that could be debated. Otherwise, at some point changes in the system will have happened, and we will not have had much say.

RITA RICARDO-CAMPBELL, Hoover Institution: I have two brief points. First, catastrophic insurance was lost in 1965, when Medicare and Medicaid were established, primarily through trade union opposition. Now trade unions have been less active in this area, and it may be worthwhile to try again, because catastrophic health insurance would be more desirable than what we have.

Second, I have been impressed by the diversity of the choice among plans in the federal FEHBP. A recent *Washington Post* article compared premium rates by the plans. The one thing that stood out is the emphasis on fees. In the case of HMOs and PPOs, the fees for families were three and, in some instances, four times that for individuals. Where the family is changing, as in California, the premium differentials may be influenced.

HAROLD S. LUFT, University of California, San Francisco: I weigh in somewhere in the middle on this choice question. We should encourage as much choice as possible in the style of delivery systems. We should limit choice, however, when various delivery systems—providers, insurers, and the like—are using the structure of the coverage and the benefits to risk select. We probably cannot second-guess them, but many things come to mind. The eyeglass example is an obvious one, as well as coverage for psychological treatment and substance abuse.

Let the carriers and the providers get together to figure out how to deal with adverse selection. Since this group understands the business, they know which plans are getting the high-risk people. Let them design ways to limit the manipulation of the benefit coverage. Manipulation of benefits must be limited in some way. I do not think we need much limitation, though, on the choices available in the delivery system. And we should not use the term *choice* as some political code word that means different things to different people.

WILLIAM J. DENNIS, JR., NFIB Foundation: As time goes on, we will get better at finding individual cases of risk, as the studies of genetics, for instance, become more sophisticated. We will get much better at cream-skimming the low-risk people. Would some sort of Dutch system such as Warren Greenberg described eliminate such selection of risk to a great extent?

MR. GREENBERG: Yes. What we could do is limit the purview of insurers to avoid the high-risk individuals, as best we can, by devising a system to adjust for risk. As difficult as it is, this approach would help avoid risk-selection competition among insurers. If we could figure out how to do that, then we would have choice based on all kinds of other criteria, such as the degree of cost-containment, quality, and convenience that consumers desire.

RICHARD KRONICK, University of California, San Diego: The question of whether we want the choice to buy a package of benefits that does not include medically necessary care is a question to which I think most of us would answer no. We all want to buy a package of medically necessary care.

The question that Clark Havighurst brings up is, How can we have choices when there are different definitions of what is medically necessary? That, of course, is unknown. It is important to have choices among provider groups that may either explicitly, in Clark Havighurst's suggestion, or implicitly in the current world give us choices of what is medically necessary—for example, under what conditions do we need an MRI or angioplasty. That is very important, but none of us are likely to make choices to not buy things that are "medically necessary."

HENRY J. AARON, Brookings Institution: I agree that choice matters. What I have tried to suggest, however, is that certain aspects of it really do not matter much, while others are very important.

With respect to the technical point that Roger Feldman and Ted Frech raised, I am not arguing about decision making under uncertainty, but I do argue that the judgments we make at one time may not be the ones that we later wish we had made.

With respect to variations in insurance benefits, benefits can come in different shapes. There are differences in cost sharing, for instance, which offers real consumer advantages if people's desires can be matched with cost sharing.

If we sacrifice some benefit choice, though, we would not have lost a great deal relative to other objectives of health care financing reform. We would have lost something. I am not taking an extreme position on this. But to the extent that welfare gains or losses are implied in particular benefit packages, we risk big gains or losses that we would not as a society want to accept. Therefore, I believe we are better off with a relatively uniform basic benefit package than with a varied one.

Another issue is whether we link financing of insurance to the provision of care. In my view, we can separate these two. We can reimburse physicians and have different methods of contracting with hospitals arranged by Prudential, Blue Cross-Blue Shield, or Kaiser. Therefore, we could get the benefit of the ability of HMOs, for example, to get price discounts. This is an issue of who shares in the cost between providers and payers.

MARK V. PAULY, Wharton School, University of Pennsylvania: In my commentary, I did not intend to stake out a position but to point out how critical it is to understand how much variation in preferences there really is among Americans. Even though it is difficult to document the true degree of variation because of the effects of risk selection and tax incentives, I believe it is necessary for understanding what we want to do.

Steve Zuckerman said he was not persuaded that we are talking about restricting choices on very meaningful dimensions. I completely disagree. Some dimensions I think are not so meaningful. I believe, for example, that deductibles are useful but not immensely so. And the degree of managed care and strictness is probably important, but not enormously consequential.

But I think the most meaningful dimension of choice is one that we know almost nothing about: the rate of introduction of new technology. That, after all, is what is driving health care costs. That is what we are arguing about—how much can we constrain new technology, how much do people want it to be constrained, and how different are they in their preferences for it?

I have a prospectus for an HMO I would like to start up; our slogan will be "Last year's technology at last year's premiums."

Jack Meyer said choice is a much more burning issue among economists than among the public. We economists, he said, are not as worried about greater equity as citizens are. I think that is wrong. It is not polite for people to talk about how they really feel about equity, but even some of Robert Blendon's surveys (for example, "Views on Health Care: Public Opinion in Three Nations," *Health Affairs* [Spring 1989]) suggest that they are not so keen on helping out the poor.

If we had better evidence on how much good more generous coverage would do, we might be able to persuade the majority of Americans to be more concerned about the poor. But I think what most people are worried about is that the government will tell us what we can and cannot do for ourselves or our family when we are sick, even with our own money. That is my own perception.

Warren Greenberg wants to limit the purview of insurers to avoid high-risk individuals. So do I. I think the way we do that is let insurers charge the price they need to to cover the cost they expect to bear. Then make transfers to high-risk individuals as part of the social obligation to ensure they can afford the insurance premium that the market generates.

PART FIVE

The Politics of
Health Policy Reform

Commentary

Dave Durenberger

Public opinion makes clear that the problem facing Americans is not universal access to health care or, as it was in 1988, long-term care. The problem is cost.

The experience of a Washington couple, Lew and Carol Olsen, exemplifies the problem. In 1989 Carol delivered a healthy eight-pound baby in a Washington hospital. The cost of her pregnancy—without complications—was over $7,000. That same procedure at the Mayo Clinic in Rochester, Minnesota, costs $2,400. That same procedure in 1934 to deliver me—apparently a difficult birth—was $31.

The answer to cost is coverage. Traditionally about 12 percent of Americans have been unable to pay their doctor and hospital bills, even when medical costs were low. But doctors and hospitals had been able to carry these people. Now we are more concerned about the uninsured. Why? Because we fear the future—a future in which we may be financially unprotected against very high medical costs.

The politics of health care and health care reform is a volatile subject, as the pollsters have shown, because it is about life and death, pain and suffering, and billions of dollars.

A cartoon by Jerry Fearing of the *St. Paul Pioneer Press* shows a doctor assessing an uninsured patient while his relatives are saying, "Help him! Do something!" In the next scene, the doctor points a large needle called "Universal Health Service" at the relatives, and they are all running out the door.

My experience is that when you translate the problem of costs into coverage and you ask people to take responsibility, they all run out the door. My unscientific sampling shows that Americans are upset about the national health system but are satisfied with their own part of it and their own doctor. This is an example of wanting to go to heaven, but not wanting to die to get there.

Four elements are necessary for health reform. The first is a common understanding of what the health care problem in America is. Unless we understand the problem, we cannot solve it. Second, we need a vision for the future—a vision that no one has yet provided. The third is a proper set of values and a way to adjust our current values to match them. For thirteen generations Americans did not need to deal with values, since each generation was able to leave their children better-off. My generation, unfortunately, is the first to leave our children less well-off. A chapter on values in the National Commission on Children report (1991) is boggling the minds of politicians in Washington. How could liberals, conservatives, Democrats, Republicans agree on values? But values are an important ingredient. Fourth is the capacity to change. If ours were the British system and we could convince John Major that change was needed, a month or a year later the change would be made. Change is much more complicated in a pluralistic system. To reform the political capacity for making expensive and difficult changes, we need trust.

Education reform and health reform can be compared because both are cost-driven, both lack quality, and in both quality is difficult to measure. The public is unhappy about education, and it trusts Republicans to get the job done. But the people who will actually reform education are the teachers, the teachers' unions, and the school boards— those who would not trust Republicans farther than they could throw them. They trust only Democrats. So a Democratic president is needed to push it.

But in health care, it is just the opposite. Although we are unhappy about the costs of the system, the polls do not show that Americans trust Republicans to get the job done. The public trusts Democrats with this issue of health care, not Republicans.

Yet the people who will fix this system—not politicians and commentators but doctors, nurses, insurers, and employers—do not trust the Democrats to fix it. They trust only Republicans.

The time is approaching for President Bush to speak on this issue. The Congress, as Neil Newhouse mentioned, got burned on the catastrophic health insurance issue. We had thirty-five votes in the Senate to keep catastrophic insurance. I actually had 45 votes, but ten members said they would give me their votes if I had close to fifty. So I don't buy the notion that the Congress could not change Medicare. But the so-called health leadership got burned because we led everybody to a good result, but the people did not appreciate it.

The Democratic leadership has no cosponsors for its health care proposal because of the leadership's history with catastrophic. Have Lloyd Bentsen and Dan Rostenkowski learned from that? You bet they have. This time they will produce a leadership package that is limited, practical, and agreed upon.

Another problem is the deficit. The federal government goes $1 billion deeper into debt every day. The single-payer Canadian system is not the answer. None of the proponents of the Canadian model can answer the cost question. How do we pay for it? Responsibility in America today says we should promise only what we can pay for. The cost problem is one more reason why an incremental approach is needed. The incrementalists believe in the marketplace and in trying to get the market to work. The buyer in the health market does not control the three elements of cost control: need, quality, and price. The sellers control all three.

In the interim, we can change that by putting prospective prices on hospitals and doctors and by introducing managed care into the system. But those things will go only halfway to solving the cost problem in America. This system will work when the sellers of services have incentives to provide only what the payer needs, at higher quality, for a price that better reflects the value of the service.

Such changes, however, will be difficult to legislate because of the nature of medicine. That is the difference between $7,000 for a normal birth in this town and $2,400 at Mayo.

Reference

National Commission on Children. *Beyond Rhetoric: A New American Agenda for Children and Families.* Washington, D.C.: U.S. Government Printing Office, 1991.

Bill Gradison

Health care is increasing in salience as a political issue. My colleagues report in their districts that the number one issue is the economy, followed by health care. This is a rising public anxiety: I have health care and can afford to pay my bills today, but can I do it tomorrow?

People are aware of health care's escalating costs and are worried about its effect on their future. We are spending more and enjoying it less. In battling these costs, however, the public views are simply unformed. Despite this, intensified political debate is far more likely to create confusion than to lead to consensus because it lends itself to very powerful negative advertising.

As Representative Sander Levin's survey shows, the public would welcome as much health care as others are willing to give them free. Reality sets in when the price tags are examined, and every comprehensive plan—every one—is costly. If it is comprehensive—not a little incremental plan to deal with the small group reform or the tort system but the actual goal in some reasonable period of universal health coverage in this country—it is not cheap.

With some notable exceptions such as the Pepper Commission, recent plans do contain specific financing, although in frankness in some instances the financing falls far short of what would be necessary to pay the bills. One estimate for the Russo plan sees a $100 billion shortfall a year. But nonetheless, there is a recognition in these plans that they have to be budget neutral.

Putting a plan together is difficult. I have been working on mine for a year, and it is not finished. I have great respect for people—regardless of their political party—who will put a plan on the table and will match it with a financing system.

Every comprehensive plan is subject to major political criticisms. Some of these criticisms are analytical and objective, and some are unrestrained politics. Despite their charms, employer play-or-pay plans, for example, can be criticized as risking job losses for low-wage employees, lacking horizontal equity for low-income workers versus low-income nonworkers; in economic terms they are a tax on low-income workers. They can be attacked as a foot in the door—and a big foot at that—for mandates of all kinds.

Employer play-or-pay plans are likely to be expensive to the government since employers are likely to pay rather than play for workers whose health care costs are expected to exceed the costs of the tax. Otherwise employers would take care of them themselves. Criticisms of mandates in general, which, as Sandy Levin has said, are critical for small businesses, have a more direct political appeal.

Underlying the criticism of play-or-pay are the taxes needed to subsidize those workers covered by the pay option plus the taxes needed to provide coverage for the unemployed uninsured. That every proposed employer mandate is also an employee mandate is not much appreciated. I have yet to see one that does not require the employee to come up with 20 percent or more. Workers may not understand that, especially those who prefer to have the cash for other purposes or who feel they are immortal and immune from health care costs.

Similarly, the Canadian-style single-payer approach is vulnerable, not only for its costs but also for the prohibition on competing private health insurance and the rationing by queuing, which is inherent in it. Wait until the governors really take a look at the Canadian plan. I predict they will explode when they see the impact of a Canadian plan on their budgets. They are complaining now that health care, Medicaid, consumes about 15 percent of their state budgets because of the mandates we have written. The average Canadian province pays 35 percent of its budget for health care under their glorious system.

My late mother-in-law used to say, "Money isn't everything, health is 2 percent." This is a valuable insight into the problem that we face. I am especially concerned about the lesson of the Medicare catastrophic law because it started and ended as the Stark-Gradison bill, and it has had a chilling impact on the decision-making process.

I want to read a statement by a representative of the United Auto Workers, which typifies this conflict: "We cannot support any legislation which would require the majority of workers and retirees who already have health insurance coverage to shoulder a larger tax burden without receiving any additional benefits."

Ridiculous. The whole exercise is to figure out how to take money from the haves, who are those higher-than-average-income individuals who have health insurance, and their employers, in order to pay for the have-nots.

When the savings and loan issue broke wide open, I received a letter from a constituent that said it all. He said, "The taxpayers should not pay for bailing out the savings and loans, the government should."

Moving the health care issue from the back burner to the front burner, as the Democrats seem likely to do, carries the risk of getting fingers burned. Once the presidential candidates get specific about health care, their plans will be vulnerable to tough, effective, negative advertising—especially on the tax side.

I do not know what President Bush's health care proposal will be, but it certainly will not be the Canadian plan, it will not be an employer mandate, and it will not be a single-payer plan. Whatever he proposes will be roundly criticized by the Democrats, but that process in 1992 could easily poison the well in 1993 and beyond, perhaps for Bush's entire second term if he receives that term. Why would that happen? Positions taken now could be polarizing and would make compromise even harder to achieve than it is right now.

One final point: health polls rarely focus on cultural factors, but cultural factors limit our political flexibility in reshaping our health care system. Americans have, for example, a strong desire for first-dollar insurance. Folks who have it do not cheerfully give it up. It is probably the principal explanation for labor unrest in the United States today. Americans have a traditional preference for fee-for-service medicine. It is changing, but still that is the predominant system today. Americans have an expectation of perfect medical outcomes that borders on a belief in immortality. Americans have confidence in the ability of science and technology to improve the human condition. If they do not get a perfect baby, it is the doctor's fault or it is the hospital's fault or it is the drug company's fault; it is not just one of those tough breaks that happen in life.

Americans are impatient people. Their impatience in waiting for health care services borders on hostility. Think about your own experience waiting for service that you were going to pay for or your insurance company was going to pay for. Most people will not wait much longer for a bypass operation if the doctor says they need it than they are willing to wait for a Big Mac at McDonald's.

Finally, with regard to cultural factors, much of what we think of as health care costs in this country is a result of factors—cultural, sociological, or whatever—that are unrelated to medical care but push up the costs: drugs, homicides, obesity, bad diets, alcoholism, smoking, and a lot of other things. In other words, something has got to give, but taking into account those constraints does limit our options. We will end up with a health care system that is distinctively American: it will be very complicated and expensive.

Karlyn H. Keene

To put the issue of public concern about health care into a broader perspective, consider this simple question: What is the most important problem facing the country today?

This question has been asked for decades in the public opinion polling business, and recently it has been asked monthly by some of the major pollsters. While you think about your answer, let me tell you how that question has been answered by Americans recently.

When the question was posed by Gallup and ABC News/ *Washington Post* in the period from 1979 to 1981, about 70 percent of Americans spontaneously mentioned high inflation as the most important problem facing the country. When that question was asked in 1982, during the recession, about three in ten said high unemployment, five in ten high inflation. When the question was asked in October 1989 at the time of President Bush's speech on drugs, 63 percent of us said drugs constitute the most important issue facing the country today.

By contrast, after 1981 in the Gallup and the ABC/*Post* polls, health care or health has never been mentioned by more than 3 percent of the American people as the most important problem facing the country today.

This "most-important-problem" question is an indicator of political intensity. When you ask Americans if there is a national health care crisis, as Gallup did in June 1991, 91 percent respond Yes. But the broader most-important-problem question shows far less intensity. The question is more telling as an indicator of the political potential of an issue than of whether the system is in crisis.

Most polls show that Americans are concerned about the cost of health care, but that, too, should be put in context. This does not mean that Americans are ready to embrace a major, costly new federal program to enhance current coverage. I have never seen the public more firm about holding the line on what government should do.

This analysis contradicts conventional wisdom. A number of polls suggest that Americans want President Bush to turn his attention from foreign affairs to the domestic agenda and to do more to solve our problems. Cartoons that show the president being welcomed home offer anecdotal evidence that Americans feel he should come back to America and deal with the problems here. The commentary in much of the editorial and opinion pages echoes a new assertiveness about domestic policies.

But I read the public mood differently, and this might affect the health care issue. Polls are a very blunt instrument. They can tell us some general things about the electorate. They are not very good at giving us specifics. They also reveal ambivalence. In many different areas, Americans are of two minds about policy. We want a strong and assertive military, yet we are reluctant to send troops anywhere. We applaud those efforts to increase women's opportunities in the work force, yet we worry about the effects of women's involvement in the labor force on young children. We want to get government off the backs of business, but at the same time we want to be protected from the excesses of business. These are examples.

So we have an "on-the-one-hand–on-the-other" mood in many areas of public opinion, including the question of what government should do, particularly the federal government. We are a rich and powerful country and we want government to do many things.

In 1938 when the Gallup Organization asked whether government should be responsible for providing medical care for those who do not have it, 80 percent of us indicated that government should have that responsibility. When Gallup asked that question in 1991, once again 80 percent of us said this was government's responsibility—an indication that the public sees a strong role for government.

That is one dimension of the public opinion picture. But equally powerful is the view that government, and particularly the federal government, is too big, too intrusive, inefficient, and ineffective. ABC and the *Washington Post* pollsters regularly ask Americans how much of every dollar collected by Washington in taxes is wasted. In the past five years when that question has been asked, the median response has been that nearly 50 cents of every dollar collected by Washington is wasted. Concern about waste makes Americans skeptical of an enhanced government presence in many areas—including health care. Add to this Americans' real concern about the cost of new government efforts. When Americans were asked by the polling firm of Mellman and Lazarus how much they would be willing to pay to cover those who do not have health insurance, 30 percent said $50 but not $100; 19 percent said $100 but not $200; 9 percent said $200 but not $400; 4 percent said $400 but not $500. Three in ten said they would not pay $40 a year.

So we are pulled back and forth between these two views of government, depending on economic conditions. When we feel that we and our families are doing well, as we did in 1985 and 1986, we want government to do more. When we and our families are uneasy about our current financial situation, we want government to do no more than it has been doing and perhaps a little less.

Polls on reducing pollution, solving problems in education, or correcting the abuses and inefficiencies in the health care system show that Americans say they think that more money should be spent on these problems. But these polls are misleading, because the questions are not followed up with the qualifier, "if your taxes have to be raised." When that phrase is added to survey questions, as is done occasionally, many Americans still say, Yes, we should be doing more, even if my taxes have to be raised.

But we have to go beyond even these responses to public perceptions of the cumulative effect of the total tax burden Americans face. The anecdotal evidence is revealing. In man-on-the-street interviews in New Jersey after the Florio tax rebate in 1991, individual after individual suggested to interviewers that the rebate was not going to help them because other taxes were going up.

We have to put attitudes about what the federal government should be doing, even in an area of great concern like health care, into that broader context of the cumulative tax burden that we feel government is placing on us. That burden is large.

About a decade ago the Public Agenda Foundation asked a large focus group about different popular social programs—extending coverage for women, infants, and children's feeding programs, providing long-term health care for the unemployed. They found that only a minority would spend more than $25 a year on these popular programs. The public feels stretched and burdened by taxes they believe are rising.

What does that mean in terms of the health care issue in particular? There are many areas of concern, but the data suggest that Americans want to be cautious about what the federal government should do.

Adding to this is another powerful new current in public opinion: Americans are feeling greater and greater distance from the national debates that policy makers are involved in, so they will not be providing much specific guidance.

Who is in the driver's seat politically? When the issue of health care is asked about, broadly and generally, the Democrats have a significant advantage over the Republicans on virtually every question. But if the subject turns from concern about health care to an economic concern, an issue of costs, the Democratic advantage may dissipate. One of the major changes we have seen in survey data over the past decade is in the public perception of the Republicans as better economic managers.

The political dynamics of this issue are unknown. The public is not going to be providing a great deal of specific guidance to health policy analysts about what the federal government should be doing in this area or how much the federal government should spend to repair or expand the current system.

Sander M. Levin

Recently I took a comprehensive health survey in my congressional district. It was a serious effort, and we had the help of the leading professional health surveyers. The district I represent is suburban and urban, proportionally more suburban, and is rather typical of districts in this country.

When the initial results came in, we were rather perplexed. After spot checking, however, the answers quickly leapt off the page. In a ranking of national priorities, health care was listed first by 51 percent of the approximately 9,000 respondents. Immediately following health care was waste of government money, chosen by 49 percent. Incidentally, homelessness was chosen by 12 percent. Then we asked people, "Are you satisfied with the health care services you and your family receive?" Seventy percent responded "very satisfied" or "somewhat satisfied." Then the next question was, "Today if there were a major ailment in the family, do you think you would have adequate health coverage?" Only 40 percent said no, 34 percent agreed, and 26 percent were not sure. When we asked them how they thought costs should be lowered, overwhelmingly they favored physicians' accepting lower fees, employers' accepting more responsibility, and insurance companies' accepting more regulation. It was overwhelming; four or five to one gave this response.

We asked, "What do you think about higher health insurance costs for the same amount of coverage?" Only 6 percent thought that was a good idea. Higher income taxes, even if dedicated only to health? Only 25 percent thought that made any sense. A slight majority favored excise tax increases earmarked for health care.

One other question's response was interesting: "Are you worried that if in the future a major ailment occurs in your family, you will not have adequate health care coverage?" Sixty-four percent said they might not be able to pay for the health care—and only 14 percent were sure they would have adequate health care.

These figures accurately reflect the data we have heard from Karlyn Keene and Neil Newhouse. I draw two conclusions relating to the presidential campaign and to what we are doing in Congress. Presidential candidates do not win or lose the White House because of the health care issue. But an underlying economic security issue exists in this country, and health care is an important piece of it. The White House can be won or lost depending on how that economic issue runs in this country and how the people respond to it.

The main issue in health is not the 37 million uninsured. Some discussion will take place concerning the 25 percent of American children in poverty—the underclass, those left out—and the ramifications for the rest of America. Yet, the key focus will be on what is happening to the middle-income groupings in this country—the immense stagnation in their income during the past twelve or fifteen years, and their fears for the future. Health is very much a part of that picture. If not dynamite, certainly there is a bit of dry timber in the health issue.

Do you get stalemate from today's antitax, antiwaste, and anti-government feelings? I think not. What you will see emanating from the Democratic ranks is a package that does not embrace a single-payer system—a system that cannot survive politically. It is arguably good on waste, because it is easier to control costs under a single-payer plan than under a diversified system, but the tax shift is so massive and the role of government so clear that its success is doubtful.

What emerges from the maze of antitax, antiwaste, antigovernment feelings is something along the lines proposed by the Senate and by the chairman of the Ways and Means Committee. It is a play-or-pay system with heavier reliance on employer participation and a global approach to cost-containment, with far more incentives for managed care than in the original Senate leadership proposal. It also will include reform of the Medicaid system so there will be comprehensive coverage.

The problem with play-or-pay lies in modulating the impact on small businesses so that they are not politically alienated. The only way to accomplish that is through a phased-in transition and some kind of subsidization. Any sensible proposal would provide some kind of help through risk-pool arrangements, through a general Treasury-linked provision. That is one of the puzzles to be resolved.

I think there will be a great deal of discussion in the Presidential campaign about health care as part of an attack on economic issues with an effort in the House and Senate to at least have a package pieced together for consideration on the floor. The future will tell how important this issue is for the Presidental race.

The unemployment figures came out this morning. Unemployment is now 9.8 percent in Michigan. If we project the present national unemployment rate for another nine or ten months—and the present stagnant growth rate might very well continue that long—we see how incendiary the health insurance issue can be. Increasingly, more Americans are going to ask questions they were not asking in the mid-1980s: not only, Will my kids be able to buy a house? Will I be able to educate my kids? Will we be able to take a vacation? but also, Are we going to have basic, adequate health care coverage in the years ahead?

Neil Newhouse

When Americans believe things are going in the right direction, they reelect incumbents. It is a status quo election, as were 1984 and 1988, to some extent. When voters believe things are going off track, however, they make changes by throwing incumbents out of office. Currently, less than 33 percent of Americans believe this country is headed in the right direction, and 57 to 65 percent of them believe things are off on the wrong track.

Americans are frustrated and in a mood for change. I think the Democratic presidential candidates have accurately interpreted the frustration that has risen between what people saw as a tremendous military success in the Persian Gulf by the administration and the lack of action in this country on domestic issues.

Americans do not believe that the same kind of effort is being put into education, environment, and health care in this country. Domestic problems are not being solved, which makes them anxious for change.

I would like to talk about the health care issue in that context. The key issue is the cost of health care, not the 37 million Americans who are underinsured or who have no insurance, but those who are paying increased premiums or who can no longer get health insurance when they change jobs.

These problems hit different income levels and different groups of Americans across the board. A recent *New York Times* poll asked, "Have you or anyone else in your household ever decided to stay in a job you wanted to leave mainly because you didn't want to lose health care coverage?" A third of Americans making between $15,000 and $50,000 a year said yes: those are the middle-income voters that the Democratic presidential candidates are trying to win.

Beyond that, 50 percent of Americans who make more than $30,000 a year reported that their employer has cut health benefits or required employees to contribute more. This issue affects higher-income Americans, those more likely to vote Republican. The more this issue impinges on the Republican electorate and the Republican base, the more potential it has to affect the next election. The most partisan voters, not just one party's electoral base, are hit.

In the 1988 presidential election between Bush and Dukakis, just 9 percent of Americans considered health care or health care costs as most important to them in making their voting decision. These voters were poor, black, Hispanic, and uninsured, and they voted for Dukakis by about a three-to-one margin. That demographic analysis does not described a swing voter group in the next election cycle, but the higher-income voters are.

Health care issues in elections are most salient when cost becomes the issue rather than the uninsured and when they hit the Republican coalition, not just the Democratic.

I think Congress is very cautious on this issue, because lawmakers were burned on the catastrophic health care bill several years ago. They are acutely aware of the repercussions in their districts and states.

In addition to the mood in the country, I sense a very strong anti-incumbent feeling. Anti-incumbent hostility is so powerful that Congress has a 33 percent approval rating while George Bush has much higher ratings. If the Democratic leaders of Congress try to challenge President Bush on some of these key issues, they would not have the credibility that the president has.

Although Congress has low approval ratings and the public lacks faith in the federal government to solve problems, ironically over 50 percent of Americans look to the federal government to help solve the health care problem. On one hand, voters say they want to throw all the incumbents out of office because they are not doing the job. On the other hand, voters believe we need the federal government involved in this issue.

We should also consider that there will be a villain: health insurance companies, doctors, or hospitals. One of those three—maybe all three—will be pointed out by either politicians, political candidates, or the administration as the group to take the lumps.

In the early days of the 1992 presidential campaign, for example, former candidate Bob Kerrey asked: "Are you willing to take on the American Medical Association? Are you willing to take on the insurance industry? Are you willing to take on vested interests out there that may have given to your campaign?"

Villains are already being singled out on this issue and will continue to be as we proceed to sort out this issue over the next four or five years.

Finally, the chapters and commentary in this book are far ahead of where the public is right now. The public is simply uneducated on this issue, and health care will not become a true voting issue until Americans have an informed opinion on it.

As Karlyn Keene states, only 2 percent of Americans believe that health care is a key problem; therefore, it is not a major issue. In some cases the percentage may be misleading: 1 percent of Americans see abortion as the most important problem facing the country, and yet 20 percent of Americans identify themselves as single-issue voters on that issue. Just a few years ago 28 percent considered crime and drugs the most important problem facing the country. As a Republican pollster, I looked high and low for Democrats in favor of crime and drugs. And lo and behold, we had a very difficult time finding those candidates.

It is clear to some extent what Americans want out of a health care system: they want the same excellent standards they have received in the past, they want to maintain access, and they want to cut costs by half.

Health Reform Politics

Discussion of Part Five

NORMAN J. ORNSTEIN, American Enterprise Institute: I will start with a rather depressing question. Americans are not particularly complaining about the services provided in the health area; they like the services. The anxiety level to which Bill Gradison refers is about the costs of health care. Almost any solution will bring bad news to people. It will be about cutting services, raising taxes, or offering no further improvements in the level of services. People are looking for good news, if any news, from the government.

Add to this the public's distaste for having government do anything and the public's belief that government cannot do much right, and it becomes difficult to get out of this box. In a presidential campaign it is difficult to do more than offer soothing comments: that we understand voters' anxieties, or that we have vague plans that avoid specifics. Basically these plans say you must either pay more and get nothing more for it right now, or you must pay more and probably get a little less for it. It becomes difficult to make any move, even an incremental one, in this area.

Are we not really waiting for some kind of an explosion to occur before we get anywhere in this area?

DAVE DURENBERGER, U.S. Senate: Lloyd Bentsen has addressed that concern in terms of triage. As soon as we have sensed a consensus on the problem and we have an opportunity to target some villain to solve it, then we ought to do so. And we are there now. We need small-group insurance reform.

We have identified the rating or pricing system for insurance as being unfair; some people pay substantially more than others for the same product just because of where they work and the size of the group.

There is a consensus about that in state legislatures and in Washington. And the villain is the insurance companies. We have to pick on somebody big, and our Republican-side pollsters tell us to spend 1992 picking on the insurance companies and we will do well.

In addition, we face the issue of administrative costs. The people who invented the estimate of $100 billion in administrative costs did not get it right. The cost is much smaller, but it is still a problem.

So people on both sides of the aisle will recognize this, and I hope that in 1993 Congress will pass legislation to address it.

BILL GRADISON, U.S. House of Representatives: We have a crisis-activated system. The question is, How bad must the crisis be to activate it? It varies throughout the country. It is popular to criticize the health insurance companies, but as an economist, I find it difficult to understand how health insurance can be inexpensive if health care is expensive.

Take a look at West Virginia. Blue Cross-Blue Shield went belly-up, leaving tens of millions of dollars worth of unpaid bills from hospitals and doctors, who are now demanding payment from the policy holders.

My greatest fear is that we might wait until things are so critical that action is imperative. Such action, in the urgency of the situation, would necessarily be highly centralized and highly regulated. It would be preferable to act before there is a crisis.

Fortunately, as the states emerge from this recession, it is unlikely that they will wait for actions to be taken by Congress. The pressures on them are as great as those on Congress to deal with this issue. A number of states have already acted, in spite of the difficult economic circumstances they face.

The more states that deal effectively with the health care issue, the less pressure there will be to impose a central, national solution. And the dimensions of the problem vary enormously from state to state.

In Minnesota, Dave Durenberger's state, about 6 percent of the population lacks health insurance. In Ohio, my state, it is 9 or 10 percent. In California, 6 million lack health insurance—20 percent of the population. In Texas and New Mexico, it is around 25 percent.

In our federal system, things do not stand still, and if we continue to wrangle we may find solutions here and there. That is what happened in Canada, starting in the middle 1940s in Saskatchewan.

SANDER M. LEVIN, U.S. House of Representatives: Perhaps it is unwise to inject a note of optimism, but I will do so. First, we should not be too harsh on ourselves, the American people. We are no different from others in waiting for crises; possibly we are better than some nations.

Second, although the focus is on the large, middle range of our society, some attention is being effectively paid to those who fall outside of it. It will have some impact. Having 37 million uninsured is disgraceful enough to paint the picture wide.

Many Americans can understand the dynamite contained in 37

million of their fellow citizens who have no insurance coverage. We can explain it in economics alone.

A third point concerns the immense waste in this system. The administrative costs for health insurance are unacceptable. Whatever one thinks of a single-payer system, Medicare is considerably cheaper to administer than are the other insurance programs of this country. We should pay attention to that.

In terms of duplication of services, some economic rationalization can go on. There has been immense waste and some corruption in the health care system. And one can talk about more effectively running a diversified system.

Are we going to wait for the ultimate crisis before we move? Maybe so, but maybe not.

MR. ORNSTEIN: We have talked about taking care of the 37 million who are uninsured. We have talked about portability of benefits for those who are worried about leaving or losing their jobs. We have talked about some form of safety net, of catastrophic care for everybody, to guard against the possibility of some awful illness wiping out a family. And there is the broader issue of cost-containment, along with comprehensive change.

In this menu, are there some items on which we will be moved to act sooner rather than later, assuming we do not act in a comprehensive way? What is the incremental road map to which we can look forward?

CONGRESSMAN GRADISON: First, I do not question the accuracy of that study about portability, but it has not asked enough questions. Many people do not want to leave their jobs because they do not want to walk away from a pension before they become vested. Health care is not the only factor that deters people from changing jobs.

Second, the insurance industry is on trial. The question of insurance reform, particularly in the small-group market, offers a major challenge but is feasible. There is a will to do it on the parts of both the insurance companies and the people in government. Some progress could be made in a relatively short time—perhaps a year or two—in dealing with a piece of the problem.

CONGRESSMAN LEVIN: It is easy to caricature employer mandates. But it makes common sense to Americans for more people to be covered through their employment.

In Germany they have more of an employer-based system than we have, and it is complicated. But if you ask Americans whether we should emulate the mandated employee coverage of Germany, increasing numbers are saying yes. And we are going to emulate it. I defy anybody to suggest an alternative to a single-payer system, other than employer mandates. What other approaches are there?

CONGRESSMAN GRADISON: There is an entirely different avenue, which some have called an empowerment approach. It would use refundable tax credits related to income to enable the individual to have a means of payment. That approach could be combined with a requirement on the employer to make health insurance available but not necessarily to pay for it. That combination would offer the advantage of access to the system through groups without mandating that the employer pay the costs.

I am not trying to sell that approach. It could be debated. But it is a different avenue, which many experts are looking at.

CONGRESSMAN LEVIN: Right, and we will have that battle, and perhaps sooner rather than later.

SENATOR DURENBERGER: I agree with Bill Gradison on small-group reform. But I will add two additional points. One plan now on the table and about to be implemented is the resource-based relative value scale. The projections indicate that in the next five years, Medicare income for doctors in Miami will go down 31 percent. But in Minnesota they will remain about even, on average. Thus there is no justification for the fees being charged in Miami—and not only in Medicare.

The changes that will occur in the practice of medicine alone under this pressure are enormous, if we are smart enough to reward them in some way.

Second, look at Oregon. One of Yogi Berra's famous remarks is, When you come to the fork in the road, take it. And Oregon is taking it. I do not interpret Oregon's policy as explicit rationing, even though it is sometimes called that. The biggest problems in health costs today are the growth in intensity and the cost of procedures. In Oregon they are taking the cost for each person and flipping it on its side to see how many people they can cover with the available money. There are 720 procedures, and perhaps they can afford only 580. This is important for what it is doing to make people think differently about each health dollar.

CONGRESSMAN GRADISON: It is interesting that people talk about a minimum-benefit package but do not define it. My challenge to people is to ask, When you talk about a minimum-benefit package, what do you leave out? Almost nothing is left out.

In the case of Oregon, there is a recognition that in a world of limited resources, we cannot do everything. It is an attempt to save what would be left out. The amazing part of the Oregon effort is that its leader is an emergency room physician who is the president of the state senate. I have always believed that the last people in America who would put their fingerprints on rationing would be politicians.. Significantly, however, he has just announced his plans not to seek reelection.

MR. ORNSTEIN: I have one question for our polling people. Mr. Newhouse, you referred to a series of potential villains, and we have heard some talk about those who will be made to bear a greater burden. Looking through the menu of insurance companies, employers, doctors, which group is likely to take the greatest hit?

NEIL NEWHOUSE, Public Opinion Strategies: I agree with Mr. Gradison that insurance companies are the most vulnerable. But this is not a one-way street. They are going to fight back. The villains have the resources to wage their own campaigns. As Constance Horner has said, a national health care system would have the efficiency of the post office, the compassion of the IRS, and the cost-control of Pentagon purchasing. Imagine advertising that would be used by a local health care clinic that serves the public the way the Department of Motor Vehicles does.

Our villains will not lie down and take it. They will fight back. More than anything else, this battle will inform the public—or maybe ill-inform the public—about the issue and will draw the battle lines. Informing the public is difficult for the government to do, and the press may not do it very well either. So the people with the most to lose will do most to draw the battle lines.

EDWARD BERGER, Institute for Health Policy, Georgetown University: In terms of state initiatives, one that has been given less visibility is Hawaii's. That state has had long experience with a mandated employer-based system.

In the Canadian experience, after Saskatchewan took initiatives with both their physician-payment and hospital-payment systems, it was easier for the federal government to move ahead for the entire country.

I am intrigued to see what lessons we might learn from our own history. In 1968 and 1969 there was a crisis in health care with two components, cost and access. The Republican president in 1970 and 1971—Richard Nixon—found it to his advantage to embrace health care, as well as population and family planning, as a presidential issue. He assembled a health care package that included two proposals for national health insurance.

Besides the increase in the national expenditure for health care and the concern about the deficit, what makes things different now? What should we learn from that experience?

410

CONGRESSMAN GRADISON: This leads to a marvelous health care Trivial Pursuit question. Who was the only president of the United States to recommend to Congress, in writing, an employer-mandate plan? Of course the answer is Richard Nixon.

The difference between his plan and the current play-or-pay plans was that his was mandate-only. It did not include a pay provision for the employer, although there was a 35 percent employee contribution. It was dismissed out of hand by the leaders in the Congress because it was not comprehensive—it would not deal with the whole problem. Things have changed today. President Bush will not recommend such a plan. If he did, it would be quickly embraced by the Democrats. That indicates the direction in which the debate is moving.

And we have had some movement. As a member of the fifteen-member Pepper Commission, I was impressed by the fact that some of the more comprehensive changes were not even put on the table in the private conversations, which were the vehicle in which we did most of our work. The sense was that they are not appropriate for our country right now.

Some people look only at the proposals for play-or-pay or for a single-payer plan, for example a Mitchell plan or a Russo plan. Their tracks do not meet. The AFL-CIO group that met to propose a recommendation was split down the middle, between the employer mandate and a play-or-pay proposal. So it is unrealistic to say we are moving toward a compromise just because so many plans are under consideration. But we have made some progress in the discourse since the early 1960s and 1970s.

CONGRESSMAN LEVIN: Of course, if we leave out the deficit we are leaving out about 50 percent of any issue.

C. EUGENE STEUERLE, Urban Institute: The lessons from the Medicare catastrophic experience are often misstated. As Congressman Gradison has said, most of our major actions are taken in reaction to crises. But with Medicare catastrophic, there was no crisis at all. A secretary of Health and Human Services started pushing hard for action and led on this issue.

CONGRESSMAN GRADISON: The crisis came after, not before. It was a self-made crisis created by the Congress!

MR. STEUERLE: That is right. It was also pushed forward by the lack of a domestic agenda, which says something about how the desire of the Congress or the administration to do something—anything—can at times overwhelm other forces working against legislation.

But a second lesson is this: had the original catastrophic bills—the Reagan bill, or perhaps some of the early drafts of the Stark-Gradison bill—been adopted they probably would have been sustained. The attempt to move beyond incremental reform and add a fairly monstrous and elaborate tax structure really led to its demise. Might those lessons not offer some guidance for how future reform should proceed?

CONGRESSMAN GRADISON: This is what happened with the catastrophic bill. The Ways and Means Committee approved something very close to the president's plan. It went to the Democratic leadership of the House. Claude Pepper, Jim Wright, and others said, "This is too bipartisan, and we want to add a drug benefit." And the Ways and Means Committee was told to add a drug benefit or else it will be added by the Energy and Commerce Committee, or on the floor.

With hindsight, we can see that adding that large increment of cost—and an uncertain cost, as well—had a lot to do with the requirement for a larger income-related premium and the corollaries that followed from it.

One other element is directly relevant. Approximately 6 million Medicare beneficiaries did not feel they were being offered anything by the catastrophic bill that they were not already getting free. I am not referring to medigap. One could argue that they would pay less for medigap if catastrophic coverage came along. But I am referring to government employees, military retirees, and people with generous health care plans. These people said, "Why should we pay anything for this? We are not getting anything from it, not even a lower medigap premium." And they were right. I do not know how to answer that question today. What are we going to give them?

CONGRESSMAN LEVIN: The catastrophic bill could have lived anyway. The basic mistake was to say that people who have a family income of $45,000 a year are rich. If we say that, we will have to retreat. Had we started the schedule we eventually adopted earlier, for half of the impact on midincome families with $35,000–$40,000 income, the catastrophic bill might have survived.

CONGRESSMAN GRADISON: But the kind of comprehensive plans being discussed—for example, the Pepper Commission recommendations—would have increased federal costs alone by $66 billion a year in 1990 dollars. They could not be implemented without tapping the middle class. There are not enough rich people in America, regrettably, to foist it off on them and on the corporations.

412

CONGRESSMAN LEVIN: Perhaps not, but it was too heavy a burden for what they were receiving.

JACK WERNER, private consultant: I have been in the health economics business for 20 years, and I was involved in a national commission on the cost of medical care 20 years ago. I have looked at health care systems in other countries, and I would not like to see our system go the way of a single-payer system and lose the benefits of a pluralistic system. The cost of medical care, however, will drive us to a single-payer system unless we do something about it.

I see no mystery in understanding the cost of health care. The basic causal factors are:

1. the diffusion of technology, for which we pay too much
2. too many hospital beds—the data on empty hospital beds show a figure about the same now as fifteen years ago, even though the patient days and admissions have fallen considerably
3. a supply of doctors that has tripled in the past few decades
4. a continuing, rapid rise in compensation and wages in the health care sector
5. a continuing increase in drug costs as the government provides monopolies for drugs

Is our political system capable of addressing these significant cost factors? We cannot address the cost problem by tinkering at the margin. We are going to impose some major changes on some of the larger stakeholders now in the system. I favor the private sector, but it is not capable of solving these problems without a concerted effort on the part of the public sector. Can we get consensus in the health care sector to address these problems?

SENATOR DURENBERGER: The answer is yes, we can reach such a consensus. That is why in my introductory remarks I pointed to the four ways in which we will solve this problem. The first is reaching a common understanding of the problem. We could not have put together this collection of health policy research even a year or two ago. The research and analysis now being written and talked about is helpful to all of us in putting things in perspective.

Second, we are beginning to develop several distinct visions of the future. This is the way the American political process works.

Third is the issue of values. In this era we are able to discuss values. We can start with simple ones, like not pulling the plug and rationing, or with the more difficult question of consumption versus investment in health care. We have discussed these issues for ten years, but we have

413

not yet applied our values to these basic choices.

The fourth step in approaching a solution is our increasing capacity to change, especially at the local level. As Congressman Levin has pointed out, the deficit and the lack of confidence in government have combined to make change at the federal level difficult. The change is going to come at the state and local levels, in places like Minneapolis–St. Paul. There we have five bone marrow centers, though we need only one or two. We have more magnetic resonance imaging facilities than we need. But we have done much to change the way the market works.

It is only a matter of time until we have the information and knowledge to allow the private sector to have a true effect on health costs.

A NOTE ON THE BOOK

This book was edited by
Cheryl Weissman, Dana Lane, and Ann Petty
of the staff of the AEI Press.
The text was set in Palatino, a typeface designed by
the twentieth-century Swiss designer Hermann Zapf.
Publication Technology Corporation, of Fairfax, Virginia,
set the type, and Edwards Brothers Incorporated,
of Ann Arbor, Michigan, printed and bound the book,
using permanent acid-free paper.

The AEI PRESS is the publisher for the American Enterprise Institute for Public Policy Research, 1150 17th Street, N.W., Washington, D.C. 20036; *Christopher C. DeMuth*, publisher; *Edward Styles*, director; *Dana Lane*, assistant director; *Ann Petty*, editor; *Cheryl Weissman*, editor; *Susan Moran*, assistant editor (rights and permissions).

Printed in the USA
CPSIA information can be obtained
at www.ICGtesting.com
JSHW011520221024
72172JS00014B/113